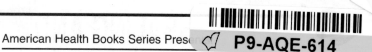

NATURAL HEALING AND PREVENTION SECRETS

**BY THE EDITORS OF
AMERICAN PUBLISHING CORPORATION**

NATURAL HEALING AND PREVENTION SECRETS

IMPORTANT NOTICE
This manual is intended as a reference volume only, not as a medical guide or a reference for self treatment. You should always seek competent medical advice from a doctor if you suspect a problem.
This book is intended as educational device to keep you informed of the latest medical knowledge. It is not intended to serve as a substitute for changing the treatment advice of your doctor. You should never make medical changes without first consulting your doctor.

Printed in the United States of America 0 9 8 7 6 5 4 3 2 1

ISBN NO. 0-9638596-1-7

NATURAL HEALING AND PREVENTION SECRETS

TABLE OF CONTENTS

Accidents

* 19 Things You Should have in Your Medicine
Chest for Emergencies 3

Acne

* An Acne Diet that Will Surprise You..7

Age Related Diseases

* 4 Ways to Strengthen the Gland that Controls Age Related Diseases.......8
* 5,000 Year Old Medicine Fights Aging...9
* Exercise for Independence with 15 Minutes a Day...........................9
* Free Government Publications on Staying Healthy as We Grow Older.....11
* The Nutrients that Can Prevent and Fight Back Age-Related Blindness....11
* The Truth About Some Popular Anti-Aging Drugs..............................12
* 3 Anti-Aging Nutrients that can Reverse Aging,Improve Memory, and
Fight-Off Disease...13

AIDS

* 3 Keys to Prevent Getting Aids from Common Medical Procedures.........14
* 5 Things You Need to do to Prevent Getting AIDS.............................15

Alcoholism

* A Home Program to Break the Alcohol Craving................................17
* What a Good Treatment Program Should Have................................18
* Why a Single Drug can Cut Your Need for Alcohol...........................19

Allergies

* 9 Leading Causes of Allergies and What to do About Them..................20
* Allergy Relief Tips..23
* A Simple Diet that Can End Allergy Misery.....................................24
* Emergency Treatment for Acute Allergic Attacks.............................25
* Why it is Hard to Spot an Allergy—Allergies Many Faces...................25
* Food Allergies and What to do With Them......................................26
* The Type of Clothing That Could be the Cause of Your Tiredness,
Headaches, and Other Health Problems...30

* What the Clothing Industry Doesn't Want You to Know About a Big-Selling, but Harmful Fabric..30
* Why You Should Not Buy Colored Toilet Paper................................30

Alzheimer's Disease

* 2 Vitamins that can Prevent You From Getting Alzheimer's Disease........31
* Alzheimer's Promotes Confused Thought, But Some Diet Changes May Help..31
* Amino Acid Help for Alzheimer's..32

Anemia

* A Diet Plan to Counteract Anemia..32

Anger

* Natural Mind-Control Secrets to Get Rid of Guilt, Fear, Worry, and Anger Feelings..33

Angina

* Relief From Angina Pain with Lysine and Vitamin C................................35

Ankle and Foot Pain

* How to Fight It Whether it's Deep or Shallow................................35

Anxiety

* 12 Fights Against Fear and Anxiety Without Drugs................................36
* 13 Natural Stress-Reducing Foods..41
* Relief from Anxiety Attacks Without Drugs................................41
* The Major Anxiety Treating Drugs and What they Do................................42

Arm and Leg Pain

* The Causes and Cures of Arm and Leg Cramps................................43

Arterial Blockage

* The "Miracle Food" that Fights-Off Hardening of the Arteries................44
* The Incredible Vitamin that Fights Off Highly Toxic "Free Radicals" that Block Arteries..45

Arthritis

* 5 Step Plan for Pain Free Food Preparation................................45
* 12 Ways to Rid Yourself of Arthritis Pain................................47
* A Few Diet Changes to Relieve the Discomfort................................50
* Common Beverage that Can Make Arthritis Worse................................50
* Finger Joints Hurt—It Might be the Way You Read................................51
* 3 New Arthritis Healers that Really Work................................51
* Prevent Arthritis by Losing Weight..52

Asthma

* Safe Ways to Handle a Deadly Disease...52

* 2 Hints to Cutting Attacks of Asthma..52

Attitude

* 10 Tips to A Happy Life...53

* Use Your Mind to Improve Your Health.......................................55

Backache

* 4 Exercises to Relieve the Aching Back.......................................56

Baldness

* The Nutrient that Might be a Solution to Baldness.......................56

Bedwetting

* What Not to Eat...57

Bladder Infection

* A Honeymoon Disease that Affects Most Women.........................58

Blood

* Lab Tests and How to Read the 15 Measures They Give You.................59

Brain Power

* A Vitamin that Will Increase Your Mental Performance.................64

Breathing Problems

* 3 Types, and What, If Anything, You Can Do................................64

Bruises

* Household Treatment to Minimize Bruising...................................66

Bulimia

* A New Cure Using Just a Pill..66

Bursitis

* Natural Way to Get Rid of Pain in Your Shoulders, Knees, Hips,
and Ankles...67

Cancer

* Cancer Screening—A Schedule for Early Treatment....................68

* Colon Cancer Surgery that will Leave You Normal.......................69

* Foods that Fight Off Cancer..70

* 5 Secrets to Lower Your Risk of Getting Cancer By 75%.............70

* Deadly Prostate Cancer--Use the Natural Detection Secret.............72

* Detect and Treat Breast Cancer-What Every Women Should.............72

* Foods With Indoles-Proven Cancer Preventers............................74

* How to Cut Colon Cancer Risk by 50% with Aspirin....................74

* Life After Cancer...75

* Mineral That Cuts Your Risk of Colon Cancer by 30%.................75

* Prevent Colon Cancer With Exercise-Get the Facts.................................76
* Saccharin or No Saccharin—Decide for Yourself....................................76
* Stop Cancer Cells—A Spice that Inhibits Cancer Cells..........................77
* Supplement to Avoid Cancer from X-Rays..78
* The Cervical Cancer Vitamin C Prevention Diet....................................78
* This is in Your Medicine Cabinet, and It Can Cut Your Risk
  of Getting Colon Cancer by a Full 50%...79
* 7 Skin Blemishes, Bumps, and Rashes That Could be Early
  Warnings Signs of Cancer..80
* Trace Mineral Cuts Breast Cancer Risk by 72%...................................81
* Vitamin Protection from Cancer, A Simple Combination that Works..........81
* Vitamin Proven to Lower Cervical Cancer Risk by 80%.......................82

Cellulite
* Treatments that Work, and Ones that Don't..82

Chest Pain
* Try Safe and Effective EDTA Chelation Therapy Instead of Surgery,
  and 94% Effective...83
* Two Nutrients That Can Relieve Chest Pain...84

Childhood Emergencies
* First-Aid for Choking in Children..85
* The First Step to Take in the 6 Most Common Situations......................85

Childhood Nutrition
* A Good Diet in Childcare—Don't Bet On IT!...90
* Free Nutritional Guides for Your Children...90
* Iron Supplements Can Poison Your Child...91
* Should Milk be in Your Baby's Diet?...91

Chronic Fatigue Syndrome
* Doctor's Aren't Sure What's Wrong With You? The "Mystery Illness"........93
* Symptoms of Chronic Fatigue Syndrome..93
* Treatment for CFS...94
* What Causes CFS..95
* Why Your CFS Can Affect the Heart...96
* How to Gain Energy—Naturally...96
* Fight Chronic Fatigue and Aging at the Same Time..............................96

Circulatory Disease
* Diet Tips to Improve the Circulation...97

Clothing and Health

* Your Necktie can Choke You...98

Colds and Flu

* A Common and Dangerous Cold Medication to Avoid.............................99
* 3 Alternatives to Treat Colds..99
* 4 Cold Symptoms and What to do About Them.....................................100
* 4 Questions About Colds and Flu that You Should Know........................102
* 8 Foods and Drinks that End a Cold or Flu Faster.................................104
* How to Avoid the Common Cold...105
* When to Get Your Flu Shot and Why...106

Constipation

* Foods That Help You Stay Regular..106
* The Beverage that can Ease Pain in Joints, Fight Constipation,
  and More..108

Cramps

* 7 Secrets to Relieving Menstrual Cramps...108
* Causes and Cures of Muscle Cramps...111

Depression

* Natural Way to End Depression—Four Ways to Talk Yourself Out of it....112
* Non-Drug Depression Control..113
* People Call it a Miracle—All We Know is it Can End Depression...........114

Diabetes

* 4 New Ways to Get Rid of Diabetes...114
* 5 New Ways to Manage or Cure Diabetes...115
* 6 Step Plan that Can Reverse Diabetes..117
* 20 Natural Ways to Control Your Diabetes and Lesson Insulin Needs....119
* Diabetes Breakthrough—Get Rid of Insulin Shots................................124
* Diet Tips for the Diabetic..124
* How You may be able to Reverse Diabetes in the Future........................125
* Get Off Diabetes Pills With Chelation Therapy......................................125

Diagnosis

* What to do If Your Doctor Can't Tell You What You Have.......................125

Diarrhea

* 4 Natural Remedies, and a Few Traditional Ones..................................127

Digestion

* Diet Changes to Calm the Upset Stomach...129
* Natural Way to Improve Your Digestion
  and Get Rid of "Nervous Stomach"...130

* New Study Reveals Foods that Help You Stay Regular...........................130

Divorce

* To Avoid Divorce Avoid Psychologists..131

Dealing With Doctors

* 3 of the Biggest Lies Doctors Tell You...132

Doctors

* 5 Questions You Should Answer Yes About Your Doctor.........................133

Earache

* New Method of Handling Ear Problems Mean Quicker Cures.................136

Eczema

* You Probably Cause It, and You Can Probably Cure It...........................137

Electricity and Health

* Is Your All Electric Life Good for You?..138

Emergencies

* The 19 Things You Should Have in Your Medicine Cabinet
  A Handy Checklist...139
* Why Hospital Emergency Rooms are Bad for Children..........................142

Endometriosis

* A Mystery Problem Women Should be Aware of....................................143

Energy

* 4 Tonic Teas to Pep You Up...144
* Burn Fat for More Energy, Here's How...145

Exercise

* 3 Tips to Safe Exercise...145
* 4 Secrets to Prevent Skin Problems When You Exercise......................146
* 6 Week Plan to Get In Shape for those Over 40...................................147
* 8 Step Plan to a Good Exercise Program...149
* A Key to Happiness and Healthy Living..151
* Checklist for Putting Together Your Own Program of Exercise...............152
* Don't Like Going to a Club to Exercise—You Don't Have To.................155
* How to Make Your Exercise Program Work for You...............................156
* Like to Exercise Early—Watch Out for Back Injuries.............................156
* Sore Muscles—2 Vitamins Can Make the Difference............................157

Eye Problems

* 93% of the Nearsighted May Be Able To Do Away With Glasses............157
* Nutrients to Fight-Back Age Related Blindness.....................................158
* See Specks Crossing Your Eye When you Read, You Have Floaters.......159

* Sore, Irritated Eyes? A Home Remedy that Gives Fast Relief................160
* 2 Vitamins to Cut Your Risk of Cataracts by 50% or More......................161

Fatigue

* A Simple Nutrient to Cure Fatigue and Increase Performance................161
* 9 Rare and not so Rare Causes of Tiredness...161
* What to Eat to Charge Your Batteries...164
* Setting Yourself Up for a Good Night's Sleep...165

Feeling Good

* 5 Tips to a More Satisfying Life..167
* 6 Natural Secrets to Feeling Good...168
* 8 Ways to Stop Negative Feelings from Spoiling Your Day......................170
* For a Long Healthy Life Find Some Friends...173

Fertility

* Turning Back the Clock for Successful Pregnancies..................................174

Fever

* When is a Fever Not a Fever?..174

Food Poisoning

* 81 Million Americans Each Year - What to Watch Out For.......................175
* 10 Causes and Symptoms of Food Poisoning..176
* How to Avoid the 7 Most Common Types of Food Poisoning.................178
* What To Do for a Poison Free Picnic..179

Foot Problems

* The Common Way to Relieve Foot Pain—That Doctors Overlook............181
* Type of Shoes to Prevent Corns, Bunions, and Hammertoes.................182

Gallstones

* Dangerous New Surgery for Gallbladder Removal that Can Increase
  Your Chance of Serious Injury..182

Gout

* Isn't Gout Extinct?—Then Why Have I Got It?..184
* Simple Plan that Gets the Gout Causers Out of Your Diet.......................184

Grief

*Steps to Dealing With Grief...185

Gum Disease

* A Natural Way of Curing Gum Disease, With No Side Effects.................190
* 2 Ways to Prevent, or Get Rid of, Gum Disease..190

Hair Problems

* Dull Gray Hair—Here's How to Make it Shine...................................191

Halitosis

* How to Sweeten Your Breath With Your Diet................................192

Hayfever

* 6 Ignored Secrets to Controlling Your Hayfever............................193

Headaches

* Clothes that Can Cause Headaches and Tiredness.......................195
* The Vitamin to Avoid if You are Taking Aspirin...............................195

Healing

* How to Heal Faster from Cuts, Scrapes, Bruises, and Surgery.............196

Health Care

* Free Health Care—Where to Look to Find It................................197

Health Insurance

* Cut Your Rates by Nearly 50% With these Tips............................198

Hearing Loss

* Need a Hearing Aid? Where to Get Information to
  Find the Good Ones..199
* Worried About Your Hearing—Avoid Noise................................199

Heartburn

* 4 Keys to Avoiding Heartburn...200
* The Sleeping Position to End Heartburn.................................201

Heart Attacks

* What to do If You are having a Heart Attack............................201

Heart Disease

* 2 Natural Approaches to Fighting Heart Attack and Stroke..............202
* 3 Ways to Beat Heart Failure..202
* 8 Pains That Could be Warning Signs of a Heart Attack................204
* 50 Milligrams Daily of this Supplement Can Cut Your Risk of a Stroke,
  Heart Attack, or Related Death in Half...............................205
* 4 Healthy-For-Your-Heart Eating Secrets.............................205
* 4 Vitamins and Minerals That Protect You Against Heart Disease,
  and Can Even Reverse It...207
* A Blood Pressure Medication Without Side Effects?...................208
* Heart Blockage—Protect Yourself After Angioplasty?.................209
* Heart Catherization? Is it the Right Test for You?..................209
* Heart Problems? This Reduces Stroke by 79%,
  says a Harvard Doctor...210

* How the "Over 40" Woman Can Lower Her Risk of Heart Disease..........210
* If You Take Saldane, You Should Never Take
These Two Drugs With It..................211
* Is Angioplasty the Right Treatment for You?..................211
* Is It Worthwhile Exercising to Prevent Heart Attacks?..................212
* New Study Reveals Nutrient that Can Reduce Your Risk of a
Heart Attack by 36%..................213
* Prevent Heart Attacks..................213
* Risk of Heart Attack and Healthy Cholesterol..................214
* Smoker's Beware—Trying to Stop Might Give You A Heart Attack..........214
* The Vitamin That Helps You Prevent Killer Heart Disease..................214
* What Effect Aspirin Really has on Heart Attacks..................215

Hemorrhoids
* Non-Surgical Treatments You Need to Know About..................216

Hernia
* A Problem Which Deserves Conservative Treatment..................218

High Blood Pressure
* Lower Your Chance of Needing High Blood Pressure Medication by
Simple Dietary Changes..................219
* 2 Natural Ways to Lower Your Blood Pressure Up to 53% in
Only Eight Weeks..................220
* 2 Ways to Protect Against the Effects of High Blood Pressure..................221
* 46% Cut in Risk of High Blood Pressure with Fruit..................222
* What Household Spice to Use to Lower Blood Pressure..................222

High Cholesterol
* Amazing New Research Shows Nutrient that
Helps Lower Bad Cholesterol..................223
* Chinese Food Lovers' Cure for High Cholesterol..................224
* Cholesterol Warning: Popular Drug that Increases Death From
Non-Cardiac Problems..................224
* Does Margarine Protect Against Cholesterol? Maybe Not..................224
* Natural Ways to Lower Your Cholesterol Without Drugs..................225
* No Cholesterol Foods That Are Actually Bad for You..................225
* The Real Reason People have High Cholesterol
It's Not What You Think..................226
* What Your Doctor Probably Misses from Your Cholesterol Report
You Need to Know Total Cholesterol Divided By HDL..................227

Household

* Eliminate Toxins from Your Dishwater.................................227

Immunity

* A Vitamin to Maximize Your Immune System...........................228
* Kick Your Immune System Into High Gear..............................229

Impotence

* A Diet to Help, and Its Simple Too...................................229
* Natural Remedies to End Impotence and Premature Ejaculation
  Plus Increase Sexual Desire...230
* Simpler Treatment Which is Closer to Natural........................231

Incontinence

* Prescription Drugs May Cause Your Problem...........................231

Infertility

* The Latest Views on Curing Infertility..............................232

Injury Secret

* Use this Ice-Then-Heat Treatment for Best Results...................233

Insomnia

* 6 Tips to Stop Insomnia...234
* How Sleep Loss Affects Your Health..................................236
* Jet Lag or Changing Shifts, Prevent Insomnia With a Pill............236
* Natural Cures for Your Sleep Problems...............................237
* Relax Tension to Overcome Sleeplessness.............................238
* What to do About Chronic Insomnia...................................238
* What to do About Temporary Insomnia.................................240

IQ Boosters

* 6 Types of Food Which can Increase Intelligence.....................240

Kidney Pain

* 2 Things You Must do to Save Your Kidneys
  Or Even Reverse Kidney Disease......................................244

Kidney Stones

* Diet Changes to Help You Get Rid of Them............................245
* Prevention With A Nearly Free Beverage—In Your Home Now,
  and Also Effective for Urinary Tract Infections and to Ease Joint Pain,
  Fight Constipation, and Avoid wrinkles..............................246

Knee Pain

* The Common Cause and What to do About It............................247

Longevity

* 5 Natural Ways to Purify Your Body—Get Rid of Toxins that Cause so Many Health Problems...249
* Birthdays Can Shorten Your Life—But Who Are They Worse For?.........250
* Foods to Eat to Beat Disease, Reverse It, and How to Stop It From Attacking Your Body..250
* 9 Tips that Can Add 10, 15, even 20 Healthy Years to Your Life.............251
* Recovery Secret—How to Imagine Yourself Healthy Again.....................252
* Natural Life-Extension Secret that can Add 10 to 1 Years to Your Life.....253
* Regain Good Health, Vigor, and Have Abundant Energy.........................254
* Strengthen the Natural Disease-Preventing Organs in Your Body............255
* The Type of Hospital to Avoid—Your Chances of Dying are Increased 25%...256

Loneliness
* Is it More than Being Alone?...256

Looking Good
* Crowning Your Way to a Better Smile..258
* Feel You Look Older Than You Are—Here's How to Look Younger...........259
* Facial Fitness Exercises to Erase Wrinkles?...260

Loss of Appetite
* What to Eat to Stimulate Your Appetite...260

Low Energy
* Want More Energy? 20 Natural Foods that Boost Energy.......................261

Low Self-Esteem
* 12 Ways to Feel Better About Yourself..262

Low Sex Drive
* 2 Vitamins Known to Help Athletes..264
* A Couple of Diet Changes that Can Change Your Life.............................265

Medication
* Foods to Avoid with Your Medicines..265
* 10 Popular Drugs that May Harm You—and Why....................................266
* How to Get Free Medicines, Even Expensive Prescriptions.....................267
* How to Read a Prescription Chart Tells You What All the Scribbling Means..267

Memory Loss
* Drugs to Avoid that Cause Short-Term Memory Loss..............................269
* How to Improve Your Memory in One Hour by Up To 50%.......................270
* Once-A-Day Natural Secret That Will Relax Your Nerves,

Sharpen Your Mind, and Boost Your Spirits..............................271

Menopause

* Estrogen for Menopause—Some Risks to Consider.....................272

* It Might Just Be the Best Time of Your Life.............................273

* Menopause Relief—Natural Secrets that Work.........................273

Migraine Headache

* 14 Million Missed Diagnoses in the United States.....................274

Muscle Cramps

* The Home Remedy Your Doctor Probably Doesn't Know About...............275

Muscle Pain

* Natural Ways to Get Rid of "Morning Aches" in Your Body.......................276

* 3 Simple Stretches that Relieve Muscle Stiffness in Seconds.................277

Nausea

* An Herbal Secret Which Prevents Nausea.............................277

Neck and Shoulder Pain

* A Guide to the 5 Minute Cure You Can do Anywhere.............................278

Nervousness

* This Free, Once-A-Day, Natural Secret Will Relax Your Nerves,
  Sharpen Your Mind, and Boost Your Spirits.............................279

Nightmares

* Nightmares Scaring You as an Adult—Not Uncommon.........................279

Nosebleeds

* The Best Way to Treat a Nosebleed.............................281

Nutrition

* 6 Healthy Choice Answers You Should Know.............................282

* 9 Nutritional Myths that Can Hurt Your Diet.............................284

* Avoid Chewable Vitamin C for Your Teeth.............................287

* Calcium for the Bones!—Take It the Right Way.............................287

* Guide to Building a Low Cal Salad to Fit Your Diet.............................288

* For the Best Juice Get the Best Juicer—What to Look For.....................288

* How to Store Vitamins to Keep Them Strong.............................289

* Liver! Should You Eat it—Why and Why Not?.............................289

* Magnesium, the Overlooked Miracle Nutrient.............................290

* 20 of the Best Sources of Magnesium.............................291

* Tap Water Taste Good? It May Not be Good For You.............................292

* Big News—Take Time Release Vitamins for Poor Nutrition.....................293

* If Your Food Tastes Bland, You Need Zinc.............................293

* Message in Your Vitamins With Exercise.................................293
* Should Iron Supplements be In Your Diet?.........................294
* The "30 Plus 40 Plus 50" Rule for Good Health......................294
* The Vitamin That Can Make You Sick If You Overuse...........294
* Trouble Getting Your Iron, Maybe Your Blocking It?..............295
* What to Avoid to Keep Your Body's Vitamin Levels High.......295
* What is A Recommended Daily Allowance?.........................296
* What to Put in Your Tea So Your Body Absorbs More Calcium and Iron...298
* Why Pink Grapefruit is 20 Times Better for You Than White Grapefruit...298

Oily Hair and Skin
* A Hint that You have too much Oil in Your Diet, and What to do About It..299

Osteoporosis
* A Drink a Day to Keep the Doctor Away................................300
* New Ways to Strengthen Brittle Bones.................................300
* 7 Foods That Strengthen Brittle Bones.................................301
* Osteoporosis and Contraceptives—What is the Connection?.................302
* Osteoporosis and the Older Female....................................303
* Caffeine Effects and Osteoporosis.....................................303
* Stop Bone Loss With 1,500 milligrams of This Mineral Daily.................304

Overactive Children
* Diet of Foods to Avoid Calms 63%......................................304

Overweight
* Build Muscle and Lose Weight With this Nutrient....................305
* Don't Yo-Yo, even If you Hate Your Weight...........................305
* Guide to Building a Low Cal Salad to Fit Your Diet.................306
* Here is Why Your Teen-ager is Dieting.................................308
* New Weight Tables Revised Upward 5%................................308
* Revised Weight Table—MEN - Age 25 and over......................309
* Revised Weight Table—WOMEN - Age 25 and over.............309
* The Amazing Natural Supplement that Will Speed-Up Your Body's
  Fat Metabolism Function for Faster Weight Loss.....................310
* To Lose Weight Permanently—Cheat on Your Diet.................310
* Want to Lose Weight—Turn Off the TV................................311

Pain
* A Household Chore that Relieves Shoulder, Arm, and Hand Pain.........312
* A Breathing Technique that Stops Pain Dead in It's Tracks....................313
* Nature's Miracle Pain Reliever—Rub on Your Pain for

Fast Effective Relief..314

* Pain Control After Surgery can Protect You From Cancer.......................315

Phobias

* 5 Secrets to Ridding Yourself of Fear..315

PMS Problems

* What Men Can Do to Help Women Cope with PMS..............................318

* PMS Relief—Natural Secrets that Work..319

* The Nutrient that Lessons PMS Irritability, Anxiety, Crying, Pain,
  and Water Retention..319

Pregnancy

* 4 Exercises to Make Your Pregnancy Easier..320

* 4 Secrets to a Healthy Pregnancy and Baby...321

* A Simple Way of Preventing High Blood Pressure During Pregnancy....322

* A Vitamin to Help Morning Sickness..323

* Avoid Lead Poisoning Your Baby by Avoiding this Natural Nutrient.........323

* Protect Against Birth Defects with a Nutrient..324

Premature Ejaculation

* One Drug to a Better Sex Life..324

Prescription Drugs

* 10 Most Used and What to Watch Out For...325

Prostate Problems

* Diet Changes that can Help...327

* What to do If It's Cancer..327

Psoriasis

* A Natural Oil that Can End this Skin Problem, and Available in Health
  Food Stores...329

* A Nutrient that Moisturizes Flaky, Cracked, Callused,
  and Itchy Skin "Magically"..329

Recovery Secret

* Doctor's Proven Way to Imagine Yourself Healthy Again—It Works.......330

Relaxation

* 7 Relaxation Methods for a New Life..331

* 10 Second Secret for Tension Control..332

Sexual Desire

* 2 Foods that Will Increase Your Sexual Desire, or Your Partner's..........333

* 8 Secrets For Better Sex After Age 40..334

* Male Sexual Performance Too Low—This May be Why...........................336

Sexually Transmitted Diseases
* The Forgotten Disease that 30 Million Americans Have...........................337

Shingles
* What You can do About Shingles—Can You Prevent It?........................338

Sinus Problems
* Runny Nose Bothering You—Drug Free Way to Control It.....................339
* Sinus Pain—Natural Relief Without Drugs..339
* Your Cold Might Really Be a More Serious Sinus Inflammation.............340

Skin Problems
* Better Skin Care From Your Refrigerator...341
* Dry Skin? A Nutrient that Almost "Magically" Moisturizes Dry Skin.........341
* Some Hints to Get Rid of Freckles..342
* Natural Wrinkle Removers and Why They Work.....................................342

Sleeping Problems
* 2 Natural Secrets for Good, Restful Sleep Every Night..........................343
* Use Daily Rituals to Overcome Sleeplessness......................................344
* What to do If Body Pain Prevents Sleep..345

Smoking
* 5 Alternatives Ways to Cure this Addiction..345
* 5 Step Plan to Break the Tobacco Habit..348
* A Painless 7 Day Plan to Stop Smoking..350

Snoring
* 10 Cures to Snoring So You Won't Go Crazy...351
* Some Simple Cures to do at Home..354

Sore Throat
* On What to do, and Why You Shouldn't Let it Bother You......................355

Stomach Problems
* 9 Causes and Cures of Stomach Pain..355

Stress
* 3 Exercises to Relieve Your Stress..359
* 13 Natural Stress Reducing Secrets..360

Strokes
* The Antioxidant Vitamin that Can Help You Prevent a Stroke.................362
* The Vitamin Supplement that Cuts the Risk of Dying from a Stroke......362

Summer Health
* 10 Summer Health Hazards to Watch Out For..363

Surgery

* How to Tell If You Need Surgery Or Not—20% of All Surgery is Unneeded...366
* Is Your Surgeon Experienced Enough to Operate on You?...................367

Thyroid Problems

* Alleviate Thyroid Problems and Disease Without Harmful Drugs...........368
* What are They and What Some of the Best Treatments Are..................369

Toothache

* Herb that Relieves Toothache Pain.......................................370
* How a Slice of Cheddar Cheese After Meals Can Prevent Plaque, Tooth Decay, and Gum Disease...370
* How to Whiten Your Teeth Without a Dentist..........................370
* What A Gum Surgeon May Never Tell You..............................372
* Natural Ways to Save Your Teeth Without Surgery....................372

Toxins

* 5 Natural Ways to Purify Your Body, and Get Rid of Toxins that Cause so Many Diseases and Illnesses...................................373
* Harmful Toxins from Your Dishwasher?—How to Eliminate Them..........375

Ulcers

* Does Aspirin Cause Ulcers?Sometimes...................................375
* Heal Chronic Ulcers With this Combination Treatment..................376
* How Licorice Tablets Can Help You Get Rid of an Ulcer................377

Underweight

* No Sympathy and Little Help—Here's Some.............................378

Urination Pain

* A Test You Can Use in Your Home to Prevent Infection.................379
* Secrets to Prevention forWomen.......................................379
* Your Pain May be the Price You are Paying to Treat Your Cold.............381

Vaccination

* Shot and Test Reference Guide—A List of Vaccines and Screening Tests You Should Get, At What Ages, and How Often................................382

Vaginal Infections

* Ever Had a Yeast Infection? Here are a few Diet Hints...................... 383

Weight Loss

* 7 Questions and Answers to Help Lose Weight While You Eat Fast Foods..384
* 10 Ways to Lose 10 Pounds...387

* 11 Foods that Lowers Cholesterol While You Lose Weight....................390
* A Miracle Pill for Weight Loss Is It Safe?................................393
* 10 Secrets for Getting and Staying Thin................................394
* Lose Up to 14 Pounds in 7 Days................................396
* An Amazing Herbal Tonic Tea to Lose Weight and More........................398
* Chocolate or Carob Candy Which is Best?................................398
* Mineral Weight Loss Miracle Pill What is It?................................398
* Snacking Diet Lets You Lose 5 Pounds a Week................................399

Wounds

* Cure a Simple Cut on the Fingers With a Band-Aid................................400
* Wound Healing Secrets—How to Recover Faster from Accidents, Cuts,
    Scrapes, Bruises, and Even Surgery................................401

X-Ray Defense

* Supplement Which Neutralizes Free Radicals................................402

Format of the Book

This book presents its "health secrets" in a unique manner. The Table of Contents and the Index have been combined into an expanded Table of Contents. The main topics are alphabetical, and the information relating to each of the topics are included under each of the main topic headings. In the few cases in which more than one topic is discussed in an area, the main topic headings refer to the initial set of information.

Also left out of this book are chapters, since dictionaries and encyclopedias do not have chapters, there is no reason why a book arranged alphabetically should have chapters either.

Each topic area may be looked-up directly in the Table of Contents, and those discussions of importance can then be examined for advice in natural methods of influencing and preventing disease under each category. The areas covered are broad, and include both ancient wisdom and new research. They are meant to be reminders as well as informers of what can be done with simple, in many cases household, substances. While not every remedy will work for every case, every piece of information included is based upon medical practices or medical research, and most of it will stand up to the test of time.

INTRODUCTION

Why We Have to Look Out for Our Own Health

Have you ever been sick? Or had a sick relative or friend? Everyone has, and everyone has been touched by their friendly doctor or hospital. While we are often helped by going to the doctor, many times we pay our money, but are told that nothing can be done. Sometimes, even, the drugs we are given to make us well just make us sicker.

That is the reason for looking for ways to prevent disease before we become sick, and for ways of strengthening our bodies when we do become sick. By helping our bodies to be healthier, we are sick less often, and therefore, we recover much faster.

Do you know that even cancer patients who are thought to be dying sometimes recover. The recovery is called a remission, and even doctors don't know how it happens, but one thing we do know about remission is that the body does it on it's own, not the medicines the patient is being given.

The more we are able to care for ourselves, the more we are in control of our lives, and being in control of our health is a big step in gaining control of our lives. The hospital and the doctor's office can be impersonal places that a person finds himself in.

The essence of this book is that most of the time we can do things to help ourselves be more healthy, and we can always do things to help ourselves to recover from diseases when they do occur.

These hints may or may not save lives, but they are certain to give every-one a chance of caring for themselves, and of keeping their bodies healthier and happier. Good health is the absence of disease, and the more we can do to give ourselves good health, the better off we will be.

A blessing of good luck and good health to all who seek natural healing.

ACCIDENTS

19 Things You Should have
in Your Medicine Chest for Emergencies

The nature of accidents are that they happen unexpectedly. Furthermore they do not become emergencies unless they are also serious. In this sense a serious accident becomes an emergency, but not all emergencies are accidents. A heart attack is surely an emergency, but is never an accident. In spite of the difference, if you are fully ready for the emergencies caused by accidents you will also be ready for most of the emergencies which have other causes as well.

The major classes of accidents are: automobile accidents, either being struck by an auto, or being in one which crashes; accidents in the home including falls, poisoning, burns, drownings, cuts, and broken bones of all sorts; and various accidents of lesser frequency of many types such as gunshot wounds, falls on the street, strikes of lightening, and so on. Some of these you are liable to see, and others you may never see, but you should nevertheless have some idea of what to do as emergency first aid when any accident occurs in your vicinity. And with this preparation we commence the list of the 19 things you should have in your first aid kit for accidents and emergencies.

1. A good book on first aid procedures should be your first choice. While there are many you can choose from, the Red Cross puts out a good one, and any book store will have a broader selection if you want to compare some. This little handbook will give you basic instructions for practically any emergency you may run into, as well as tips for special equipment that might not be included in our list of the 19 basic items given here.

2. Band aids of various sizes, with or without disinfectant, can be used for any minor cuts, scrapes, or punctures. The band aids should range in size from about 1/2 inch to 1 inch, and include both strips and circles. The basic use is very simple, simply clean off the injured area with soap and water and cover it with a band aid. Then replace the band aids as they become loose or dirty for a day or two, until the wound heals. An area of dry, cracked skin, or small cuts on the fingers can be healed very effectively with just band aids by covering the sore area for 2 or 3 days, or more. Keeping it covered will hold in moisture, and get the healing process well started. Generally no further care is needed.

3. Since we have already mentioned it, you should make sure that you have a good, and fresh disinfectant for wounds. The main problem with wounded areas are that the dirt that gets into them, or the nail or glass that makes them, is not a clean object, and can carry bacteria. Even a minor wound can have strep-

tococcus or gangrene bacteria from what they call gas producing bacteria. This bacteria lives all around us in the dirt we walk, and in the dirt that can get into any cut or scrape you get on your body. Disinfectants will help kill this bacteria and keep the damaged area clean. The two most common disinfectants were mercurochrome and iodine. In years past people didn't like to use iodine because it hurt when it was put on, but now it is made so that it won't do that. Nowadays many first aid kits come with a cream called bacitracin, which is probably better than the older disinfectants, and keeps better too.

4. Since we are talking about wounds the next object in your kit should be a roll of gauze for larger wounds. Gauze is sterile, and can be used to either jam into a large wound to get pressure, or to wrap a whole arm or leg that is cut badly so that bleeding can be put under control. Because you will probably use gauze only when you have a large area to cover, it would be a good idea to keep a couple of rolls with the first aid supplies.

5. Speaking of wraps, this brings up the question of what do you do for breaks. For breaks the best choice is an ace bandage. Ace bandages are the same things you get from your doctor when he wants to wrap an arm or leg that is weak and sore, and must be particularly protected. It is one of the simplest first aid items to use, and can be applied in a matter of seconds to any broken bone, including the ribs. It is also better than gauze for this purpose since it is stronger, and comes equipped with a little clip device that can be used to secure the end.

6. The next item assumes that an injury you have from an accident is also going to be painful, and you need a pain reliever that is essentially safe and effective for everyone. The first pain reliever that comes to mind is simply aspirin, and it can be buffered as well. If you have an objection to aspirin for any reason then go with Tylenol or Ibuprofen, which are improvements on aspirin, although at a slightly higher cost. Aspirin has the other beneficial affects of lowering fevers and acting as a mild sedative to induce sleep.

7. Assuming that accidents happen wherever and whenever they want to, and are not planned, it stands to reason that they often happen away from home. For this reason it is always a good idea to have a couple of dollars in change among your emergency items. While this does not appear on any Red Cross checklist, it is often the only thing that will get you help if you are in an accident in which you need a friend or family member and not an ambulance. It can also come in handy if you are stranded away from home for a while and need a little something to eat.

8. While we are on the subject of being stuck away from home, you should also have a one day supply of every prescription drug you are taking whenever you are traveling, even to your local mall or market. This, along with a list of the medication you are taking can be a life saver if you are in an accident that renders you unconscious. Imagine being in an accident where you are unable to get your insulin, if you are diabetic, or heart medicine, if you are on a cardiac program. Delays of a day in getting either of these can send you into a diabetic coma, or give you a heart attack.

9. Speaking of medicines, you should also have a selection of any emergency medicines you normally keep near you, but included in your emergency accident kit. Such items as nitroglycerin for angina, or a candy bar to bring your blood sugar level up to normal for a diabetic, which you don't need every day but might need any time are a necessity. With a little planning and a little care there is no reason to ever be completely away from any potentially life saving item that you normally have at your fingertips when you are in your own home.

10. You will also need a more general disinfectant for larger areas of the body, and even for knives and other instruments you might need to use. A simple and cheap chemical for this is hydrogen peroxide. Peroxide is available in the supermarket, and should be replaced anyway once or twice a year. When you use it you can either pour it over the affected area, or put some into a container and let the body part, or instrument, soak for a minute or two. Of course if you get it on clothing it will cause it to bleach out, so watch out that it isn't spilled on anything that you care about.

11. We are beginning to get the stuff we need into this first aid kit, but we still lack a sharp instrument. A scalpel is the best, but a sharp and clean knife is also acceptable. You may need this to cut away something you have become entangled in, or to open an obstinate medicine bottle, but knives do come in handy when you least expect it.

12. Now back to personal items. Include a list of important phone numbers, including for friends, family members, and your doctor or heath care provider. You will be surprised how you will forget these numbers in an emergency, and how valuable they will become if someone else is looking through your things trying to decide who they should call in regard to giving you help. For convenience these numbers can be placed on a single 3x5 inch card, and then sprayed with a little hair spray to waterproof it. That will prevent fading, and water damage in most cases. One of these cards should also be carried in your wallet or purse.

13. While you are at it, you can pretty well predict that any accident you have is going to ruin your clothes, and may require something to cover parts of your body. For this I would recommend a full sized blanket and/or a change of clothes for yourself. For really general use the clothes may be in the form of a sweatsuit with a zip up front. You can dress in a sweat suit and walk out in public, which you may not be able to do in a blanket, and especially in clothes that have been ripped from your body. Did you know that if you go to the emergency room of a hospital and are discharged, nobody makes any effort to see that you are dressed before they send you out the door. If you want to ensure that you have something to wear in an emergency situation, then you have better include it yourself.

14. Getting into the small tools, a pair of tweezers can help with embedded thorns, pieces of metal, and dirt and debris that gets into wounds. The tweezers should have a good tight close, and not be too difficult to work. If you are going to use tweezers on any open wound, clean them first with the hydrogen per-

oxide and allow them to air dry. Drying them with a dirty cloth will make them just as dirty as they were before you began, and you could add cloth fibers to the wound as you try to clean it.

15. Something to calm the stomach is always a good idea. If the accident involves anything that makes you throw up you may need to take a stomach calmer until you can get professional help. The big problem with uncontrolled throwing up, as with diarrhea, is that they leave you weak and dehydrated. For children, the sick, and the old this can mean a quick death as well. In a pinch milk can help, except if you have a problem digesting milk and then you get diarrhea. You are probably better off with a product like a chalk based medicine. The chalk coats the stomach, prevents the stomach acid from reacting with the stomach wall, and neutralizes excess acid.

16. If you are anywhere in the vicinity of your home, and that can mean with a couple of hundred miles of it, a cellular phone can save you in any location you may be stranded or hurt in. Cellular phones start at around $100 and go up. A good one will probably cost you $200 to $300, and you want to be sure that you can carry it with you since they are very popular for thieves. If you get a cellular phone you will also need to get a phone service since that is how they work.

17. You may also have a problem in which your body becomes sore and bruised, or you are feeling cold. For these problems, and especially if there is no one with you to give you a massage, you should have a container of canned heat. Canned heat is sold in sporting goods stores and pharmacies, and when applied to the skin it stimulates blood flow and makes the area feel hot. Do not get this in your eyes or your mouth, or you will need another kind of first aid to prevent the burning of the eyes, or poisoning.

18. While we are talking about the problem of soreness and the need to promote blood flow, you may have the opposite problem of decreasing the blood flow in order to control a fever and cool the body. Now while water will work, rubbing alcohol is more compact and works much faster. If someone is suddenly struck with a fever, give them aspirin and start making applications of alcohol. This will cool the surface of their skin, and may just save someone's life in the case of extremely high temperatures.

19. Finally we are concerned with the problem of protection from the sun. Sunburn protection is a necessity in any accident that leaves you exposed, or where you have already gotten a burn. The best sunburn lotions, spf 15 and above, will cut out virtually all of the ultraviolet radiation. For additional protection you should also have a sunburn lotion that contain hydrocortisone to relieve pain for both sunburn and skin rash.

That is the list of 19 items for an accident and emergency kit. Obviously not all of these can be carried on your person, but they can all fit into your car and your home. In cases where you are walking, hiking, or biking away from home, make up a smaller pack using a selection of the 19 above. And while there is no guarantee that the items in this list will supply every one of your accident needs, it is a good bet that it will take care of 90% to 99% of them.

ACNE

An Acne Diet that Will Surprise You

Ever wonder why you get acne, or at least why teenagers get it? Well its not quite for the reasons you think, Mainly its caused by the hormones we produce as our body matures, and the worst cases are limited to the teen-age years. If you still have acne as an adult it may be because your hormones are not acting as they should, or it could be because of a bad diet, or that your skin is being exposed to something it is allergic to. Here, though, we are interested in doing something about the acne that is caused by your diet, and we have some changes you can make that will help to cut down on the acne problem.

First, to get rid of one worry that you may have, it is not chocolate or greasy foods that cause acne. They may clog your pores and cause blackheads, but that is not acne. Acne is caused by the oils and acids that are produced by your body, and not by the oils and acids that your body is digesting because you ate them. So what you want to do is to cut down on foods that cause you to produce more of these oil and acids, and that means cutting down on processed foods and sugar.

To help your acne you have to get back to a natural diet, and with more vitamins and minerals than you probably have in your regular diet. You need more zinc, and zinc is found in lean beef. You need whole grain cereals, dairy products, peas, beans, root vegetables like potatoes and beets, nuts, and lecithin (which you get from egg yolks). You also need to eat whole grains and seafood for selenium, and vitamin A, vitamin B6. Raw fruits and vegetables, and leafy green vegetables, will give you vitamin C, and vitamin E. For an extra kick of your acne have 3 cloves of crushed raw garlic each day. Of course you can also get garlic oil capsules and avoid the breath problem.

AGE RELATED DISEASES

4 Ways to Strengthen the Glands
that Controls Age Related Diseases

A gland that controls age related disease, isn't that silly? On the other hand why shouldn't our glands affect the way we age? Certainly not everyone ages the same. Some people are healthy at 90, and others are old at 40, so something is certainly going on in addition to the number of years you have lived. Glands produce those things that keep our bodies operating as they should, and when the glands don't work right neither do our bodies. In a word, we get sick.

As you live more years you have more chances for your glands to malfunction. Naturally you are going to have more sickness the older you get, and you will have more chances to get illnesses that can't be completely cured. So maybe there is a gland that controls many of the diseases we get as we age, and maybe strengthening that gland will prevent some of those diseases, and keep us healthier longer.

The gland that most fits this idea is the thymus, and it is known to control the function of the immune system. Now you should know that if you have reached the age of 50 it may be hard to even find your thymus, since it reaches its peak of activity by around age 20 and then begins to gradually disappear. This disappearance of the thymus in older people is a good clue to why we are most susceptible to serious illnesses in older age. But the real question is what can you do to correct this thymus deficiency, and to prevent the diseases of aging.

1. The first thing that you can do is to buy a thymus extract and take it as a supplement to replace your missing thymus. A good one available in the health food store is called Immunoplex 402, and is made from the thymus glands of calves. This doesn't have to be taken all of the time, but any time you have an infection it can be useful.

2. In cases of more serious diseases such as hepatitis B, or even AIDS, a stronger form of thymus is available as in injectable. This is a synthetic form called thymosin alpha 1, and it has been found to raise T-cell levels in the body, and increase the interferon and immuno globulins that the immune system uses to fight infections. Used for hepatitis B patients, 86% were cured after being given injections twice weekly.

3. A third form of thymus is in oral form, and is called thymodulin. Oral thymus administration has been looked down on in the United States because it has been thought that the acids in the stomach would destroy the extracts. However, thymodulin has been extensively studied in Europe for many years and

---

has been found effective against hepatitis B, herpes zoster, whooping cough, chicken pox, and mononucleosis. These effects are significant enough that oral thymus drugs are standard in Europe.

4. Now that you have been given the three main forms of thymus, you have to know that you should not take it alone. When you are taking thymus in any form you should also be taking a good vitamin and mineral supplement. The proper levels of vitamins and minerals are necessary to produce the various substances that are needed to fight disease and infection.

5,000 Year Old Medicine Fights Aging

If you have an interest in natural ways of fighting disease then it shouldn't come as any surprise that some people were fighting aging before the Romans founded Rome. Of course any medicine around that long has a good track record, if we can just find out what it has been used for all of those years we should know pretty well what we can do with it today. Well, in the case of the Ginkgo biloba we apparently have found a winner. The ginkgo is probably the oldest tree on earth, and its use in Asia is known to go back for thousands of years, perhaps as many as 5,000. While we don't really know everything it has been used for over those many years, it is now being used in Asia and Europe by over 5 million people to counter the physical effects of aging.

Now this is a very undefined use since we undergo many changes as we age, it is useful if we also know which effects of aging we can expect to counter by using it. First of all it acts by increasing the blood supply to the brain and protecting the tissues from damage by free radicals. The aging processes which are offset by these effects are better memory, alertness, and attention. In fact the worse off you are the greater the effect that it has. It may be that improving circulation automatically improves the oxygen supply to the heart, muscles, and internal organs, and keeps them healthier and more disease free. It also helps the eyes from degenerating as well. Now just think of the people who usually die youngest, of disease, in American society today. A great many of them are smokers, and smoking decreases the supply of oxygen throughout the body, as well as introduces many toxins into it.

If this has convinced you to begin taking ginkgo, you can get it over-the-counter in a 24% ginkgoloid tablet. The standard dose is three of these 40 mg tablets daily. If you are going to Europe you will either have to take your own supply or get a prescription while you are there.

Exercise for Independence with 15 Minutes a Day

To become dependent upon others, no matter how loving, when you get older is often a slippery road to a board and care facility or nursing home. And while it looks inevitable because so many older people are in that situation, it is

---

not at all incurable. If you are still independent, or nearing that decision point of whether or not you can take care of yourself, there is something you can do that can add up to 15 years to your independence. That something is exercise.

Now you will ask what exercise, you have lived 70 years without exercise and can't see yourself out running miles at your age, or peddling a bike down the highway either. The truth of it is that you don't have to do either of these things, and you can be helped at 70, or 80, or even 50. Age is not as important as getting out there and doing it as early as you can. The fewer problems you have when you begin, the better off you will be over time.

The benefits of exercise for seniors have been investigated by researchers at the University of Toronto, in Canada. They have found that even a modest exercise program can add 10 to 15 years of independent living to the aged. They also found that it doesn't matter what type of exercise you do, as they all give the same benefit. You can always walk, or swim, or play tennis, or whatever you can find enjoyment and interest in. The only guideline you must follow is that the exercise is done atleast every other day (or more), and that you keep it up until you begin to sweat.

It will probably be the part about doing it nearly every day that is most discouraging to anyone not committed to exercising already. But that is where the flexibility of the program comes in, if you don't like to walk all the time then find something else you like to do occasionally and put that in. In fact find 6 things you like to do and you won't have to repeat the same pattern for years at a time. You will still have an excellent exercise program that will give you all of the benefits of exercise, and little of the boredom of repeating yourself every day.

Of course everything must have cautions, and exercise is no different. Exercise done to excess can injure you, or it can just be so hard that you get discouraged and don't go on with it. The rule of thumb is that while a little stiffness is fine while you are active, you should not have pain from the exercise that carries over more than one day afterwards. Also, while you are exercising you should not have pain in your chest, back, or knees. And when you are doing the exercise you should keep it down to where you can still speak comfortably to anyone with you. Don't exercise yourself until you are completely out of breath.

Now for those of you who are competitive, take your time. Take whatever activity you are doing and whatever level you are doing it at, and don't try to improve more than one percent a month. What? That is too slow! Nonsense, one percent a month will increase your ability 12% a year, and every year. Ask any professional athlete if he would be happy to improve 12% every year, and all of them over the age of 20 will say they would be thrilled.. Give yourself time and keep working and you will get to be as good as you can be.

Getting started is the hardest part, and has been put off till the last. To start, if you are doing nothing now, go out with a small 15 minutes a day. Just 15 minutes a day and in two months you will see benefits in how you feel and what you can do, but you need to keep it up. Of course you want to increase your time as you get in better shape, and after 3 to 6 months you should be up to 45 minutes a day, 4 or 5 times a week. If you can't quite reach this level, then just do as much as you can as often as you can.

If you take some effort to take care of your body now, it will help to take care of you later. Only you can put this effort into keeping your body flexible, strong, and capable of taking orders from you when you need it to do something, even taking care of yourself.

Free Government Publications on Staying Healthy as We Grow Older

One of the most difficult problems in staying healthy at any age is finding reliable information at a reasonable price. The government happily offers more than 60 publications on staying healthy for the older American, entirely free of charge. To get a list of the publications, or to find information on a specific problem, you can call, toll-free, 1-800-222-2225, weekdays, from 8:30 A.M. to 5 P.M., EST. This is the National Institute on Aging (NIA) hotline.

The Nutrients that Can Prevent and Fight Back Age-Related Blindness

Poor eyesight just seems to be something all older people have, and we tend to think that there is nothing you can do about it as you get older. Fortunately this idea is dead wrong, and there is quite a bit you can do about it. Furthermore, you are the main one who has to act if you want to prevent your vision from getting worse over the years. Don't worry about the charts the optometrists use as much as you worry about your own ocular nutrition, and you might just avoid the unfortunate loss of sight so many old people face.

The first nutritional step to take in preventing the loss of your eyesight is to have a good nutritional supplement program before you have any problem with your eyes. These supplements should contain a liberal amount of anti-oxidant vitamins like vitamin E and vitamin C, as well as B-complex. Establish this as part of your living plan as young as you can, and keep it up as long as no problems develop. When you do have a medical problem in spite of the nutritional program it will be time to take additional nutritional steps for correction.

Since our main interest is in your eyes, you should know that the eyes have their own nutritional needs and that they may not be met with a normal supplement plan. When you are younger and in good health the eyes will get all of their proper nutrients from the foods you eat and the supplements you take. But when you are older you may not eat quite the same, and you may have a problem absorbing the nutrients you take into your body as a result of some other medical problem.

At this time the eyes may need additional supplements of an amino acid called taurine, which serves to stabilize the cells in the photoreceptors of the eyes. This stabilization protects the eyes from the effects of ultraviolet light, and free radicals. In animal studies, animals who were deficient in taurine developed degenerative changes in the photoreceptors, in the same way as many people whose condition is improved by taking taurine supplements. Even children on taurine deficient diets showed abnormal retinas, and the condition was corrected by adding additional taurine to their diets.

Flavonoids are another class of nutrient our eyes need that is found in many plant foods. The specific flavonoids we need to concentrate on are found especially in blueberries and grapes, as well as in many other fruits and vegetables. They are called anthocyanosides and they help especially with night vision. If you have any problem with your night vision you should look into supplements for this flavonoid, as well as increasing fruits and vegetables in your diet. They have also been found to cut down on bleeding in the eyes of diabetic patients, which is one of the major factors in deteriorating vision of diabetics. In a study of 60 patients with a serious vision deterioration condition called macular degeneration, who were given this anthocyanosides, half had improved vision.

Don't ignore your vision any more than you would ignore any other part of your health. Treat yourself with proper nutrition and you can prevent, or limit, changes in your eyes with aging, or that accompany diseases such as diabetes.

The Truth About Some Popular Anti-Aging Drugs

Drugs to fight the aging process have been around for many years, and some people do seem to look and act many years younger than their age, but do the two have anything to do with one another? So far as is known there is no drug that stops or reverses aging, though there are many things your can do to stop some of the effects of aging. The claims that drugs such as gerovital, which is a preparation of procaine, is an anti-aging drug are rather silly. This drug is also known as Novocaine, and has no obvious effect on aging. It is used by dentists across the country, and acts as a mild anti-depressant as well as pain reliever.

The anti-aging drug GH-3, which was introduced in Rumania in 1956, is even more of a problem. Although claimed to be highly effective, it has been controversial since its introduction, and seems to have no more effectiveness than gerovital.

The true anti-aging prescriptions are to be found in those people who live long and healthy lives in the world. To be one of those you need to maintain a

---

moderate exercise program, cut to a minimum any bad habits you have, and it is not a bad idea to take some vitamin supplements, no matter what the doctors say, they do not hurt you and can save you a lot of illness when anything does attack your body.

3 Anti-Aging Nutrients that can Reverse Aging, Improve Memory, and Fight-Off Disease

While it would be wonderful if there were a magic pill that would cure all of the ills of aging, the truth is that there isn't. Aging is a continuous process, just like life, and if we don't age in one way, then we age in another. And of course the term isn't used to refer to people who go from 20 years old to 30 years old, it usually refers to those around 60 and above. Anyone who is 60 or 70 or 80 years old can expect little more than to be referred to as an aged, or aging person. While that can be insulting, since no one likes to be put into a box which deprives them of opportunities, it at least gives a focus to certain types of information, and the nutrients listed here fall into one of those types of information. So for some hints as to nutrients which may reverse aging, improve memory, and fight off disease, sample what is offered in good health.

1.   For a nutrient which is always thought of as having the ability to reverse aging we turn to vitamin E. Vitamin E is discussed many times in this volume, but this is the first time it is presented as the "antiaging" vitamin. And why do we call vitamin E the antiaging vitamin, because it has the greatest ability to get us out of our easy chairs and into an active lifestyle again. The reason so many older people spend their time sitting is because the circulation in their legs decreases they are more prone to leg cramps after minimal exercise, or even after no exercise at all. If you give in to this sitting lifestyle you eventually develop a condition called claudication in which the blood pools at the contact points where you sit, and your legs may then ache all of the time. In order to fight aging you have to remain active, and to do that you have to use your legs. You can use them very vigorously as in dancing or jogging, or more gently as in walking or gardening. But to be healthy you have to get up and move. Vitamin E does this for you. Of course it also has the effect of fighting free radicals, as does vitamin C, but that is another story.

2.   The best way to keep your memory sharp at any age is to use your mind. Your mind and memory are put to the greatest use when you are communicating by talking, writing, reading, playing games, or learning something new. It is put to the least use when you are simply in an environment where things are going on around you that you are not directly involved in, and where you have no role in the outcome, such as watching television. But even assuming that you are staying involved in everything that goes on around you it is still possible to lose some of your ability to remember because of a nutrient shortage in your diet. The

memory nutrient has been designated vitamin B12, and it is found abundantly in green vegetables. The problem as we age is that our digestive system makes it harder to digest roughage such as we get in leafy green vegetables, and we cut down on our total diet as well. Consequently we end up with nutritional deficiencies in certain items, and vitamin B12 is one of those most commonly deficient as we age. The solution is simple, increase the B12 foods in your diet, take supplements, and if your need is more extreme get B12 shots from your doctor. If you have been feeling a little dull mentally over a few weeks or months it will seem like you have just awaken' to a new world where you can again be your normal self.

3. Disease is such a broad term, especially when it refers to older people. Disease is anything that limits our activity by interfering with the function of our body. Naturally there is no one medicine or nutrient that can either cure or prevent all diseases. But there is a nutrient that is a great help in the case of many diseases, and it is something we can depend on. The nutrient is vitamin C, and in sufficiently large doses it may cure colds and the flu, help blood flow through the body, and relieve body pain and fevers. If this isn't a nutrient that can help to cure the diseases of aging, then I guess that one doesn't exist. The daily therapeutic dose of vitamin C is 2 to 3 grams, and if you are actively ill, up to 5 grams. Doses should be spread out over the day, and natural sources can supply a large amount if you choose foods just for vitamin C content. An added bonus of vitamin C is that it helps wounds and surgeries to heal along with preventing and curing many of the daily ills of older Americans.

AIDS

3 Keys to Prevent Getting Aids from Common Medical Procedures

The greatest risk of getting AIDS from a medical procedure is that you will get it through a blood transfusion. The risk is not especially great since only one in 250,000 units of blood are contaminated with the AIDS virus (a risk comparative to some forms of cancer), and of course you only have to get it once. Because of what AIDS is, and what it can do, it is worthwhile for you to take whatever precautions you can to prevent yourself from being exposed to AIDS contaminated blood. If you can follow the three keys below you can certainly lower your risk of getting AIDS through a blood transfusion to much less than one in 250,000.

1. Prepare for your own surgeries by setting up your own personal blood bank. You do this by going in periodically and having your blood withdrawn and

stored at the hospital where you are going to have your operation, or where you are likely to be treated if no operation is planned. Since you will then be getting your own blood in transfusion you can't give yourself anything you don't already have. The problem in this is that if we don't plan for an operation, and we have to have one as an emergency because of some accident, then we probably won't have any of our own blood stored. You can cover this by going to your local hospital on a regular basis anyway and having blood taken and stored, but it would have to be done regularly from year to year because hospitals aren't going to just store your own blood for you for a very long time. The best bet for this method of avoiding AIDS is only if you have some idea that you are going to have an operation requiring blood, and it will be sometime in the future so you can go through the blood drawing and storage process. The hospital you use should have use a process called cell savers. In this procedure your own blood is collected during surgery and circulates it back into your body, which cuts down on the amount of blood you would need in transfusion.

2. Get to know something about your doctor, and don't choose one who recommends surgery first, before trying other therapies. For one thing, many medical treatments can take the place of surgeries, and sometimes cure problems just as well. If you are in an emergency situation you may not have this choice, but for most surgeries you will have a warning of several months to a year or two. In these cases get to know as much as you can about your doctor, and then do as recommended above and set up your own blood bank. Of course you also have to know if your doctor will work with you on this, and avoid those who won't when you are not given an explanation that satisfies you.

3. Look into the practices available to save your own blood that is lost in surgery, and re-using it for transfusion. This is a very specialized process, but it can keep you from being exposed to AIDS. You are going to have to question your doctor as well as look into the hospital practices, which your doctor can do if he does not know already. The procedure is called "cell-salvage," and salvages your own blood cells during the operation.   If you can follow any, and preferably all, of these pieces of advice you can save yourself from exposure to AIDS through blood transfusion. Of course if you are in the hospital for an emergency and are told you will be given a transfusion don't refuse because it may very well be your own chance of survival.

5 Things You Need to do to Prevent Getting AIDS

You get AIDS after first getting the HIV virus from another person. If you want to prevent yourself from getting AIDS then you must not get the virus in the first place. If you do get infected, you still might want to prevent yourself from getting AIDS by taking care of yourself very well, and doing all of the right things.

1. Since most of the time AIDS is gotten through sex, the first thing you

must do is practice safe sex. For someone not infected with HIV, safe sex is never having sex with anyone who has HIV. If you don't know, then at least use a condom, and if you are a woman use an anti-spermicide cream, and make sure your partner uses a condom too. No one who is not infected should ever have sex with anyone you know is infected. If it is a new relationship, and you don't know each other very well, then you should both take precautions. If you are using a condom and it breaks or slides off, then stop and clean up. This may not be as much fun as just having a good time with someone, but it could mean your life a few months later. If you have been with someone for at least a year, and been tested a couple of time, you will have very little risk of aids and can feel pretty good about stopping the use of condoms so long as both of you are faithful.

2. Stay away from needle-sharing, if you are a drug user. This is the second highest risk area, and most of the drug users who share needles probably have AIDS. If you don't believe this, just ask around and find out how many have died from AIDS, you will find the numbers larger than those who have died of overdoses, and also everyone scared of AIDS. Whatever the other problems of drug use, no one should have to die of AIDS just because they have a drug problem. If you are a needle user, then use your own. If you share needles, then clean them with heat or bleach. If you don't take these precautions then prepare yourself to die from AIDS, because that is probably what is going to happen.

3. Look into what AIDS is, and what you can do about it. There are a lot of publications that deal with AIDS, and a lot is published every year. If you don't keep up with what is going on then you don't know where the new sources of infection are coming from, or how to avoid them, This is information that everyone should have, but especially if you or your companion are having any sort of casual sex, or are involved in needles and drug use. Never depend upon word of mouth for information that is this important.

4. If you may have been exposed to HIV the first thing you should do is to reduce your level of stress. Stress reduces the effectiveness of your immune system, and can send you on the road to full blown AIDS. To reduce stress you should look into getting social support for yourself from a group, or professional of some sort. AIDS is so scary to most people that your judgment will be affected, and your emotions torn apart. By being able to share these feelings with others, and getting their opinions, you will be able to relieve a lot of this anxiety. Professionals in this area are usually able to answer all of your problems, since they hear them from every patient. And don't be afraid to ask for help since you will find a lot more understanding than you might think is out there. If your fears prove false, then you can go back to your normal life. But if you do have HIV or AIDS, then stay in the program for the support and comfort it will give you. Friends and family often do not know how to handle a disease like this as well as a group of strangers who share the same experience.

5. And especially if you have AIDS, or even if you do not, maintain a healthy diet and exercise program. All of the long-term AIDS survivors have been active physically and very diet conscious. While it is not known why AIDS breaks

out in some HIV patients and not in others, it is known that diet and exercise do help raise the effectiveness of the immune system. On diet use fresh fruits and vegetables, cut down on fats, sugars, and alcohol, and get plenty of rest and relaxation. All of these things should be done every day. If you can't keep to this program100%, then at least stick to it as much as you can. The better you are physically the better able you will be to resist disease, even AIDS.

This completes the 5 things you need to know to prevent AIDS. They won't all work for every one, but if you take them seriously you will increase the chances that you will not get AIDS, and that you will live a longer and healthier life.

ALCOHOLISM

A Home Program to Break the Alcohol Craving

Alcoholism was long thought to be something we did just because we wanted to. But eventually it has been shown to be the result of a physical craving which requires medical attention as well as just making up our minds to stop drinking. Unfortunately many doctors still try to correct alcoholism by just telling their patients to use willpower, and not surprisingly they are usually unsuccessful.

This old fashioned approach is still being used, even though nutritional studies have long shown that the alcohol craving is actually a problem of vitamin and mineral malnutrition. Animal studies have found a direct relationship to the levels of nutrition and the percent of rats that become alcohol dependent. At a level equal to our RDA's, 10% of the rats were alcoholics, at 1/3 RDA, 1/3 of the rats were alcoholic, and at 3 times the RDA, only 1/100 of the rats were alcoholic. This seems like pretty good evidence that alcoholism in humans can also be both caused and cured by the amount of nutrients we have in our diets.

If you have a problem with alcohol, and this means a craving whether or not you are an alcoholic, try a doubling of all of your RDA's, and increase your intake of water or fruit juices to the 8 glasses a day that all diets recommend. If that doesn't do it then double the RDA's again, to 4 times the normal RDA, and continue with the water intake level. Along with the nutrient change you should also increase the amount of fresh fruits, vegetables, and juices you have each day. Begin by having one serving of these with each meal, and in between meals as well if you need a snack.

If you are already an alcoholic,and your craving is out of control, then you are going to have to correct it at a more aggressive rate. Go immediately to 3 times the normal RDA for your nutrients, and also do the 8 glasses of water and fruits, vegetables, and juices. While we can't guarantee that this will cure your craving for alcohol, it is a fully natural way of going about it that has a very good chance of success, and that you can carry out yourself.

Once your alcohol craving decreases you can cut down your nutrient levels to perhaps 2 times the RDA, but not so low that you again begin to crave alcohol. Continue the natural foods diet, and you can decrease your water intake levels somewhat, but not below 4 to 6 glasses a day.

In a study of this diet 32 patients with high blood pressure were watched for 7 months. The damaging behavior of this group was that they all smoked or drank to excess, and controlling their addictions was a matter of life and death. At the end of the 7 month period 80% had stopped their destructive behavior spontaneously.

If you have decided to go on this diet to control alcoholism there are 2 additional nutrients that should be added to your diet, which have been found to reduce alcohol craving. The nutrients are L-glutamine and L-carnitine. The L-carnitine will help to protect your liver from alcohol damage and helps to improve fatty acid metabolism. Doses of 2 grams daily of L-glutamine and 1 gram daily for L-carnitine. Exercise is also recommended as you dry out since it helps in the metabolism of nutrients and strengthens the immune system.

What a Good Treatment Program Should Have

A good alcoholism treatment program should have everything you need to cure you. But what is it that you need to stop you from drinking? Is it lectures about drinking from ex-alcoholics? Maybe, but you will probably need a lot more than that if you are going to stop abusing alcohol permanently.

The people who like the counseling approach do not like to here it said that alcoholism is something your body demands that you do because of a chemical imbalance. But it is partly true anyway. If there were no alcohol there would be no alcoholics, while certainly true, does not help you live in a world where the fruits in your kitchen make alcohol all by themselves. We have always had to live with alcohol, and for the most part we have been able to do so without becoming addicted to it. Truly primitive and isolated cultures do not have alcoholics because they do not have enough alcohol around to make them out of the members of their society that would like to become alcoholics.

But if alcoholics are made and not born, then what is the best way to unmake them so that no one is an alcoholic? There is a clue to the answer to that question in the body chemistry of the alcoholics themselves. All alcoholics have very poor nutritional balance. If looked at outside of the alcoholism they are malnourished in minerals, and have low blood sugar. These conditions are not only

---

found in all alcoholics, but they get worse whenever he doesn't drink for more than a few hours at a time. This produces craving for alcohol, and salty snack foods—junk snacks. It is this combination of body imbalances and craving needs that produces the alcoholic, and gives the clue to what is needed in a good treatment program.

To begin this treatment program you must first dry out the alcoholic. This will take a few days to a few weeks, but it will unmask all of the other craving as well. The recovering alcoholic is attracted to all sorts of foods which sustain his addiction until he can get another drink, but these have to be resisted.

Once the drying out has gotten under way real well the alcoholic must be given a balanced diet with high nutritional value. With proper nutrition, and abstinence from alcohol, the craving will gradually pass away. Foods to avoid more or less permanently are sugars, salts, fats, refined flower, and caffeine drinks. None of these has much nutritional value and all make it harder to quit drinking. If you go to AA, or some other support group, you would do best to skip the coffee and donuts that are usually given along with the meeting.

To complete the program you also need to take a supplement for the essential fatty acids, which alcoholics are also low in. Fish and flaxseed oil tablets twice each day will supply all of these that you need. If you eat fish each day you can do away with the tables. And if you follow this simple plan, you can join the 75% of those who have tried it and found that it cuts out the alcoholism, as well as any craving or desire for alcohol as long as you stick to it.

Why a Single Drug can Cut Your Need for Alcohol

Why become a life long member of AA to break your need for alcohol if you can do it with just a simple prescription drug. The drug that does this for you is called naltrexone, and to work effectively it has to be combined with changes in your behavior as well. The success rate is in the 23% to 54% range, since this method is rather new the numbers haven't settled down as yet. Now why it works, the most apparent effect is that the drug and behavior changes stop the alcohol from producing the "high" that alcoholics crave, and in so doing cut the overall desire for alcohol at all. This is not an over the counter treatment, and you will have to go through your doctor to find out if you are a candidate for it and to get the medication and program. But it's still a lot simpler to do than many of the alcohol treatment programs that have been around a long time.

ALLERGIES

9 Leading Causes of Allergies
and What to do About Them

Allergies are always caused by things which are outside of our own bodies, and they are a reaction of our immune systems to being exposed to those outside things. Nobody really knows why you are allergic to some things and not to others, but if you have allergies the question becomes just what is it I am allergic to, and what can I do about it? To help get you started on your hunt for your own personal allergy list, the 9 most common causes of allergies are given along with some ideas as to what you can do to avoid them. If dealing with these 9 areas doesn't get rid of your allergy, it just means that you are allergic to something a little less common, and you will probably have to have the help of an allergy specialist to find out what it is.

1. Food is one of the most important causes of allergies there are. This is so because we all have to eat every day whether we are allergic to our food or not. If our food allergy is very strong then it is easy to find out what food it is, and just stop eating it. You probably have friends who are allergic to milk, or eggs, or strawberries, so you know it is not uncommon. But if your allergy is not very violent you will have a much harder time finding your allergic food and cutting it out of your diet. For a place to start the foods most people are allergic to are milk, eggs, wheat, peanuts, seafood, and tree nuts. To test these eat each one and nothing else for an afternoon. If you are getting an allergic reaction then wait a few days and repeat the experiment. If this works 3 times in a row you will have good evidence that you have found one of your allergic causes, and that you should replace it with something else in your diet.

2. Ragweed pollen is always at the top of the list for causes of allergies. Ragweed, and other, pollens are released by flowering plants during the time they are in flower. To avoid ragweed pollen all that you have to do is find out when it is flowering in your area and do things to cut down exposure. Usually you only have to worry about it for a few weeks in the spring or early summer. After the ragweed has dried out though you still have to avoid going out on very dusty and windy days when you can get a fresh exposure. As soon as the ground dampens in the fall most of the summer pollen will stay settled for the rest of the winter. During the peak of the ragweed pollen season you should stay indoors and in air conditioned areas as much as possible. If you must go outside then the first hours of the morning are best since most nights are calm and pollen will have settled. Avoid all afternoon and evening exercise and gardening at this time.

3. Grass pollens are a bit trickier than ragweed pollen. Grasses will flower over their whole growing season from the spring through the summer, and that is the time when they must be cut the most often too. If you can't afford to hire someone else to cut your lawn you may have to invest in some of those surgical masks to wear while you cut the lawn. If this doesn't work as well as you want you can always resort to renting or buying a goat or some sheep to graze your grass for you. The ultimate solution is to remove the lawn completely and put the area into a rock garden. Even if you do this you will still have to watch out for your neighbors lawns, but that just means not going out at the time they cut their grass or on windy days, and that is much easier to control than your own lawn.

4. Tree pollen has been saved for the last of the pollens because it is the most variable, and has the longest season. It is also the hardest to avoid. Probably around where you live there are dozens of varieties of trees, any of which you might be allergic to. And because the trees are already up in the air when they shed their pollen it drops right down on you. Also whenever the wind blows it will spread the pollen over a wide area. In addition trees bloom at different times of the years, so that if you are allergic to more than one kind of tree pollen there may be things you are allergic to in the air all of the time. The first thing to do is find out which trees you are allergic to and get those out of your living area. That will cut down contamination of your lawn and house somewhat. Then, for other trees in the area that give you allergies, you will have to get into the habit of doing your outside activities either when they are not in bloom, or when the air is still. If none of this works for you, then you may have to move into an area where you can get away from the trees. If you are living in the city this could mean moving to the coast, mountains, or desert.

5. Stinging insects are a huge problem for many people. You can always tell if you are allergic to the bite of a stinging insect because you will have a violent reaction. If the allergy is kind of low grade, all that you will get is some swelling and redness. But if it is very violent you can get seizures and cardiac arrest. The tricky thing about allergies to insect bites is that you can become allergic to an insect bite that did not bother you before. Normally if you get a lot of bites by a particular insect, such as mosquitoes, you are more likely to become allergic to it than that you will become immune to it. This happens because any time that you get a bite the insect injects some poisonous substance into the bite area, and your immune system attacks it. When this happens enough times your body attacks the poison in such a violent way that you get sick. The solution is to find out what you are allergic to and avoid them. And if you get a lot of insect bites every year you should start wearing insect repellent every afternoon, and long sleeved clothing as well. Most insects bite in the late afternoon and evening, so you should avoid going out at that time of the day for anything you don't have to.

6. Medicines can be either life savers or poisons, depending whether you are allergic to them or not. Doctors always ask their patients whether they are allergic to a medicine before they give it to them. If you are allergic to medication, such as penicillin, and don't tell your doctor, then a single shot could kill you and

it would be your own fault. If you know that you have allergies to medication then wear a medic alert wrist band. This will tell anyone giving you medication what to avoid, and it won't matter whether or not you are conscious at the time. If you are being given a new medicine and don't know if you are allergic to it, then you should only be given the smallest amount that can be effective at first. If you have any allergic reaction then you should get something else. Self medication with over the counter drugs like aspirin should follow the same plan if you don't know if you are allergic or not. The drugs you should know about are aspirin, insulin, penicillin, and cephalosporin. These are used by so many people that knowing whether or not you are allergic to any of them can save your life.

7. Pet allergies can break up marriages, and can cause you to suffer for years because you do not want to get rid of a pet you love. Usually pet allergies are something we find out about in someone else's house. If we get a pet we usually find out before very long if we are allergic to it. Sneezing fits or nasty swelling after a scratch from a pet make it easy to see if our own pets are the problem, and make it easier to find a new home for them. Also if you go into a strange home and get the same kind of a reaction you may have no choice but to go somewhere else. But if you have a pet and your allergy is very low grade, you may decide to live with it. If that is your decision then frequent baths may take care of problems of shedding fur or dandruff, and clipping nails the problem of scratches. It can be done, usually. if it is important to you and you will put up with some extra trouble and expense. But if all of your furry pets give you allergies you don't want to live with you can usually switch your affection to fish, turtles, or birds, and get rid of the problem that way. Pet allergies are usually limited to one type of pet, or even one variety of a type, like long haired cats.

8. House pests seem like they shouldn't cause allergies since you are always trying to get rid of them anyway. But in spite of that homes have cockroaches, and dust mites, and fleas, and all of them can cause allergies. Ones that bite, like the fleas, can cause allergies directly. But the others only live around us, and our allergies are more likely from their feces. The feces come from the fact that they are living and eating close to us, and they don't go outside to use the bathroom. The feces carry the digestive products of the pests, and can be very irritating. But how will you know if you are allergic to the dust of your own house? To get a diagnosis, if you want one, you are going to have to take some of the dust to an allergist and have them test it on you. While this will tell you if you are allergic to it, it won't clean up your home, and this is where you come in. But perhaps you should start here anyway. If you have cockroaches, kill them, or have someone kill them for you. For home use there are a lot of cockroach control kits that might do the job, If you can't do the job and are tired of trying, then hire an exterminator. It will cost a few hundred dollars, but that will get your home started. Once you have gotten rid of the pests as well as you can, then clean everything, even shampoo the carpets. Dust mites are another problem since they are too small to see. But cleaning everything thoroughly and keeping it clean should take care of the pest feces problem.

9. Household molds are a similar problem, but one that will be limited to

any damp areas around your house. You are likely to run into household molds in the kitchen, bathrooms, and laundry. They are not even that hard to see if you look around. In areas that stay wet most of the time you should be able to see blue, green, yellowish, black, or white molds. Even if you can't there might be some in cracks and crevices. Again clean all of these areas well with a disinfectant, and try to dry them out. If you can't dry them out then at least clean and disinfect them on a regular basis. If that doesn't get rid of the molds it will at least cut down the amount so much that it probably won't bother you any more.

Remember that all allergies are a result of the amount you get of the thing you are allergic to. There is always a level that is safe for you, and no matter what you do you can't make the world 100% clean. If you learn your limitation and live within them, then you should be able to live just as comfortably and happily as any one else.

Allergy Relief Tips

If you seem to have colds every spring, or have a chronic runny nose over the summer, or feel "a little sick" after eating certain foods, then you probably have an allergy problem. Most people are allergic to many things, but don't know what they are unless they have gone to an allergy doctor for a diagnosis. Allergies can come at any time of the year, and can be very severe or very mild in what they do to our bodies. Just because most people have allergies, it does not mean that most people know what to do to help themselves feel better, or how to protect themselves from allergy attacks. Aside from going to a doctor for allergy treatments, what can be done to relieve and protect us from our allergies?

1. A few simple precautions can protect you from most allergy attacks. In the spring and summer, when most people are bothered by allergies, it is best to do outside activities in the morning when the air is calm and the grass damp. Doing things outside on windy days is generally bad in the spring and summer because of the dust and pollen in the air.

2. A lot of things we are allergic to are in our own homes. What detergent we use to wash our clothes, what kind of pets we have, and even the dust that comes up when we clean the house. We can often avoid allergy attacks from these sources by the way we clean or wash, such as changing the cleaning agents we use in our homes. If you seem to have a lot of little colds through the year, it is a good bet that what you have are allergies, and short of having a doctor run a series of tests on you to see what each of them are, just try changing your cleaning agents, vacuuming more often, or even giving your pet a bath every week or so and see if anything changes.

3. Of course you will have an even bigger problem once you have an allergic attack. It is hard to know what to do if we are coughing or sneezing, and our eyes are running. Simply taking a shower can often relieve this kind of attack

because the water washes off the things that we are allergic to. Simply washing our faces can often have the same effect when the allergy is all in the head.

4. If you like sports but suffer from allergies, there are still many sports that you can participate in safely. Water sports of all kind are usually allergy free since there is not a lot of pollen around swimming pools. Indoor sports like weight lifting and aerobics also get you away from the outdoor causes of allergic attack. For things you like to do outdoors like biking, running, and tennis, there are often indoor versions that will give you the same workout. If you have to do them outdoors then keep it early in the morning, and never on windy days at any time.

When the allergies persist, the simplest thing to do is to take a decongestant, antihistamine, or aspirin or tylenol. The decongestant will help stop coughing and sneezing, which is what most persons are bothered by. The antihistamine will help with watering and itching of the eyes and skin, and the pain relievers will relieve general body ache.

A Simple Diet that Can End Allergy Misery

If you really suffer from your allergies, there may be a diet plan that can set you free. Using diet to escape allergies is based on the idea that a lot of allergies are caused by either the foods you eat, or that your body becomes sensitive to things around you because of the foods you eat. This adds up to pretty much of the same thing, but gives a simple plan for relief, You should only try this diet plan though if common treatments like histamines don't seem to do much good.

The diet is based on two ideas; the first is that you are allergic to some of the foods you eat, and the second is that the combination of the foods you eat make you susceptible to allergic reactions to other things around you. To solve both problems you can use the same approach, with the first objective being to find what you are allergic to and get rid of it from your diet, and the second being to find what combinations you are allergic to and get those out of your diet.

The solution lies in a simple diet in which you eat one type of food at each meal; say fruit at breakfast, vegetables at lunch, and protein foods at dinner. But you need to keep each meal to as few of these foods as possible at each meal. Of course you can rotate what type of foods you have at each meal, and you need to vary any given food over a period of 3 or 4 days so that you are not eating the same things every day.

To make sure you get a proper diet choose your foods from these food groups; for protein use meats (3 1/2 ounces per day is sufficient, and legumes (beans and peas); for vegetables choose from the mustard class (greens, cauliflower, cabbage, and broccoli), nightshades (potatoes, eggplant, and tomatoes), and composites (lettuce and artichokes); and for fruits chose from melons, berries, and stone fruits (peaches, nectarines, and plums).

If you have a type of food at one meal and react allergically then don't repeat it again for several days. If you do this 2 or 3 times and always have an allergic reaction, then cut that food out of your diet. The same thing goes if you have combinations of foods. For the most part once you have gotten rid of the individual foods you are allergic to you will not have any combinations to deal with either.

Emergency Treatment for Acute Allergy Attacks

Acute allergy attacks can be life-threatening and require an emergency rescue service, but they can also be treated at home if you are prepared. Giving yourself emergency treatment should only be done if you know that you are highly allergic to something, such as bee stings, and also should only be done if you do not think that you can get conventional medical help in this kind of emergency. But if you keep these things in mind, having the ability to treat yourself in these situations can very well save your life.

The treatment is given through a product called an Epi-Pen Auto-Injector, which is about the size of a pen and injects a drug called epinephrine into your body. The device can only be obtained through a prescription, so you will have to talk this over with your doctor. The injection is almost painless as the epinephrine enters your body to stop the agent from attacking your body by closing down the blood vessels. While this is not something that you can take lightly, with proper use it can be a lifesaver.

The cost should be in the $45 area, and it contains only a single dose, so use it only when you are sure of what you are doing.

Why it is Hard to Spot an Allergy

The Many Faces of Allergies

When we think about allergies we usually think of the most common symptoms that we have, or that our friends have. That would be runny nose and sneezing as most common, or swelling up if it is a food allergy. More serious allergic reactions, such as to penicillin, do not usually come in our way, and when they do there are always doctors around to tell us what we have.

But in the case of the normal allergies we have at home, we just don't

---

usually go much beyond food allergies and allergies to things floating around in the air. Unfortunately for our bodies that is not where allergies end. Asthma is very closely associated with allergies, and 80% of the asthma in this country can be cured by removing the allergic foods and airborne particles from around the asthma sufferers.

Allergies do not just come in the form of asthma and sneezing, it is also believed that 5% of the rheumatoid arthritis in this country is caused by food allergies, and maybe 50% of our whole population run across foods that they are allergic to on an occasional basis. This makes the whole idea of allergies, and especially food allergies rather scary. If you have a 1 in 2 chance of being allergic to something that you eat, then how can you ever be certain that your cold and flu symptoms aren't just allergy attacks?

That is where the problem of allergies many faces comes in. Allergies can fool you into thinking that you have diseases that you don't, or can give you diseases all on their own because allergies attack particular areas of the body. And depending upon what area is attacked you might have muscle pain, headaches, problems with digestion, or breathing problems. Each of these could be caused by an allergic reaction to one thing, or each one can be caused by some different allergic substance.

Because of the many ways that allergies can attack us, and the many allergies that we can have it is extremely difficult to find out what we are allergic to or what to do about it. But sometimes we can help our own case by keeping a diary of our allergy attacks, and general aches and pains, along with the weather, and what we are eating and drinking. While this is not an exact science, it can go a long way toward solving our allergy problems and of protecting us. Even if we find that we are allergic to something that we can't avoid, we have good information to take to our allergy doctor so that he can give us a program to cure the allergy. In most cases that is the best that we can hope for.

Food Allergies and What to do About Them

While you may know quite a bit about what pollens and plants you are allergic to, since they give you hayfever every year, do you really know if you have any food allergies and what they do to you? Unless your allergy gives you the same symptoms when ever you eat the food, and there is nothing else that gives you these symptoms, you probably don't even know what allergies you have. That is the problem, because it is often harder to identify our food allergies it is also harder to cure them.

As it turns out, food allergies are also much more common than they were in the past. Before modern food marketing some foods were going in season while others were going out of season the year around. We ate strawberries for 3 months, and then watermelons for 2 months, and oranges for 3 months, and so forth. But usually only a limited variety of fruits and vegetables at any given time. If we were allergic to one of the fruits or vegetables in our diet, then you would have the allergy for a month or two, and it would clear up. Now everything is different, we can eat the same things all year around, and many of us do. If we like apples or strawberries, they are locally available everywhere throughout the year, although the price may go up and down quite a bit. If you are allergic to a fruit or vegetable that you like, and you eat it all year around, then you will be sick from it all year, and it will act like any other chronic disease and cause long term changes in your body like arthritis, or chronic muscle pain.

Part of this problem of increasing allergic reactions is that we build up a sensitivity to certain foods when we eat them every day. Suppose we eat something that gives us a very mild allergic reaction, but we eat it every day. Eventually we are going to start having very violent allergic reactions that will cause permanent changes in our bodies. If this seems strange just look at people who suddenly begin to have violent allergic reactions to bee stings. They may have had one or two stings before, but had no particular reaction. Suddenly on the next sting they are in a life threatening situation and may have to go to the hospital to save their lives. This is because allergies are caused by our immune systems attacking our own bodies. The first time your body runs into something it is allergic to it doesn't respond very strongly because it takes time to get its defenses ready. The next time though it is all ready, and it starts taking blood and oxygen from other parts of your body to fight the allergen. If this happens very often it injures those parts of the body where the battle takes place, and may also injure those areas where all of the weapons were taken from. So you can get aches and pains, fevers, runny eyes and nose, and so on and on.

Allergies are also very particular as to who they attack. You can be sitting in a room with just your family members, and each of you can have a different food allergy. While some allergies can be inherited, most are caused by the reactions of our bodies to our own particular diets. If you are never exposed to something, you can't be allergic to it, but one exposure can make you allergic. Other times it can take 100 or a 1,000 exposures before you develop an allergy.

One of the huge problems with finding food allergies is that they may not show up until a full day after you eat the food you are allergic to. If you have a complicated diet, and most of us do these days, you won't ever find one of these delayed allergy foods just by watching your diet and seeing when you have allergy attacks. And this brings us to the plan to find the allergic food.

To find the allergic food, or foods, you are going to have to keep a diary of everything you eat or drink, as well as of when you have allergic attacks. Of course you don't have to do this if you don't have any chronic problems that may be allergy related, and you can stop now. But if you have allergies, get yourself a nice clean notebook, because this may take a while and you will need some room to write.

Now you are going to go on a special diet for 7 days, in which you give up everything in your diet except what is on the list below, and write down each of these that you have as well. Mix up the combinations, but stick with this food selection as these are all foods which do not commonly cause allergy attacks. If you are right, and your aches and pains, or whatever is caused by a food allergy, then the symptoms should go away in the 7 day trial period. If they don't go away then you are suffering from a disease caused by something other than a food allergy, and you should look to other causes.

7 Day Food Allergy Plan

1. Apples	11. Cucumbers	21. Potatoes
2. Artichokes	12. Ginger	22. Rice
3. Bananas	13. Green beans	23. Spinach
4. Bean sprouts	14. Honey	24. Squash
5. Beef	15. Lamb	25. Tapioca
6. Beets	16. Melon Lentils	26. Tuna
7. Canola Oil	17. Mustard	27. Turkey
8. Carrots	18. Pears	28. Turnips
9. Celery	19. Peaches	29. Veal
10. Coconut Gelatin	20. Pork	30. Zucchini

Now that you have completed the 7 day diet plan, you should know either that you don't have a food allergy or that you do. If you do it is time to start introducing all of those foods you gave up to follow the anti-allergy diet. You want to introduce your old foods slowly and in small quantities, not in the same amounts as when you were living off of them. Of course you continue to eat the anti-allergy diet for the major part of your needs. Each of the old foods should be given 2 days before going on the the next one. That is because of the 12 to 24 hour delays some food allergies show.

If you find a food that gives you a reaction within one day, then you are probably allergic to it and it needs to be taken off of your diet. Then wait an additional day and again start reintroducing foods from your original diet one at a time.

When you have finished you will have a list of foods that give you allergic reactions, but you may not have to give up all of them forever. It is always possible that the allergy foods will have to be given up forever, but oftentimes giving them up for 3 to 6 months will be enough for your body to have gotten over its allergic reaction. This is because these particular chronic allergies were the result of eating the same foods every day. When you stop eating these foods over a period of time your body can lose some of its sensitivity to the food, and its ability to produce an allergic reaction.

At the end of a minimum 3 month period you can introduce small amounts of the foods from the allergic list, for two days at a time, the same as before, and see if you have any reaction. If you don't, then you can introduce as a permanent item in your diet, except that you should pay attention whenever you eat it.

If you did get a reaction, no matter how slight, put that food aside and test again in another 3 months. If you do this 3-monthly tests three times, this is 1 year after you have cut the food from your daily diet, and you are still getting allergic reactions then you can be pretty sure it will have to be permanently removed from your list of acceptable foods. Of course you can test again later on, say once a year, but don't be surprised if you never get to the point where you can eat this particular food without care. Chances are it will have to be permanently removed from your list of acceptable foods for your personal diet.

For your personal use, here is a list of the foods most commonly thought to cause allergies. These are the ones that you should watch carefully any time that you take a look at your diet.

Allergy Causing Foods

1. Sugar Additives
2. Chicken
3. Chives
4. Chocolate
5. Citrus
6. Coffee/tea
7. Corn
8. Eggs
9. Milk
10. Oats
11. Onions
12. Peas
13. Peanuts
14. Soy
15. Tomatoes
16. Vinegar
17. Wheat
18. Fermented food

The Type of Clothing That Could be the Cause of Health Problems.

What the Clothing Industry Doesn't Want You to Know.

Do you have a problem with constant fatigue, headaches, and other non-specific health problems? It could be that your clothing is poisoning you. The poison is formaldehyde, and it comes from the permanent press type clothing that so many of us like. The formaldehyde gets into the clothes when they are given the permanent press treatment, and it is mostly found in linens, and polyester and cotton fabrics. Now these are some of the biggest selling fabrics you are going to find on the market, so it is no wonder that the clothing industry doesn't put warning labels on the clothes they sell.

The problem comes with making the fabrics permanent press. To do this the material is put through a formaldehyde resin treatment. If they lose the resin they are no longer permanent press, so you can see that as long as the clothing stays permanent press it is going to emit the formaldehyde.

The most common symptoms are fatigue, coughing, watery eyes, and general respiratory problems. And the only real defense is to buy natural, untreated, fabric clothing. You should also stay away from clothing that is labeled as easy care, or no iron, although it may or may not mean that it was treated with the formaldehyde resin material.

I suppose the one hope in all of this is that the fashions are much in the natural and rumpled look right now, so there is at least not quite as much pressure to permanent press clothing anyway. But if you have been buying permanent press, and haven't noticed anything, then you can probably conclude that at least you aren't sensitive to formaldehyde fumes. However, most people are, and most are going to show symptoms at times during the year.

Why You Should Not Buy Colored Toilet Paper

While colored toilet papers will never be thought of as one of the big risks in life, they are still to be avoided for your health and comfort. Actually more for your comfort than for your general health. The dyes used in colored toilet papers can cause allergic reactions when applied to an exposed portion of your raw anatomy. Now this is not an especially prevalent reaction, but when it does it may leave the sufferer wondering for a long time what is going on. But you can avoid the problem altogether by just sticking with uncolored toilet papers, and at the very least switching to uncolored ones when you develop any kind of a rash or tenderness on your private parts.

ALZHEIMER'S DISEASE

2 Vitamins that can Prevent You
From Getting Alzheimer's Disease

The New Jersey Neurological Institute has linked high levels of vitamin A and beta-carotene to lower risks of Alzheimer's disease. These are anti-oxidants that have been used to slow the effects of aging, and they seem to work equally well in slowing the effects of Alzheimer's disease too. The Institute even suggests that you take these vitamins to prevent Alzheimer' in the first place. While they don't spell out the exact affects, it is well known that free radicals in the body are given the credit for many of the things we think of as natural results of aging. Also vitamin A and beta-carotene are recommended for other anti-aging affects. So taking them to counteract Alzheimer's just seems like a good and sensible thing to do.

Dosage and source are important with vitamin A. Do not take over 5,000 IU (International Units) of vitamin A for any purpose or you risk getting sick from having too much in your body. Also for older people the supplements are better utilized than the natural sources. Finally, if you are not already on some sort of vitamin A, beta-carotene, supplement plan, then talk to your doctor before you begin. An new drug, and vitamin supplements qualify as drugs in this sense, and should be cleared for dosage so that they don't clash with medicines you are already taking.

Alzheimer's Causes Confused Thoughts,
But Diet Changes May Help

Of course the confusion that results from Alzheimer's disease is caused by changes in the function of the brain, and to a certain extent medicine prescribes drugs that are able to counteract these changes. But if drugs can counteract some of these changes then why can't diet help too?

Well, the answer is that diet can help, perhaps not as much as the medications you are given, but diet can still play a very positive role. To begin with cut down on both white flour and salt. And increase your diet in raw fruits and vegetables, and fresh juices. Then for supplements, or in natural foods if you can find them, increase your nutrients in vitamin B, vitamin C, vitamin E, calcium, magne-

---

sium, zinc, and lecithin. There you have it, a few simple dietary changes that should at least help out the memory of alzheimer's patients.

Amino Acid Help for Alzheimer's

Amino acids make up the proteins that our bodies use to keep our cells and muscles in good shape. And there is one of these amino acids, EDTA (ethylene diamine tetra-acetic acid) which helps some Alzheimer's patients to live more normal lives. The benefits which have been reported for some patients include better memory function, better comprehension when talking to people or reading, and an increase in levels of motor skills. Now while Alzheimer's is still incurable, if these effects work for any significant number of Alzheimer's patients, then there is hope for them of a much longer life at a much more socially involved and pleasant level.

ANEMIA

A Diet Plan to Counteract Anemia

Anemia is not usually thought of as a diet problem, but diet can certainly influence your chances of recovery. If you develop anemia you should first cut out all coffee, tea, chocolate, and alcohol. To boost your vitamin levels you need to increase your intake of raw vegetables, vitamin C, and zinc. In order to get more iron in your diet you need more meat, fish, poultry, whole grain cereals, peas, beans, lentils, green vegetables, nuts and seeds. And for copper you need seafood and legumes. This diet will go a long way to helping your blood get back into a proper balance.

ANGER

Natural Mind-Control Secrets
to Get Rid of Guilt, Fear, Worry, and Anger

These deadly emotions can cripple you and make you unable to control your life. Many evils are done when you don't know how to get rid of these emotions, but keep them bottled up inside until they just boil over in a self-destructive eruption. Families are broken, jobs lost, and friends alienated just because of temporary emotions that, once they have passed, seem to be very unimportant themselves. No important decisions should be made when you are in a highly emotional state, and these secrets of mind-control will help you to control yourself, and your own destiny. The principal is to let your emotions teach you about yourself and about the problems you are dealing with.

1. Allow discouragement to exist, for a time, in your life. Discouragement is a personal defeat of something you are trying to accomplish, but it is just a signal that some effort you have made has not worked out. You only become discouraged when you have put your hopes and dreams into something, and then been rejected. This could have been a social relationship or a job application, but in either case the end of one effort is simply your cue to form new plans and go on to another goal. Discouragement is a sign that your current path is ended, and that you should redirect your next effort in a new way.

2. Allow yourself to be fearful, as fear breeds caution, and caution breeds change. Fear can be immediate and focused, in which case you will know what the danger is and can deal with it specifically, or it can be vague and undefined. It is only when fear is undefined that it becomes an emotional burden that threatens your ability to function in the world. Don't deny your fear, but realize that it is real and a signal of something that you feel inadequate to deal with. To overcome fear you will need to express it, and the best way to express it is through a close family member or a friend, someone who will give you moral support and join with to solve the problem producing the fear. Much of fear is really a feeling of being alone, and that no one cares for you. If you have the support of others you will rarely suffer fear that you will be unable to deal with.

3. Talk about your feelings to others. This is one of the very best ways of resolving both fear and discouragement, for it brings in the resources of others who are sympathetic to you in those problem areas which are most troubling to you. While in most cases only you can solve your own problems, it is also true

---

that most problems you will face are much less unsolvable if you have the chance to express them to someone else. Occasionally your listener will give you good advice, or be able to solve the problems for you, but most of the time just being able to express your thoughts will allow you to see the true solutions to the problems that concern you.

4. Exercise your strong emotions away. While it might seem a bit peculiar, exercise by itself is capable of clearing up strong emotional problems. Emotions, while they may seem to be in the mind, are actually part of your body chemistry, and exercise changes body chemistry to get rid of the things causing the emotions and replacing them with chemicals which make you feel good. It may take a regular exercise program, if you are constantly in situations that cause strong emotions, but it will work for from a few hours to a few days to relieve whatever feelings you are having that are interfering with your life. Besides anger, exercise is an excellent way to deal with grief and despair. The exercise does not have to be extremely vigorous, but can be as simple as a walk of a half hour or more, but it can also be something very active if that appeals to you. It is also something that you can do if there is no other person to whom you can talk to, but it works best if combined with other forms of dealing with your emotions.

5. Express your feelings through drawing or painting. This is to give them a visual definition, and it works best when you are not completely certain what your feelings are or how to define them. Many times, when there is a tragedy involving many children, the news will feature their drawings as an expression of what they are feeling. This is because it is such a good way to get things out of your system, and doesn't even require you being able to talk about your emotions. These expressions can be fully understandable to you, and totally hidden from anyone else. They give you a private way to see your problems, and define them in such situations as where the other people in your home are the cause of the feelings you are dealing with. You can also dispose off the drawings afterward, when the feelings have passed, and symbolically destroy what it was that was destroying you.

6. Compose a poem about your grief. Don't worry if you can't rhyme, most poets don't rhyme anymore anyway. A poem is an emotional way of expressing your emotions. Poems are meant to speak to the emotions, and so for a good avenue of resolving emotions. You can also express all that is in you through a poem. Also a poem can be as long or as short as you like, since there is no minimum requirement. The poem will allow you to arrange the feelings of your grief into a visual form which can also be expressed out loud if you wish to do so.

7. Express your anger in a letter to the person making you angry, but then tear it up. Anger is not a long term emotion like grief, which can take a year or more to get over. Anger usually goes on for no more than a few days, but can be very intense and all-consuming over that time. When you compose a letter you can say all of those things to your tormentor without fear of reprisal, and express everything you need to. Many times you may have done this in a private diary,

but to use a letter and then destroy it is a means of saying all that you must and then destroying it and the person who has aroused the emotion in you in a safe manner. You can do one of these every day if you have the need, particularly if its something like a job that you can't afford to quit, and every day you can tell your boss off and destroy those feelings, and there will be nothing he can do about it where one word face-to-face would get you fired.

ANGINA

Relief From Angina Pain with Lysine and Vitamin C

According to Linus Pauling, two time winner of the Nobel Prize, you can relieve angina with a few simple vitamins. In fact taking these vitamins can prevent or reverse angina and blockage of arteries. We get angina because the arteries become blocked with plaque, and as less and less blood comes through them the heart gets starved for oxygen.

Taking 6 or 7 grams of vitamin C, and six grams of L-lysine, spread out over each days can relieve the symptoms and maybe reverse the disease. Together these vitamins stop plaque build up, and can attack the blockages themselves. While its a good idea to discuss this combination with your doctor before you start it, you can also write to the Linus Pauling Heart Foundation at 299 California Ave., Suite 320, Pale Alto, CA 94306, and they will send you all of the information you need to take this wonderful combination for treating angina.

ANKLE AND FOOT PAIN

How to Fight It: Whether it's Deep or Shallow

Ankle and foot pain can vary from a mere irritation to such severe pain that you can't even walk, and the type of treatment you give will depend upon what's causing the pain. For instance, a surface pain may be caused by irritation on the ankles and feet from walking. This kind of pain is very easily corrected since all that you have to do is take your shoes and socks off and put your feet up for a few hours. If you want to take a little more action you can soak your feet in warm water.

If your pain goes a bit deeper, say because your ankles are bruised, or your feet have blisters, you need to take a little more aggressive action. Again start by soaking your feet. If you have blisters, drain them, and then cover them with a band aid for a couple of days. If you don't drain them and you continue to be active the skin will tear and you may be put out of action for a day or two. If the pain is from bruises to your ankles or feet you can apply a little cortisone cream to relieve the irritation, and put soft pads in your shoes or wrap your ankles with an ace bandage if you want the support. These conditions are essentially never treated by a doctor, and unless you have a medical condition that would warrant it, such as hemophilia, there is no reason for you not to treat yourself.

But having gone through the simple sources of ankle and foot pain, lets say you have a medical problem that is causing it. Some of the medical problems in this area, and these are all definite ones for which you would need a doctor's care, are diabetes, ingrown toenail, and phlebitis. The one common element to all of these, once your doctor has done what he can, is that you get up and go out and use your legs. Walk, bike, or swim, but stay in motion. Do you realize that they get surgery patients and new mothers up the day after their big events and make them walk the halls of hospitals because it helps them to heal faster. If it is good enough for our medical establishment, and all of the people in our hospitals, it should be good enough for the rest of us too. Besides, if you force yourself to do it a few times you will suddenly find that it is something you are looking forward to rather than dreading.

ANXIETY

12 Fights Against Fear and Anxiety Without Drugs

When there is fear and anxiety without a direct and appropriate cause it is called a phobia, and the easiest way to cure a phobia has always been with a pill. But if you don't want to take a pill every time your heart races at the thought of speaking before a group, or you look out of a high window, then you need some non-drug approaches to dealing with your fears. Fear causes anxiety, and anxiety stops you from living a full life doing the things you want to do. In its extreme form it pretty much stops you from doing anything, and then you are in a prison of your own making, but one that you can't control no matter who made it.

Of course fear can be a good thing too, like when it makes you jump out of the way of an oncoming car, or when it keeps you from going down a dark alley where a bunch of strangers are lurking in the shadows. But that is not the kind of fear and anxiety that should be treated, because it is more likely to save your life than to cause you problems.

Just because these fears and anxiety attacks are unreasonable does not mean that they are not fully real. Your body goes through the same changes it does every time you deal with a real threatening situation; your heart pounds, your pulse races, the muscles tense, the stomach tightens, hands become clammy, you get a cold sweat, and your skin and scalp may get a prickly sensation.

In spite of all this, and the fact that 24 million Americans suffer from it, it is still true that doctors don't really know what the cause is. Perhaps that is why they are so quick to prescribe drugs, or recommend that you see a psychiatrist when you don't respond to their treatments. If you think that you suffer from a phobia, then you probably do. There are three categories that phobias are divided into. These big 3 are:

1) snakes, dogs, height, and public speaking

2) social phobias which include crowds and public spaces

3) is agoraphobia, or the fear of open spaces, and which a person who is cooped up in their homes for over 10 years is very likely to run into.

If you suffer from any of these, or know that you have an unfounded fear that is interfering with your life, look over these 12 methods of coping with phobias and find the ones that apply to you. Always keep in mind that this is your life, and that you have to take control of it if you want to be a happy and healthy person.

1. The first of our drug free treatments for anxiety and fear is to be used at the first signs of an attack. When you feel your anxiety is beginning to build, you may be able to cancel it out by doing something to take your mind off of the thing that is scaring you. It can be something as simple as counting to 1000, or it can be somewhat more complicated like imagining you are in Hawaii. The idea behind it, and this works, is to get the intense concentration of your thoughts off of the trigger and put it working on something neutral or pleasant. For many people this will work just fine to put yourself in a frame of mind where you can work logically and normally. If you don't think about a disturbing thought then it can't scare you, or give you any other emotion. So what you are trying to do is to produce a pleasant emotion, or a neutral emotion, in place of the one causing the attack of fear and anxiety.

2. But what do you do if a simple distraction like counting doesn't get rid of the anxiety? In that case you can go to the next step of self therapy, which is simple shock treatment. An example of a simple shock is giving yourself a slap in the face. You might also just keep a rubber band on your wrist, and just give it a snap when you feel panic coming on. A little pinch on the arm might do just as well too. The whole idea in this maneuver is to focus yourself on reality which is different from the imagined threat that you are facing. If you have never tried this approach, you may be pleasantly surprised at how often it can stop an attack. Of course this is the same approach that is used in the first non-drug method of stopping an anxiety attack, but by actually giving your body a little physical pain you change your body chemistry slightly, and it is often enough that it simply interrupts

the processes you have to go through to develop fear.

3. But let us suppose that you aren't satisfied with these methods, and would like to try something else. For this approach you need to get into your imagination, and this is appropriate since it is your imagination that is giving you anxiety in the first place. Consider the approach to use if you are afraid of crowds, and you find yourself in a crowd, what do you do? You can consciously shut out the crowd around you and imagine yourself on a desert island. If you are alone, and that is what frightens you, then imagine yourself in a place with many people, like Disneyland. The idea behind all of this is to take whatever situation you are in that terrifies you, and instead imagine that you are in a different place that is completely safe and secure, and it should be as nearly opposite the frightening one as possible. If you don't think that you can do this just think about the last time you saw a movie you liked, or read a story that absorbed you. When you did these things you experienced the feelings of love or danger that were told in the story and forgot about your surroundings, and you can do this anytime that you want with a little practice.

4. The first 3 methods were silent and personal, and now you are ready for a noisy and public one. When you get the first flutters of fear, start talking to your self. Tell your self that there is nothing that can harm you here, that you can handle anything, that you will be fine, and that you are calm and well. This approach works quite well in many cases. It both reassures, and it distracts, you from your fears of the terrible event or setting that you are in. Fear is a powerful force, but you have to buy into fear before it can have any power over you. If you resist it consistently enough you can often defeat it as a control of your life. Even firemen, who enter burning buildings, cease to fear what they are doing and concentrate on what they are trying to accomplish. If you questioned a few of them you would find out that they first started to overcome their fears by talking themselves out of it. Of course as you talk, you are only talking to yourself, and it doesn't matter if anyone else hears you or not, just so long as you do hear what you are trying to say.

5. An approach to use when you aren't actually in an anxiety situation is to start a journal. Of course it doesn't really have to be a journal, it can be just a bunch of scraps of paper you can look at from time to time, but some organization does help. What you do is get your journal or notebook and sit down in a calm and secure place, and you begin to write. Write down all of the things that bother you, how you feel about them, what you think caused them to scare you, why they shouldn't scare you, and anything else that is a special concern to you. Now you don't do this just once, but you need to do it every day, and it doesn't matter if you don't have something new to say each time. Over a few weeks you should find that your feelings and thoughts have changed, gotten better maybe, and that you have more clearly defined what is the real problem. Maybe fear of crowds is really just a fear of running into one type of person in a crowd, and you can work around that by being mainly in crowds that are seated like at a movie theatre. The better you can define the trigger for your anxiety the better you can whittle around the edges, and eventually defeat the problem.

6. Now while both talking and writing are fine, they both require you to think, and if you can't think because of the fear and anxiety you are experiencing there is still something you can do. You need to get a mantra. A mantra is a short sentence of 3 to 6 words that you can easily repeat. The catholic practice of repeating the "Hail Mary" is a mantra, even though it is also a prayer, and so is the Lord's prayer. The most famous users of mantras are the priests in India who sit around repeating prayers all day, every day. With a few repetitions the mantra is able to cause you to have a state of calm since it locks out all outside influences. Of course since you are trying to deal with a fear causing situation you can use a mantra that talks about that fear, such as "this too shall pass," or "crowds can't hurt me." You can make up your own or use someone else's, it doesn't really matter. Just so long as you can recognize that what you are going through will not last forever, and that it can be accepted without fear, so long as that fear is inappropriate, a mantra can dispel your fears.

7. Sometimes we can't get through our anxieties alone, and then we need to find someone to talk to. You need someone who will listen to you as long as you need to talk. It can be a friend, but if you don't have one there are many help-lines in cities that will have a volunteer on the other end who will let you talk. When you get this chance let out all of your problems in this area. Tell them what is scaring you and why. What you hope to do about it, and if it is getting better or worse over time. Talk face to face or on the phone, and if you can do it face to face then physical contact can be very soothing. Healers are always saying that they can cure illness with their touch, but even if they can't their touch still brings comfort to the sick who may have very little human contact. Being humans most of us crave contact, but we are often afraid to give or receive it because of the threat that it may not be lovingly given or received. But when you are in need it is time to take a chance, and most of the time you will be able to find a friend or family member who will give you a hug, or back rub, or a pat on the arm and let you tell of your fears, anxieties, and phobias as long as you need to.

8. Of course talking to just one other person can exhaust both the other person and you. Pretty soon you can run out of things to say, and they can run out of the ability to listen to you patiently. When this happens you need to go into a support group. Support groups make up the people who participate in group therapy sessions with psychiatrists and psychologists, but they can be less formal than that. Some are even offered through the public schools as night school classes, and you can form your own group if you know some other people with the same problem. In these groups you sit around and share experiences, get sympathy and understanding from others in the group, and hopefully learn to understand and deal with your own fears yourself. The reason you may want to do this with a trained group manager is that it is easy to get off the track or to end up with one dominant person doing all of the talking, and in both cases you will get less and less out of it if that happens. A manager will keep things fair and keep the group on track.

9. This brings up another point which is just as important as finding a listener or a group, and that is how do you know when you should do this? The

answer is probably when you can't control your life, in spite of dealing with the problem alone, and it interferes more and more with who you are. Of course you are going to have to pay some attention to what anxiety is doing to you, as well as how to handle it. But when you do seek outside help, take some care. Not everyone, amateur or professional, is well suited to treat the problem you have. Some are better and some are worse, and some are no good at all. If you can get recommendations from friends, relatives, or a doctor who knows you, go with that first. But if you can't then go and try out a few without giving them your full commitment. Remember that you may be working with this person for years, and that it will be expensive. You want to be as certain as possible that you are going to get the treatment you need when you go in and spend your time for help.

10. Now we have gotten you into some therapy, but you still have to deal with the anxiety attacks whenever they are triggered. One means you haven't tried yet is physical movement. Now this taps into your basic human, and mammal, system of surviving threatening situations. When any of us is threatened our natural animal response is to fight or run. When we stand our ground we are fighting, and ideally we always want to fight and we always want to win. But when we can't, the next best thing is to move away from the threat. This will not only eliminate the threat itself, but it will change your body chemistry by giving you adrenaline and oxygen. If your anxiety is of a more chronic nature, so that you are never completely free of it, then take up an exercise program to help control it. Jog, walk, or run on a regular, or even daily, basis. The more physical activity you can get the calmer and more in control you should feel all of the time.

11. An even more subtle way of handling anxiety is by changing your diet. It is true that caffeine, sugar, or alcohol can either excite your emotions, or give you a case of depression that can also cause anxiety. People with this problem are commonly allergic to more foods than those without them, and this may be because anxiety and fear change the way your immune system works. Exercise tends to get your immune system working more normally, but cutting out foods which you are either allergic to, or which bring on the problem is an immediate step that needs to be taken. If you aren't quite sure what to do then at least get rid of the stimulants and depressants. These are often the triggers that put you on the road to a fit of anxiety.

12. And now we come to the ultimate method, and that is to face and challenge the causes that create your fears and anxiety. What ever it is that is causing your problems you need to face them. If it is crowds, then go into crowds, and if it is water than go swimming. Psychologists call this desensitizing through exposure, and it works in many avenues of our lives. Public speakers use it to learn to relax in front of a crowd. Just as you can learn to do anything, you can also learn not to be afraid when you are in a situation that has scared you many times in the past. Remember the old saying that familiarity breeds contempt, well that is just as true of fearful things as it is of the secrets of being a magician. This is the end of your therapy in any case, because to rid yourself of your fears at some time you are going to have to face and defeat them. When you can do this successfully, you are cured.

13 Natural Stress-Reducing Foods

Since many of us tend to eat more when we are under stress, it is only reasonable that we should eat foods that will relieve our stress. The foods on this list are not only good to relieve stress, but they can also help to prevent it if you know that you are going into a stressful situation., but first a few foods that you should cut down on at these times. Cut back on sugar (you don't want to be hyper), tea, coffee, and alcohol. The tea and coffee tend to add to nervousness since they speed up the heart rate, and the alcohol is a depressant that can make it harder to deal with stress in the best manner.

Your diet of 13 stress-reducing foods begins with high fiber foods, and niacin, which are found in beef, poultry, milk, fish, whole grain cereals, peas, beans, lentils, mushrooms, nuts, and seeds. You also need to increase your intake of vitamin E, calcium and magnesium. In addition to these basic foods you can also use teas to calm you down. These calming teas are made from chamomile, lime flower, and passion flower. This is not a diet you would normally have to stay with all of the time, but if you have a personality that tends toward anxiety, it wouldn't be a bad idea to make a permanent shift in your regular diet to include this items.

Relief from Anxiety Attacks Without Drugs

Anxiety attacks are not just the feeling you get when you are worried about something, they are much more serious then that. With anxiety attacks you get a racing heart, weakness in the knees, sweating palms, and pretty much an inability to act. Anxiety attacks are not good survival methods for your body to use, since they pretty much prevent you from doing anything useful.

Most of the time sufferers from anxiety attacks have been given drugs, but UCLA has developed a method of treating these attacks without drugs. They use what they call cognitive behavioral therapy. What this really means though is that you get exposed to many anxiety producing situations in a controlled setting, and after a few days you get used to the thrills and your heart stops pounding.

But does this work, you may well ask, and the answer is yes, at least for some people. When it is used, it is 67% more effective than drug therapy, but that is only when it can be used of course. For one thing you have to be very highly motivated, and your anxiety attacks cannot be so sever that they are totally unbearable. While this puts it beyond the reach of many sufferers, it also makes it available for most of those who have anxiety attacks and who need treatment.

The Major Anxiety Treating Drugs and What they Do

There are only 3 main anxiety treating drugs used in the United States: Prozac, Halcion, and Xanax. And because there are only 3 they all get used quite a lot. But before you use one of these, or any other drug, don't you think it would be a good idea to find out how the drug works? You want to know what it does to your body to cure your disease, or relieve your symptoms. You also want to know if there are any side effects, and if those side effects are dangerous. There may be a lot of other questions about drugs you want to know, but if you know the answers to these two at least you will have a start on looking after your own well being when it comes to taking medication. So if you are taking, or are considering taking, one of these drugs for anxiety, then read their summaries and pay close attention to anything about them that concerns the drug and its use.

Halcion: this is not usually used as an antianxiety drug, but primarily as a sleeping pill. It is included here because it is a close chemical cousin to the main drug used to treat anxiety, Prozac. In spite of its relationship to Prozac (both are benzodiazopine drugs), Halcion should never be used for anxiety, and should only be used as a sleeping aid under a doctor's supervision. And why, you may well ask, the answer lies in the side effects. Patients who used it for any length of time often developed a peculiar kind of amnesia, the day after taking Halcion to sleep they could not remember what they had done on that day. They would function normally, as far as anyone could tell, but then they could not remember what they had done. Halcion also has other less well defined behavior altering side effects, and a Dallas jury decided in 1991 that it was partially responsible for a murder. I would steer clear of Halcion except under very special circumstances, and many people have already done so since 1990.

Prozac: this is the nations best selling antidepressant, and is another benzodiazopine like Halcion, although without the side effects. Prozac has been used very successfully for mild depression since it was introduced in 1987, although some controversy has arisen since its use was expanded to severe depression. The problem arose after the first time that Prozac was used to treat 6 cases of severe depression, and it was reported that the patients became suicidal. The question that arose is whether or not Prozac itself can make you suicidal. In 1991 the FDA concluded that the drug was not at fault, since severely depressed patients do not respond predictively to other medications anyway, and the develop of suicidal tendencies is frequently found in severely depressed patients at all times. Consequently you may be fairly confident that Prozac is a trustworthy drug for treating depression, but is most dependable for treating mild depression. Whether or not it is really useful in treating severe depression seems rather questionable at this time.

Xanax: this is a drug whose appropriate use is for the treatment of short term panic and anxiety attacks. The FDA specifically states that it is not to be used on a regular basis to get through normal daily stress, but it often seems to be prescribed exactly for that. Rather strangely Xanax is often prescribed for such conditions as high blood pressure and depression, neither of which seem appropriate. The main side effect problem with Xanax is that it is addictive, even though it does not seem to have other dangerous side effects. So if your doctor wishes to prescribe Xanax for you make certain that it is for short term treatment of anxiety or panic disorders. Do not let a doctor give you this drug for any long term treatment plan, or for some use other than that which is prescribed by the FDA unless you are fully satisfied as to the reasons.

ARM AND LEG PAIN

The Causes and Cures of Arm and Leg Cramps

Aside from simple muscle soreness, one of the major reasons for arm and leg pain are muscle cramps. Muscle cramps are caused by lactic acid which builds up in the muscles during exercise. The lactic acid is produced naturally by your muscles when you are exercising, but it only becomes a problem in certain situations. To remain near a normal level lactic acid needs a lot of liquid in your body, but if you are sweating a lot and not drinking enough your body liquid level can fall too low and leave you with a lactic acid overdose in the muscles. When this happens, and it can happen hours after you have stopped exercising, you will develop a violent and painful cramp that can wake you out of a sound sleep and have you up stomping around in the middle of the night until the pain goes away. Luckily these cramps do not last very long once you are able to straighten out the arm or leg you get them in. This usually requires standing up and walking around for a few minutes, or a good massage right away.

If you would like to prevent these muscle cramps as well as cure them, then drink more fluids, and eat bananas, potatoes, and dairy products. These foods will provide you with potassium, calcium, and the liquid your body needs to keep working as it should as you exercise. If you also avoid exercise during hot periods of the day you can prevent the liquid depletion that is another cause of leg and arm muscle cramps after exercise.

ARTERIAL BLOCKAGE

The "Miracle Food" that Fights-Off
Hardening of the Arteries

The arteries become blocked as a result of sticky cholesterol building up along the walls to the point that the blood can't flow through freely. In addition the built up cholesterol can break off and block small arteries that it hasn't even built up in. In either case it causes heart attacks and strokes which can kill and cripple you. In even its least dangerous forms these events will cause scaring results which will make your thought processes, and your heart, work less efficiently and make them more susceptible to serious damage the next time the blood is blocked.

To counter this blockage you need to get a diet that lowers your cholesterol as much as possible, and which doesn't promote the collection of the cholesterol along the arterial walls. The "miracle food" that best fits this prescription are the legumes. Legumes include lentils, beans, and peas and have been around in our diets for thousands of years. They have been around in the diet for so long because they are an excellent source of protein, that many people are very short of in their diets, and they supply large amounts of fiber which keeps the digestion regular. Also they contain no cholesterol.

It is the combination of the high fiber and lack of cholesterol that fights hardening of the arteries. We get most of the cholesterol in our diets in trying to get our protein through meat. And if we use meat for protein then we have to eat additional foods to get the fiber we need. But if we combine the two into meals with legumes we get the effects of both, and lower our overall calories at the same time. This makes it easier to control weight, which also contributes to heart disease and high blood pressure.

So if you want to fight all of these problems at once and continue to get your necessary protein, start making up meals through the week using the legume foods. While you may need more of it to get your protein then you would of meat, it also supplies so many more things that you will still be getting fewer calories.

The Incredible Vitamin that Fights Off
Highly Toxic "Free Radicals" that Block Arteries

The best free radical fighter that we have is vitamin E, one of the major anti-oxidants in our nutritional arsenal. The other nutrients that are also anti-oxidants are vitamin A and vitamin C, although vitamin E is superior to both in fighting free radicals. Apparently vitamin E searches through our bodies and neutralizes the free radicals wherever it finds them. Free radicals do all kinds of damage to our bodies, but they take time to build up, and with anti-oxidants they can be reversed. The free radicals actually come from our own bodies. Because our body cells are constantly being replaced they are also constantly dying. As they die their chemical bonds break up and form the free radicals. Some chemicals also cause the formation of free radicals to accelerate. The most severe are the anti-cancer drugs, which then lead to other problems. But even if we do not have cancer smoking contains many substances that can cause free radical formation, and add to the cancer causing ability of tobacco smoke. Of course there are industrial chemicals that also contribute to free radicals such as carbon tetrachloride and arsenic, but these are usually controlled as far as general population exposure.

Of course the simplest way to get vitamin E is through supplements, but the most effective natural way is by eating dishes made of nuts and seeds. These can be made into a grain and used for baking or as breakfast cereal, or you can just use them as a condiment and add them to other dishes. Kick up your vitamin E to put a dent in arterial blockages, and even cancer while you are at it.

ARTHRITIS

5 Step Plan for Pain Free Food Preparation

Preparing our meals is something most of us do several times every day whether we live alone or with our families. While meals are usually painless, except for the trouble of just doing them, arthritis can make them painful tests of determination. And aggravating arthritis doing meals or anything else just makes it hurt all the more the next time we do it. In the hopes of eliminating some of that pain, and of making meals more pleasant, here are 5 steps that can be taken to make food preparation pain free.

Step 1: Before you begin to prepare food, first prepare your cooking tools. This is especially necessary if your arthritis prevents you from holding knives, or turning knobs, comfortably. For handles of all sorts you should wrap them with foam padding. Of course padding won't help knobs, but you can use locking pliers with padding to turn the knobs. The best procedure is to use this approach if you have any problem or pain in gripping objects in your kitchen. Don't wait until your problem is so bad that you can't grip anything comfortably because that may just make it get worse sooner. You are going to have to plan this yourself since only you know what you use to cook and prepare food, but once you have set up all of the handling aids you need you won't have to mess with them very often.

Step 2. Electrify your kitchen if you haven't already done so. An electric knife or can opener takes almost no gripping, and often does a much neater and quicker job than the manual versions. Although there is more expense involved, many appliances are now so cheap that they can be purchased for under $20. Electric devices not only save the wear and tear on your sore joints, but they will help to conserve the energy in the rest of your body as well and make cooking a quicker and easier task to perform.

Step 3. For your direct comfort when preparing food get off your feet in the kitchen. Since counter tops and stoves tend to be higher off the ground than other tables, a stool of appropriate height is often the best choice for a food preparation kitchen seat. These barstools can be found everywhere, and they are compact enough that they are not that much in the way for anyone else using the kitchen. If you also have back pain you can get a stool with a back rest to help out.

Step 4. Just because some meals take an hour or more to prepare, it doesn't mean that you are going to have to spend that time straight through in the kitchen. As with any chronic problem of pain or fatigue, you are much better off alternating your period of activity with periods of rest. You will find yourself able to extend a maximum 30 minutes of constant activity into an hour or two if you take a break before the discomfort gets so bad that you have to stop. For the break you can sit in a chair, stretch out on your sofa, or even lie on the floor for a couple of minutes to support your whole body. The overall meal might take longer to prepare, but you will enjoy both the meal and how you feel afterwards much more.

Step 5. As a final step, plan your meals in advance. By planning you can cut down the number of meals you have to prepare, and the number of days in a week that you have to work hard. For instance, if you like casseroles, then make enough for the week on one day and freeze them. You can also pre-prepare cut vegetables and meats for soups and stews on a single day. You can also resort to deli foods, or home delivered pizza on occasion. Of course the ultimate job reliever should not be forgotten either—eat out once in a while even if you can't do it everyday. Every city has bargain days and early meal deals, and if you are a senior there are special meal rates available at any time in some restaurants.

In any case don't give up even though you may have severe arthritis, there is always something you can do. Sometimes you need the help of others, but by using your head and planning even that can be cut down no matter the severity of your problem. There are even meals-on-wheels programs in some cities that will bring a meal to your door if that is your need.

12 Ways to Rid Yourself of Arthritis Pain

Much of the time you tell yourself that you can live with your problems if they just did not hurt so much, and that is the main problem with arthritis most of the time. Most cases of arthritis do not kill anyone, and they would not even be especially inconvenient if they did not hurt so much. If you have been suffering from arthritis for a while you may have some perfectly good way of taking care of the pain, but it is always good to find some alternatives. If you ever run out of your regular medicine, or it becomes ineffective these methods will come in very handy. If you are just developing arthritis pain they may be even more helpful since you may not yet know the best way to control the discomfort of arthritis so that you can stay fully functional. With these thoughts in mind, here are 12 ways for you to rid yourself of arthritis pain.

1. Starting with your feet, and painful arthritic feet can hinder a lot of your activity, put cushioned pads into your shoes. This rather simple procedure will take pressure off of the arthritic joints in your feet and give you relief. These pads are inexpensive and involve no drugs, so it is a good idea to try this right away if you have any pain in your feet.

2. One of the first parts of your body that often develops pain in arthritis is the hands, and one of the most annoying things about having painful hands is that you can't even open a vacuum packed jar or can. The answer to this particular problem is to keep a nail and a small hammer handy in the kitchen, and when you need to open one of these vacuum packed containers, pound a hole in the top of it first. This simple act will release the vacuum seal and make it easy to twist off the lid. The hole doesn't have to be very large, and it only has to go through the lid slightly. Always remember to put the hammer and nail away afterwards until the next time you need it.

3. We will stick with problems with arthritic hands for now, and ways to avoid causing them pain. Coins can be a problem if your arthritis affects the use of your fingers. So when you need to get coins out of a small space like a vending machine or phone, use an aide. A good aid for this job is a pencil with a new erasure. The erasure will help you to drag the coins out of the opening and into the palm of your hand. Another good idea is to keep the coins you carry on you in a coin purse that you push the ends on to open. Then you don't have to deal with any zippers, and you can just dump the coins in and out of the coin purse into your palm as you need to.

4. Writing is always a problem with arthritic hands, and it can be both

painful and difficult to write clearly. Much of the problem is in pens and pencils though, and not really in the hands. To help use a felt tip pen or marker whenever you can since they need less pressure than a ball-point, and the fine point ones are nearly as sharp as regular pen writing. You might also consider some sort of a personal computer with a printer if you are interested in these. They are now beginning to make computers that work with voice controls, so you don't even have to know how to type to use them.

5. A lot of the difficulties with arthritis involves twisting things off and on. Everyday you may have to twist car keys, door keys, deadbolt locks, and stove knobs. All of these twisting actions can cause you pain because of the finger pressure you need to hold and twist at the same time. One solution is to use clothespins to help. You just slide the clothespin on the knob or key you want to twist and use that as a lever. In most cases this will work, but if it doesn't there is something else you can use that costs a little more, but can help you twist much harder knobs. Get an inexpensive pair of vice grips from a hardware store (cost is under 5$), and then just set them to the width of the thing you want to twist. This will give you a very big lever to push on, and won't break or slip off easily. One other good use for the clothespins is to close food bags, that way you won't have to worry about zip-locks, or twist ties.

6. If you have trouble filing your nails because of arthritis, try taping an emery board to a hard flat surface like a table top. Then you can run your nails over the emery board without the problem of holding it rigidly. Another solution to this is to get a battery powered nail care kit, which would give you a complete set of tools in addition to a nail file. If you would like someone else to give you a manicure but can't afford beauty parlor rates, then look into beauty schools in your area. These schools need people to work on, and cost very little for service. If there are no beauty schools nearby, check with the beauty shops themselves, they may have a student training night once a week, or reduced rates for certain times of the day or days of the week.

7. Wet washcloths can be a problem because of the pressure needed to wring them out well after use. One suggestion is to wrap them around a faucet and press them together with the palms of your hands to get most of the water out. You can even avoid doing this in most cases if you have a bath or shower stall that isn't sealed at the top. Get one of those indoor clothes hangers that you use in bathrooms for clothes you wash at home. Keep it up in the bathroom, and anytime you get a wet washcloth just hang it on the dryer rack and leave it. It will drip into your bath and be dry the next day. If you keep 3 or 4 washcloths ready at the start of each day, then all will be dry in the morning. If you don't want to buy one of these racks, then any one inch pole cut to length for the enclosure will do just as well.

8. Brushing your teeth can even be a problem, but a little thought can solve it comfortably. By slipping the end of the toothbrush into a foam hair curler you can make the handle much larger, softer, and easier to grasp than the normal plastic handle. You could also get an electric toothbrush, which although not as

soft as a foam curler, has a large handle and doesn't require you to do all of the work. Flossing may be even more of a problem than brushing, but you can buy those floss sets that have the floss set in a little handle. Then using a foam curler handle holder if necessary, or just the handle the floss comes with, you can finish your dental hygiene in some comfort.

9. Gripping books or magazines on the edges with your fingers can be helped by laying them flat on a table, or resting them on your open palms. Both of these solutions may make it a little awkward to read, and there is something else you can do. There are table top book holders which will hold reading matter open to a page at an elevated angle and make it easier for you to read. These devices work so well they are used by many people who need to keep their hands free, and their reading material at eye level. This completes the list of specific solutions to problems, and now we will look at some of the more direct ways of relieving arthritis pain.

10. The first medicine we want to look for is a cream or lineament to relieve the pain and discomfort directly. There are many over-the-counter forms, so you might have to try a few to find the one that works best for you. There are several made from hot pepper extract that works very well for many people, so try it and don't be discouraged by the fact that it's made from pepper. Also don't get hooked into using just a cortisone cream as they may lose their effectiveness for you over time, and you can develop an allergy to them sometimes. It is best to try and find two or more that will do the job for you and then alternate between them. This will pretty well ensure that they will continue to work for you over a long period of time.

11. Many times pain can be relieved directly by the use of cold. Of course if putting cold on arthritic joints causes pain then don't do it. But if cold is effective for you, there are several ways you can do it. Ice cubes work very well, but if not put first into a sealed container they may be messy. Using a pack of frozen vegetables will work just as well, and there are gel packs that can be refrozen that are very good. These are all good for massaging the painful area, but if you just want a direct application of cold then holding a glass of icy liquid, or ice water, is fine. You can even drink the liquid, and make the cold pack do you a double service.

12. If cold doesn't do the job, then perhaps heat will. Actually heat seems to work more often than cold for many people. You can start the process of warming painful joints with a warm bath or shower in the morning, if you like to bathe when you get up. Warming your clothes for a few minutes in a clothes dryer before dressing will help you all over. For just warming the hands try holding a cup of warm liquid at breakfast, and for the feet a nice soak in a tub of warm water before putting on your shoes should be effective.

While these 12 ways of solving the problems of painful arthritis might not take care of every one of your needs, they should put you on the path to living more comfortably pain free.

A Few Diet Changes to Relieve the Discomfort

Arthritis, like many chronic diseases, can be either hurt or helped by your common, everyday diet. If your everyday diet is made up of foods that aggravate the inflammation that makes the arthritis hurt, then it is going to get worse. But if you get rid of those foods and instead emphasize foods that relieve or prevent inflammation, then the arthritis should feel better. Before you make up your mind on this though just remember where most of our medicines come from, and indeed practically all of them in China, they come from the foods you eat, or can eat if you want to. Of course the medicines your doctor gives you has the beneficial parts of your foods in a very concentrated and pure form, but you can select the foods that will give you many of the same medicines, and right in your daily breakfasts, lunches, and dinners.

First, to get cut back on those foods that make arthritis worse, cut down on saturated fats, tomatoes, peppers, potatoes and eggplant. Now if you are asking just what foods are we really talking about, here is a little more detail. For saturated fats, you need to cut down on red meats and eggs with the yolks. Of course you may not even eat all of these foods to begin with, I don't think that a lot of people have eggplant every week, and if you don't eat it then don't worry about it. Now what should you add, or increase in your diet so that the arthritis will not get worse. Begin with fish (it has no saturated fats or cholesterol), raw fruits and vegetables, zinc, copper, calcium and potassium which are found in fruits and vegetables, whole grains and leafy green vegetables for manganese, selenium, and vitamin A, vitamin B, vitamin C, and vitamin E. For an added boost also increase your pineapple, nettle tea, and coriander tea (the last two from health food stores).

Common Beverage that Can Make Arthritis Worse

Do you wonder what you can do to prevent attacks of arthritis, or even to prevent it from developing? You might have to give up milk. Milk known to increase susceptibility in some people for arthritis attacks, and is also thought to promote the development of arthritis in some people. If you are an adult and drink milk, you might consider cutting it out of your diet. If you have arthritis already and drink milk, try to do without the milk for a week or two and see if the arthritic aches and pain decrease or go away. If the results are good then dropping milk completely from your diet could be the best thing you could do to control your arthritis. Milk is so common in the American diet, and it has always been promoted as a healthy food, that it could be one of the major causes of arthritis pain in our population.

Finger Joints Hurt? It Might be the Way You Read

Some of the most common pains with arthritis are those of the joints of the fingers. Painful finger joints can throb and make it difficult to do much of anything with your hands. But now recent research has found that some of those pains are a result of the way you read. Most of the time when you read a book or newspaper you grip the sides of the paper between the thumb and fingers. When you do this you put a great deal of strain on the joints of the fingers, but because you only do this when your finger joints are not hurting you don't realize how hard your grip is. With arthritis your joints are already in a sensitive position so that the normal aggravation you give them by holding something between the thumb and fingers is enough to cause inflammation, and a good bout of arthritic pain in the fingers.

To control this problem you are going to have to use a new way of holding reading material, other than gripping it. Now when you open a paper or book lay it open on top of your hands, or put one hand on top to keep the pages open and the other underneath for support. For books it is also possible to get a book stand that will hold the book open to the page you want and free your hands completely. Book stands can be very inexpensive, and can even be made out of cardboard at almost no cost. If painful finger joints has been one of the arthritic pains that has disturbed your life, take these hints and make yourself more comfortable.

3 New Arthritis Healers that Really Work

Three new arthritis healers, called biological response modifiers, will soon be ready for public use. These amazing drugs work by preventing our immune systems from attacking our joints, which is the basic cause of arthritis. By treating the problem at the source, we can stop, as well as prevent, arthritis in its tracks.

The new drugs are Interlukin-1 receptor antagonist, anti-CD4, CD5, and II/2 receptor antibodies, and Lodine. Lodine is actually an NSAID drug like Motrin, but is effective when other NSAID drugs stop working. Lodine also does not harm the kidneys the way other NSAID drugs sometimes do.

While you need to go to your doctor for these treatments, it is always good to keep asking about new drugs for arthritis since there are many coming out soon.

Prevent Arthritis by Losing Weight

Arthritis is not something that just happens to us, we cause it. At least in many cases we know that we cause it, and one of the most common causes is extra weight on our bodies. If you are overweight, then the extra weight you are carrying puts a lot of strain on your knees, feet, lower back, and spinal column. A study by Boston University found that an 11 pound weight loss by an overweight woman decreased her chance of getting osteoarthritis of the knees by 50%. No matter how well we might be able to handle extra weight when we are young, as we grow older we usually get more out of shape, and our muscles are less able to handle the extra weight. As the weight settles onto the critical joints of our bodies they become inflamed and develop arthritis.

The biggest danger in this, other than the arthritis itself, is that arthritis of the knees is the main reason for having total knee replacement operations. If you see a person over the age of 40 who is very much overweight, you can pretty well bet that they have arthritis of the knees and lower back, and that it will get worse as they get older. Old people do not move slowly just because they are old, most move slowly because they have developed arthritis and some have had surgeries in their joints for it.   If you want more specific information about weight and arthritis call the toll-free Arthritis Foundation Information Line at 1-800-283-7800.

ASTHMA

Safe Ways to Handle a Deadly Disease

Asthma is the scourge of those with allergies, and afflicts 15 million Americans right now. Attacks feel like all of the air is being squeezed out of your chest, and you are left gasping for a few shallow breaths. Attacks which are too sever and which go on too long kill. If you suffer from asthma you are probably willing to do almost anything to prevent and relieve attacks.

The ultimate solution to asthma may be genetic manipulation, since it tends to run in families and can be inherited. But that solution is many years away, and if you have asthma you need a solution now.

Asthma becomes more serious with more attacks you have. Each attack of asthma injures the lung and makes it certain that the next attack will be even more serious. So if you have asthma now, to cure it you have to stop your attacks as soon as possible. And then keep them stopped so that you can carry out a normal life and strengthen the lungs. Stopping the attacks is the problem if you don't know what causes them, or if none of the normal asthma controls helps you.

It is known that asthma sufferers have many allergies, and that allergy attacks set off asthma attacks. So doctors have concluded that to get rid of the asthma attacks you have to control the allergies. In the past asthma sufferers have undergone desensitization procedures with allergy doctors to control the allergies, and these work quite well. But there is information that other causes may act just as seriously against those with asthma. The inhalers that many asthmatics carry are now thought to be one of the main causes of attacks.

The reason is that inhalers use beta-agonists which allow you to tolerate exposure to things you are allergic to. If you go into a room where people are smoking, and you are allergic to smoke, you can use your inhaler and stay in the room as long as you want. While this sounds good, what it actually means is that the inhaler has made it possible for you to be exposed to something you are violently allergic to, and all that you have done is cut down on your symptoms. After you have been exposed to some of these allergic substances at a high level for a long time, it is thought that your lungs develop a super inflammation which makes you more likely to have more serious attacks of asthma.

The best defense against these causes of extreme irritation and serious asthma attacks may lie simply in cleaning the area you live in to remove anything that you have a serious allergic reaction to. And switch from beta-agonist inhalers to a use of anti-inflammatory drugs such as steroids to give your lung tissues a break from their exposure reactions. Of course you should also continue to see an allergy doctor for desensitization as well. While these steps won't exactly cure your asthma if you are exposed to things you are allergic to, they should at least cut down on the exposures as well as upon the reaction of your body when exposure happens.

2 Hints to Cutting Attacks of Asthma

Asthma attacks don't just come on all by themselves, they are caused by certain things that we do. Although you may be aware that asthma attacks are often caused by allergies, you may not know that they can also be caused by going in and out of buildings or trying to keep cool on a hot day.

1. Sudden changes in temperature and humidity are known to be culprits in many asthma attacks. Your lungs are made to work harder as your body adjusts to these changes, and the result for you can be an attack of asthma.

2. Other than going into an area where the temperature or humidity change rapidly, even a blast of very cold air can have the same affect on your asthma. If you like to sit right in front of an air conditioner in your home, or have one blowing directly on you in your car, you could be causing unneeded asthma attacks.

To solve these problems you may have to change what stores you shop at, or the time of day you shop. Also what you do on a hot day to keep cool. Try to avoid exposing your head and upper body to rapid and extreme changes in temperature, either from hot to cold or from cold to hot. While your body may take a little longer to be comfortable, a little skin comfort is not worth as asthma attack that will be a lot more painful for you.

ATTITUDE
10 Tips to A Happy Life

1. Self Satisfaction—while we are always told not to be too self satisfied,. we can never be happy unless we like our own company as well as the company of others. Being happy with ourselves is one of the real keys to a happy life, and this may simply mean indulging ourselves a little bit each day so that we can do something that is really a joy to ourselves no matter what anyone or anything else is doing to us.

2. Love Others—it is important to have someone in our lives to love; a spouse, companion, friend, or children are ideal. Loving others does not necessarily mean romantic love, although that is extremely nice, but having someone in our lives we are willing, and happy, to sacrifice for.

3. A Satisfying Job—in these days of hard to find jobs and changing work places it is often hard to find a job that we love. For this reason it is especially important to keep looking when you are in a job you don't love, and which doesn't fulfill you. There is always something that each person enjoys doing, and that should be a guide to what kind of a job you should be in. It is also important to have people you like to work with, and that can be just as important as what type of work you are doing.

4. Enjoy Touching—many people act as though they don't want to be touched. But to be truly happy you should have someone you can touch, and who can touch you. Touching may be romantic or friendly, or it can be hugs and kisses of friends and family. Someone who truly does not touch others, and who cannot stand to be touched by others, is not a happy person.

5. Live Today—don't spend your time and energy worrying about the past or constantly fretting about the future. Spend most of every day doing those things that you want to, and those that you must, do today. Look about you, people who live constantly in the past worry about things that can not be changed, and those who think only of the future can never catch up to the present. Those who live in the present do what makes them happy today, and does those things which makes those they love happy at the same time.

6. Laugh—some people say they are happy even though they never laugh, and they may be telling the truth. But laughing itself is good for the soul. A few years ago a well known writer cured himself of a serious disease by laugh-

ing. Remember that you won't be hurting while your laughing, and a shared joke is a way of showing love for those about you.

7. Exercise—while most people don't want to exercise until they hurt, even those who do so say that it feels good when they stop. A good exercise program can leave you feeling good most of the time. It is like a vacation because no one bothers you while you are exercising, and exercise leaves your body feeling better and stronger for hours or days afterward.

8. A Meaningful Life—knowing that your life is important, and that what you do has meaning, makes life itself joyful. Look at anyone who is engaged in "good work," as either a professional or volunteer, and you will see a person who knows their life has meaning. People who simply see themselves as simply a cog in a machine are unhappy with what they do and who they are, and it is only by finding a meaningful outlet for themselves that they can be truly happy individuals.

9. Leisure—life is not all work, but must also include some play to be pleasurable. Children learn most of what they know through play, and adults who continue to play also continue to learn. Leisure is a portion of time that we spend on ourselves. It does not usually pay us a wage, but pays in personal satisfaction, new knowledge, and the simple fun of doing something that we really want to be doing.

10. Give to Receive—giving to, since it is helping, others will make you happy because it allows you to bring joy and relief to those you serve. Givers often lose themselves in the process of giving, whether it is teaching reading to the illiterate, or helping out in a school library, and can always find those who appreciate the gift of themselves they have brought to relieve those in need. The direct and indirect rewards givers receive makes them happy and satisfied with their lives, and makes them better people for their efforts.

Use Your Mind to Improve Your Health

Having a good attitude about life can help you to stay healthy as well as to recover from sickness when it does occur. Not only attitude but feeling good emotionally is also important. If you are usually healthy anyway than you probably already have a good attitude and healthy emotions, but if you are sick or seem to get sick very often, its a good bet that you are feeling bad about things other than being sick. Look at your self and your life and find something that you enjoy. Spend your thinking time on that and your health should begin to improve. You can even ask your doctor, if you wish, and they will tell you how important attitude is to staying well, but you can do it on your own anyway, and get the same benefit just for taking the trouble to feel good.

BACKACHE

4 Exercises to Relieve the Aching Back

You do not have to rely on medication to relieve an aching back, if you take some time for certain stretching exercises that will do the same thing. Of course these may have to be repeated through the day if the back ache returns, but there is no reason you can't use them whenever you are able.

For all of these exercises, begin by lying flat on your back on a soft surface, with a support for your head, and then just follow the instructions.

1. Place a pillow or blanket under your knees, keeping your feet flat on the floor. Then join your hands on your stomach, and relax.

2. Remove the support from under your knees, and draw your feet, still flat on the floor, about half way to your body. Keep your hands joined on your stomach.

3. With your feet still in the drawn up position, calmly pull one knee back toward your chest, placing your joined hands on the knee cap to help pull back.

4. Now move your hands to the back of the knee and extend the foot upward vertically.

Repeat these exercises with each leg two or three times over a ten to fifteen minute period, and you will both stretch and relax your back, thus relieving both pressure and pain. This is an especially good exercise to go through when you get ready for bed at night, or just to loosen up your back if it feels tight.

BALDNESS

The Nutrient that Might be a Solution to Baldness

You've always heard that baldness is hereditary, right? So if you've been born with the gene that makes you go bald, and you're a man, you're going to go bald, right? If you have answered yes to both of these questions, you are at least half right. While baldness is heredity, there are some people who go bald as a result of radiation, chemicals, or illness, in addition to those who go bald because they were born that way. And if you are born that way—well, we all know men who were going bald but aren't anymore. So nobody has to go bald, even if their solutions are only cover-ups. If you are already far advanced into baldness, and hate it, then a cover-up, or hair transplant, is always a successful way of dealing with it, and many men do exactly that.

But if you are also dissatisfied with the idea of either a transplant or a hair piece, there is still a nutritional approach that is now in the works, and may correct the problem. Studies have found that dietary zinc is one of the mechanisms controlling our growth of hair, and in tests with animals has been found to increase hair growth. While all that we can do right now is recommend that you try it, and cannot even guarantee that it is a good treatment for humans, it is still worth trying. So get your zinc intake levels upto the minimum recommended amount, and if that doesn't work increase it to up to 5 times the recommended daily amounts. This should be low enough to prevent any side effects, but high enough to show effects on hair growth.

Remember though that this is an unproven method of dealing with hair loss. Don't expect miracles, and like any slow acting medical treatment, start keeping records of your hair loss and hair growth when you start taking the zinc. If there is no change within 6 months you can probably give it up as a bad idea, but if it does work, then keep up the zinc. And if you are on any other medication check with your doctor to make sure that there will be no side effects from taking the two together.

BEDWETTING

What Not to Eat

While bedwetting is mainly a bladder control problem that affects young children and our aged population, it can also persist into the years which is uncommon and an embarrassment. For those people for whom bedwetting is caused by neither immaturity nor illness, it may well be related to your diet. Certain foods in the diet stimulate the bladder to empty, and when that happens at night you have bedwetting. Now, although many foods might be guilty of causing this condition, most of the time it is caused by a few in our American diet that nearly everyone eats, but only a few are bothered by.

To control a persistent problem of bedwetting try cutting down on foods containing oxalate, such as spinach, strawberries and rhubarb. Caffeine also has this affect and you should cut down on coffee, English tea, cola drinks, and chocolate. In particular don't have any of these foods in the evening, or just before going to bed. The longer the time period you can put between having them and your bedtime, the less chance you will have that they will cause you any trouble.

BLADDER INFECTION

A Honeymoon Disease that Affects Most Women

While it might be cruel to call bladder infections a honeymoon disease, the fact is that many women get it for the first time on their honeymoons. And the type of bladder infection they get is usually the most common, cystitis, which is caused by infection of the urinary tract by E coli bacteria. While this is truly a shame, the truth of the matter is that women are more prone to bladder infections than are men, judging from where the source of the bacteria is.

The E coli bacteria that causes cystitis comes from the digestive tract of either men or women. In women the urinary tract is closer to the anus, the source of the E coli, than it is in men. Furthermore, since women are the receivers in sex, they have a better chance of being infected by their lovers than do men.

All in all it works out that women get a dirty deal in bladder infections. Having one bladder infection does not mean that you can't get another, and most women have several, sometimes in the same year. Women who wipe themselves from back to front might even be giving themselves the infections almost willingly, although not knowingly. Men, because of their anatomy, can be much more sloppy in their personal habits and never have a case of cystitis.

But what to do about it? There are a number of actions you can take that are preventive, and a few that may be curative. The ultimate cure is to go to the doctor and get medication to kill the E coli in your urinary tract, but even baring that there are some other things you can do. First off begin by wiping yourself from the front to the back, and at least you should cut down on the self infection. Next, go and relieve your bladder whenever you feel the need, and particularly after having intercourse. Sex is likely to give you a minor infection of E coli, and holding it in just lets the E coli multiply, thus increasing the chance that it will turn into a cystitis infection.

In the case that you are in the early stages of a bladder infection immediately increase your intake of water to 8 glasses daily. This helps to flush out the bladder, and the bacteria along with it. An added boost can be gotten by drinking cranberry juice along with the water. Cranberry juice contains a nutrient that inhibits the growth of bacteria. Vitamin C is also useful, and doses should be increased at this time.

These are the basic beneficial steps you can take if you are prone to bladder infections. If you have never had one though you may be a little hazy about what a bladder infection feels like. Well, you have a bladder infection if you have a burning sensation on urinating, and afterwards, and a driving need to urinate even when your bladder is empty. This condition develops very rapidly, so if you get these symptoms start following the suggestions given above immediately.

BLOOD

Lab Tests and How to Read the
15 Measures They Give You

If you or anyone you know has ever had a blood workup, you know that all you get back is a little piece of paper with a bunch of numbers on listing things like glucose, cholesterol, and blood gases. But have you ever had a doctor sit down with you and go over each one, step by step, so that you have any idea if they are good or bad, even when he diagnoses something out of them? Well I haven't, and neither has anyone I have ever met, so I think it is time that we let ourselves in on the secret and find out what we are paying several hundred dollars for every time our doctor tells us we need to have a blood test. And just so you won't have to look through the whole list every time you want to look something up, here is a prelist of the 15 measures that we are going to talk about: 1. Glucose; 2. Urea Nitrogen; 3. Creatinine; 4. Creatinine/BUN Ratio; 5. Uric Acid; 6. Calcium; 7. Phosphorus; 8. Albumin; 9. Globulin; 10. A/G Ratio; 11. Cholesterol; 12. Triglycerides; 13. Electrolytes; 14. Lipid Profile II; 15. Cholesterol/HDL Ratio.

There you have it, the big 15. And if you can look at these yourself, you can either tell that you're fine, or you can ask some very direct questions of your doctor to find out why some of your readings are not in a normal range, and what it means or what you can do about it. Knowledge is power, and knowledge about yourself is not only power, it is the power to control your decisions. It is now time that you got some of the power to make your own decisions, or at least so that you can participate in them.

1. Glucose: normal range is 70 mg to 105 mg, and optimal range is 70 mg to 100 mg. Glucose is a measure of blood sugar, and it is tested to look for diabetes mellitus. Glucose measurement for diabetes is taken after a period of fasting, and your doctor will tell you not to eat anywhere from 12 to 48 hours before the test. A fasting glucose level above 105 mg is taken as a diagnosis of diabetes. Diabetes means that your pancreas is not working properly, specifically that it is not putting out enough insulin to keep your blood glucose level in its proper range. Having diabetes does not mean that you automatically go on

insulin shots, since most cases are caused by a low production of insulin by the pancreas. These cases are treated with diet and exercise. When they are insufficient to keep your glucose levels normal, you will go on insulin. The older you are when you develop diabetes, the less probable it will be that you will become insulin dependent.

2. Urea Nitrogen: normal range 7 to 22, and optimal range is 7 to 15. On the charts this is listed as BUN, or blood urea nitrogen. This BUN is the leftover products from the digestion of proteins in the body. When you eat a lot of protein, as most Americans do, their BUN levels are very high. Naturally the BUN levels of meat eating Americans are much higher that those of the vegetable eating Asians on the other side of the world. The urea nitrogen products are removed from the blood by the kidneys, from where it is excreted in the urine. The kidneys work by a direct filtration method, and when the filters quit working because of kidney stones or kidney disease, we get a lot of pain and discomfort. If we get kidney failure, and the filtration no longer works, then we die from poisoning by our own food by-products. High levels of urea nitrogen in the blood are problems because it can result in kidney stones, and kidney stones can result in surgery and even loss of the kidneys.

3. Creatinine: normal range is .7 mg to 1.5 mg, and optimal range is .7 mg to 1.5 mg. Creatinine is another product of protein digestion, but it is unlike urea nitrogen because it is maintained at a constant level in healthy persons. A high or low level of protein in the diet does not change the level of creatinine in the blood, normally, but if kidney disease develops, the creatinine level will climb out of the normal range. If you are having blood tests over a period of time and your urea nitrogen level is always toward the top of the range, then watch your creatinine levels carefully, and if they also increase question your doctor closely about the health of your kidneys. If he is at all honest he will sit down and give you a discussion of everything he knows about your kidneys, and what steps he thinks you can take to help it.

4. Creatinine/BUN Ratio: normal range is 6 to 27, and optimal range is 6 to 20. Since you already know that both of these measures (see 3 and 4 above) are used to look at the health of your kidneys, you know that this ratio is another measure of kidney function. In general, the lower the ratio the better. So if you are in the hospital for kidney problems and your doctor is giving you tests and looking at this ratio, you will know that you are getting better as the ratio falls. If the ratio is getting bigger, then tell your doctor that you know your kidneys are getting worse, and see if he has anything informative to say as to alternative treatments. The lower ratios also indicate lesser amounts of toxic protein products in the blood. Americans eat 5 to 10 times the amount of protein that they need to stay healthy, so is it any wonder that so many of us suffer from kidney stones and kidney failure as we go through life?

5. Uric Acid: normal range is 2.6 to 7.2, and optimal range is 2.6 to 6.0. Now uric acid is not the urea nitrogen that comes from protein, but it is a closely related protein breakdown product that also circulates in the blood. The problem

with uric acid is that it circulates in the form of crystals, and these crystals have a tendency to collect in the joints and cause what is called gouty arthritis, which is the source of the old jokes about gout that you see in some old movies. But gout is nothing to laugh at. It hurts because it results in the joints becoming inflamed and sore. Oftentimes high uric acid levels in the blood are the result of inheritance, but they also accompany diets which have large excesses of protein, and it is not known which is the major cause. The danger of high uric acid levels, other than gout, is that it indicates heart disease. It is not known that it causes heart disease, but it certainly doesn't do you any good to have uric acid levels over 6.0, or 7.2 at the most. For optimal health, work to get your uric acid levels below 6.0.

6. Calcium: normal range is 8.4 to 10.4, and optimal range is 8.4 to 10.0. The measure of your calcium levels really tells you information about the function of your hormones. Hormones keep the calcium levels within their normal range, and high calcium diets are not going to be reflected in a high reading of blood calcium. The critical measure of calcium is not given in the blood test. What you really have to watch is the amount of calcium which is taken in, and the amount which is lost from body through excretion. If you are losing more calcium than you are eating, then that calcium is coming from your bones, and you may well be developing Osteoporosis. You can't find this out unless your doctor also starts measuring your calcium losses. The loss of calcium, and the calcium balance of your body, is influenced by your diet. And it is important how much protein you eat just as much as it is how much calcium. With a high protein diet you are more likely to have a negative calcium balance, and lose more calcium than you take in. But with a low protein diet your body is able to have a positive calcium balance, and build bone. For insurance increase your calcium intake, and decrease your protein level to 3 to 4 ounces a day.

7. Phosphorus: normal range is 2.5 to 4.5, and optimal range is 2.5 to 4.5. Phosphorus is measured because it works with calcium as a measure of blood calcium, and because it can be affected by diet, and indicate possible osteoporosis. In the case of phosphorous, it goes in the opposite direction to calcium, so if phosphorus levels go up, then calcium levels are going down, and vice versa. Phosphorus though is derived from protein, unlike calcium, and a high protein intake is going to put a greater burden on the body to process it. If this burden exceeds the body's capacity, the phosphorus level will go up, the calcium level will go down, and you will begin to develop osteoporosis. Normally diet shouldn't affect the phosphorus level any more than it should affect the calcium level, since both are controlled by similar mechanisms. If you decrease the protein in your diet, you will decrease the risk of elevating your phosphorus level.

8. Albumin: normal range is 3.5 to 5.0, Albumin is another measure of protein in the blood, but rather than measuring excess protein in the diet, it is used as an indicator of severe malnutrition or serious disease. The critical point is when the albumin level drops below 3.5. Since Americans are not commonly subject to severe malnutrition, most of the time when you see low blood albumin levels you will be looking for a severe underlying disease.

9. Globulin: normal range is 1.4 to 3.9, and optimal range is 1.4 to 3.9. Globulin is another blood protein, but it is used as an indicator of the health of the immune system. Depending upon the disease the globulin level can be either higher or lower than the normal range. Globulin is also used in the treatment of some diseases, such as adult measles, where injections of gamma globulin are used to counteract the virus.

10. A/G Ratio: normal range is .9 to 3.6, and optimal range is .9 to 3.6. The A/G ratio is a measure of the respective amounts of albumin and globulin in the blood. Although changes in each one indicate disease, the ratio is a more specific indicator of what type of disease it is because some diseases affect either one or the other, but some cause both levels to change giving you a much more sensitive measure of underlying disease.

11. Cholesterol: normal range is 150 mg to 300 mg, and optimal range is under 200 mg. Actually most doctors will start advising their patients to work to lower their cholesterol levels when they begin to approach 200 mg. The level of blood cholesterol is the single most important measure for predicting heart attacks. As your level goes above 200 mg you begin to have an increased risk of heart attack, and if it goes to 300 mg or more you would be considered capable of having a heart attack at any time. Cholesterol levels are very susceptible to diet, and that is why diet is felt to be the largest factor in controlling heart attack risk. To lower cholesterol in the blood you need to cut cholesterol out of the diet, increase the intake of fresh fruits and vegetables, and exercise. While other factors do cause the cholesterol level to go up and down, if you take these steps in your your life your cholesterol level will respond. This does not guarantee that you will never get a heart attack, but the chances that you will not are much greater, and your chances of surviving a heart attack are also very much improved.

12. Triglycerides: normal range is 35 to 160, and optimal range is 35 to 140. The triglycerides are a measure of the fat in the blood. As triglyceride levels go up, the oxygen carrying capacity of the blood decreases, and the chance of having a heart attack or stroke also go up significantly. The major factors causing the triglycerides to go up are poor diet, obesity, and lack of exercise. While any one of these may result in a high triglyceride level, it is most common to find all three together.

13. Electrolytes: the normal range and optimal range are the same. The electrolytes are made up of the charged particles of the minerals and trace elements that are in our diets. They may be either positively or negatively charged, and they do not respond directly to diet. Some of the electrolytes are sodium, potassium, magnesium, chloride, magnesium, and carbon dioxide. It is largely the balance of electrolytes that indicates whether we are healthy or not, and what the specific nature of our problems may be. One thing about diet is that they are high in sodium and low in both potassium and magnesium, they can result in high blood pressure, and aggravate obesity and diabetes. Low levels of magnesium are dangerous to those with either diabetes or heart disease. When a diuretic is being used in therapy, such as for high blood pressure, potassium supplements are usually part of the therapy, but magnesium rarely is. You must be very careful when using diuretics since both magnesium and potassium can be depleted

even though you are receiving supplements for both. If electrolytes appears on your blood test results ask your doctor if everything is in a normal range, and if it is good. If there is something not in a normal range, or it was normal but you saw changes in later tests, then question your doctor closely to see the major implications and what actions he and you are going to take to correct it.

14. Lipid Profile II: this is a measure of 3 different types of cholesterol, HDL, LDL and VLDL. The normal range for HDL is 29 to 72, and the optimal range is 45 to 85. The normal range for LDL is 62 to 145, and the optimal range is 60 to 130. The normal range for VLDL is 0 to 40, and the optimal range is 0 to 30. Each of these are portions of the cholesterol in your blood. When you add up the three measures you should get the total cholesterol in your blood, as measured in the blood cholesterol reading. HDL, or high density cholesterol, is what we call good cholesterol. It helps the body by transporting cholesterol from the cells of the body to the liver, and from which it is excreted. The LDL is the bad cholesterol, and it gets deposited in the arteries, and later breaks off and causes heart attacks and strokes. The VLDL is the portion of the cholesterol that is carried in the triglycerides of the blood. As already noted, triglycerides (VLDL cholesterol) at high levels decreases the oxygen carrying capacity of the blood. So no matter what your reading of cholesterol, you want the HDL level to be as high as possible, and the LDL and VLDL levels to be as low as possible.

15. Cholesterol/HDL Ratio: the optimal ratio is less than 3.4, and can be interpreted as a risk equal to 1/2 that of the average American for heart attack and stroke. This ratio is used as a measure of the relative level of good, HDL, cholesterol to total blood cholesterol. Since HDL makes up part of the total cholesterol, it can be seen that the smaller the ratio the larger the amount of good cholesterol in the blood. Also, as total cholesterol goes up, it will probably do so because the other fractions of the cholesterol are going up, and not the HDL cholesterol. That is why high cholesterol levels generally a high risk for heart disease and stroke. A drop in HDL also indicates the same thing, and is an equal risk.

BRAIN POWER

A Vitamin that Will Increase Your Mental Performance

Want to do better on tests, think more clearly, or just be able to answer questions when they are asked without having to take time to think them over, vitamin C can help. The University of New Mexico studied 260 educated people over the age of 60 and found that those with the lowest levels of vitamin C in their blood did consistently more poorly on tests using mental skills. This suggests that vitamin C helps the neurotransmitters in the brain to operate more effectively, and raises the activity level in memory and thought. If you are preparing for any mental activity it would be a good idea for you to take some vitamin C shortly before. For natural sources to use on a daily basis, and so you won't have to go through the day eating vitamin C tablets, in your daily diet include oranges, grapefruit, bell peppers, and broccoli. Citrus of all kinds, as a rule, is high in vitamin C, so even a glass of lemonade will help.

BREATHING PROBLEMS

3 Types, and What, If Anything, You Can Do

Breathing is one of the most basic acts we do every minute of our lives. From the time we are born, and for as long as we live, we cannot stop breathing for more than 3 or 4 minutes or we will die, or suffer serious brain damage. Furthermore, this act, that must be performed constantly, has to last for 60, or 70, or 80 years or more before it closes down.

The real wonder of it all is that most of us carry on our breathing exercise without even thinking about it most of the time. The only time a healthy person thinks about breathing is when he is exercising, or trying to hold his breath for some reason. Otherwise it is non-intrusive on the real world, and does not even exist to the point that we are conscious of it.

But for the breathing impaired, every breath is life and death, and every breath may require conscious effort. The penalty for failure is to die, and yet we cannot cure the diseases of breathing when they become really severe. But we are not going to look just at the most severe cases of breathing problems, but at the 3 most common. Of these, one is preventable, one is curable, and one is eventually fatal. In each case we will also see what the better course might be to either prevent, or treat it.

1. The one that is preventable is sudden infant death syndrome, or SIDS. SIDS can strike almost without warning, and usually does for a first baby in a family, but for later babies it can usually be prevented. SIDS takes place when the baby stops breathing, usually during a nap period, and is then not usually discovered until it is too late to do anything about it. To prevent SIDS you have to wake the baby up and get him breathing every time he stops, and this has to go on for several months at least, until he is out of danger. There is also one nutritional step you can take, though. Studies have found SIDS babies to be low in biotin, so a real preventive might lie in adding biotin to your baby's formula. Or at least look for formulas that are highest in biotin. After all, it can't hurt, and it just might be a cure.

2. The breathing problem that is treatable is asthma. In asthma the attacks are not as infrequent, and are certainly not as fatal, but the distress of the sufferer is always acute. The daily treatment method is to carry an inhaler that open the breathing passages, and the medical approach has been to desensitize the sufferer to things they are allergic to. Both work, but there are a couple of other things that can be done as well. If you are struck by an asthma attack, it can help a great deal to restore your normal breathing if you totally relax. That means right then and right there. Another natural technique to treat the wheezing and distress of asthma is to learn deep breathing techniques. If you can master taking in a full breath, and slow release, for 10 to 20 times during an asthma attack, then you may be able to do away with your inhaler. And finally for the nutritional solution, take vitamin C. It has been found that a 1000 milligram a day vitamin C plan cuts asthma attacks by 75%.

3. The breathing problem which is neither preventable nor treatable is emphysema. Emphysema kills many Americans each year, and its sufferers usually end up in oxygen tents for at least part of the course of their disease. But, in spite of the fatality of emphysema and that fact that it is incurable, it is still possible to at least stop the symptoms from progressing. Studies have found that exercise has the capacity to stabilize lung function in emphysema patients, and prolong their lives. Furthermore, vitamin A simulates the development of normal cell tissue in the lungs, and can also counteract the effects of emphysema. No one can say that either of these is a cure, and beyond a certain point they are probably both useless, but as long as you have some strength and desire to fight, these are good ways to fight. And they may just give you many more good and productive years in return for your efforts as well.

BRUISES

Household Treatment to Minimize Bruising

While bruises are initially painful, and there is nothing much that you can do about that, one of the real problems with them is the ugly discolorations they leave for days afterwards as they heal. To get a bruise in any visible part of the body can leave you embarrassed and hiding out in your home until it fades. It is nice to know that there is something you can do about it, and you probably already have it around your home. As soon as you have gotten a bruise go to your kitchen and take out the sugar. Then wet the area that has been bruised, take some sugar on your fingers and vigorously massage the sugar into the bruised area. Be sure to cover the entire area past the edges of the bruise. The sugar massage will help to limit the area affected by the bruising and prevent most of the black and blue marks.

BULIMIA

A New Cure Using Just a Pill?

Bulimia is known somewhat better as binge and purge dieting, and can be very destructive to your body. Up to now most bulimics have been treated as having a psychological problem, and have been given antidepressants and counseling as a cure. These traditional treatments have had limited success and take a long time, and now it is realized that they may have been aimed at the wrong areas.

Recent studies by the National Institute of Mental Health in Washington have found high levels of a brain hormone called vasopressin that might be the actual cause of bulimia and other excessive behavior. Vasopressin works in the brain to keep all of our body's physical needs in balance. This includes eating, drinking, salt intake, blood pressure, and mental functions. When the vasopressin levels go up or down we develop strange behavior, like bulimia, that seem to be all mental.

Now that vasopressin has been found to be a probable cause of bulimia scientists are searching for a pill or other medication that will allow us to control our levels of this hormone and find a real cure. We don't have a cure yet, but if you are being treated for bulimia, or any other compulsive type of illness, you should check regularly with your doctor on the chances of treatment for a vaso-pressin level management. You might also ask to have your vasopressin level measured to see if this is the source of your problem too.

BURSITI

Natural Way to Get Rid of Pain
in Your Shoulders, Knees, Hips, and Ankles

Most of the time we know what we have done to ourselves when we get pain in the shoulders, knees, hips, and ankles. Of course the older we are the more likely it is that these pains are related to arthritic conditions or the use of muscles which have not been kept properly exercised. Occasionally it is just the recurrence of old injuries, but whatever the cause, these pains do not respond very well to simple medications like aspirin. So what else are we to try that has little or no risk, and a high probability of success?

The most likely treatment we can try for any of these is just rest. These areas of the body are not commonly sore because we have strained the muscles in that area, but we have more likely gotten involved in arthritis or some simple bruising injury. Since these also tend to be load bearing areas of the body, going about our normal routine will probably aggravate the soreness and keep the pain from going away for a longer period.

By resting the hip, or shoulder, or ankle for a few days we give the injured portion of the body a chance to heal naturally. After an initial period of rest it can also be helpful to take an anti-inflammatory medication, and to give the area some hot packs. The anti-inflammatory will relieve the soreness, and the hot packs will increase the blood flow in the area so that it relieves pain and promotes healing.

Finally as you feel the area growing stronger and less painful you need to start giving it exercise. Do something initially that will warm up that particular part of the body without straining it at all. Eventually, and how long depends upon the degree of the initial injury and how well you have taken care of it, it will approach full recovery and you may use it fully and in a normal way so long as you are care-ful to warm the area up before each use, and you stay away from the most stren-uous activity that you put your body through.

CANCER

Cancer Screening
A Schedule for Early Treatment

If every cancer was detected at an early stage, practically no one would die from it. Cancer is most difficult to detect when it is not causing problems, but is the easiest to cure at this same time. Because cancer has many causes, and occurs throughout life, each person at high risk for certain types of cancer must protect themselves by being tested regularly to ensure themselves the best chance of early detection and cure. Good tests already exist for many cancers, and new ones are being developed for others. The screening tests are listed alphabetically by the type of cancer, along with other important information you may need. Also included at new tests which are being developed, and which you may want to watch for in the future.

1. A general health exam and cancer checkup, or physical, includes exams for cancers of the thyroid, testicles, prostate, ovaries, lymph nodes, mouth, and skin. This type of exam is for both men and women, and should be done every 3 years for adults up to 39, and every year for those over 40.

2. Breast examinations are of three types—self-examination, doctor examination, and mammography. These are only for women, with the self-exam being done monthly from the age of 20 on, the doctor exam every three years for the ages 20-39, and yearly at 40 and above, and a mammography baseline between the ages of 35 and 39. Mammography should be done every 1 to 2 years from ages 40 to 49, and every year at 50 and above. Many blood tests for early detection of breast cancer are being studied, but one of the most promising is CA 15-3, which at this time is used to watch for reoccurrence of breast cancer in treated women.

3. Cervical, uterine, and ovarian cancer screenings are also for women, and are of two type—the pap test and the pelvic examination. The pap test is for all women 18 and over, or younger if you are sexually active, and should be given yearly. If three tests in a row are negative they can be done less often, but you need to talk to your doctor to see what she recommends. The pelvic exam is every one to three years for 18 to 39, and yearly at 40 and above. It is usually done along with the pap test. A new blood test for ovarian cancer is being developed called CA 125, and while it is aimed at early detection, its main use now is to measure the effectiveness of cancer treatment.

4. Colon cancer screening is done for both males and females, and con-

sists of either a sigmoidoscopy or fecal occult blood test. Both tests should start at age 50, with the blood test done every year, and the sigmoidoscopy every 3 to 5 years, depending upon the doctor. A colon cancer stool test is being developed which looks for a gene that is found in 40% of American colon cancer cases.

5. Endometrial cancer screening is for women at menopause, who are in the high risk group. You are in the high risk group if you have a history of infertility, obesity, a failure to ovulate, any abnormal uterine bleeding, or have had estrogen therapy. The test only has to be done once, and consists of an endometrial tissue sample.

6. Prostate (male), and colorectal (male and female) cancer screening should be performed yearly on those 40 and above, and consists of a digital rectal examination—that is a gloved finger is inserted into the rectum to feel for abnormal growths. While not fully replacing the digital method, there is now a blood test called the PSA which can detect prostate cancer, in many cases, at an even earlier date.

7. Bladder cancer is not now screened regularly, but a urine test is under development which could make this part of your routine physical. The test looks for mutated p53 genes in the urine, which are produced by cancer of the bladder.

8. Lung cancer is such a deadly disease that survival is almost non-existent. However, with really early detection perhaps that can be changed. The University of Texas Southwestern Medical Center in Dallas is working on a test to detect early cell mutations in sputum.

Colon Cancer Surgery that will Leave You Normal

If you have been told that you have to have colon surgery for a tumor you may feel that you are going to have digestive problems for the rest of your life. Even if the cancer is 100% cured by this surgery you will have a medical condition that will take special care for the rest of your life. Right?

Well, perhaps not for all of you. Doctors have developed an instrument called a rectoscope, which allows them to go up into through the rectum and remove tumors that they had to go through the stomach to reach before. Although you will certainly have to work with your doctor on this, if your tumor is one that can be reached with the rectoscope then you can probably keep your normal bowel function as well as cut your hospital time and recovery time by large amounts. Of course the nearer the anus the tumor is located the better, and it cannot have gone through the rectum wall. Both the rectum and colon may be operated on with the help of the rectoscope, but there are limits as to what can be done. If your doctor isn't familiar with this instrument, then ask him for a reference to a specialist who has worked with it.

Foods that Fight Off Cancer

If you pick up any newspaper you can see a list of foods that you should avoid because they cause cancer. These lists include things like animal fats, alcohol, excess salt, and charred or smoked meats. It's a very broad list, although not particularly long, and you may feel very protected if you cut all of those foods out of your diet. But you are still creating a risk for yourself by failing to increase foods in your diet that can protect you from cancer.

Foods and nutrients that protect you from cancer always begin with fiber foods like raw fruits and vegetables, and bran. The reason that fiber foods are always included in cancer fighting diets is because they protect you in several ways. First, they give you a beneficial intake of vitamins and minerals, but that is not the main reason that fiber is always mentioned. A lot of cancer in the United States begins in the digestive tract, the stomach and intestines. When you eat mainly foods made from refined flower, sugar, and fats, it slows down the digestive process. This apparently creates pockets of cells in your digestive tract where cancer develops as the food passes very slowly through you. When you eat high fiber foods they are processed very rapidly by your body, and the fiber protects you. It isn't clear if the fiber actually scours your intestinal tract or that it just keeps things moving along, but it is known that countries where a high fiber diet is common have much lower cancer rates.

Now that you have your high fiber diet going, you also need to add some fermented foods like yogurt. This brings in beneficial bacteria that has probably been removed from most of the other foods that you are eating. Sprouted seeds are good for B-complex vitamins, and you need vitamin A, vitamin B6, vitamin C, and vitamin E. For minerals take selenium and zinc. With this diet you should cut your risk of cancer significantly, and have a longer, healthier, and more cancer free life to look forward to.

5 Secrets to Lower Your Risk of Getting Cancer By 75%

Lowering your risk means preventing you from getting cancer, not curing it once you have gotten it. And if you employ all of these methods you will lower your risk by 75%. But you are not going to find any references to going to doctors for checkups in this list of secrets, doctors are good for diagnosing cancer and treating it, but they can't protect you from getting it, only you can do that. While you look these secrets over, remember that some groups of people have high cancer rates, while others have almost no cancer. Also some have certain kinds of cancer and others have other types of cancer. If you can adopt all of the habits that result in low cancer rates in each group, then it only stands to reason that you will lower your cancer risk by 75% or more.

Secret 1. No smoking, and this means you. Smoking either causes, or is associated with more cases of cancer in the United States than any other risk factor. As long as you smoke, or live in an environment where other people smoke, you are exposed to large amounts of cancer causing chemicals, and your risk of cancer is increased. Cancer from smoking comes from the tars in the smoke, as well as many other chemicals such as benzene and formaldehyde. Even the heat of the smoke, or pipe stem, can cause cancer of the mouth and throat. Smoking protects you from nothing and causes vast amounts of cancer and other diseases.

Secret 2. Eat fiber. Americans in particular are guilty of having low fiber diets. Fiber helps your digestion to work efficiently and normally. The slower and more inefficient your digestive system is, the more likely it is that you will get stomach or colon cancer. Countries with high fiber diets from vegetables and fruits have the lowest amount of these cancers.

Secret 3. Cut out fat. Fat is the number one contributor of poor digestion, and weight gain, that we have in the United States. If you have a high fat diet, the older you get the more likely you are to have poor digestion, cancer, and high blood pressure. Fat is more important than sugar in this regard because sugar at least is carbohydrate, what you get in grains anyway. Fat has no value in our diets except to give us calories, and unless you are burning 5,000 calories a day you have no need of those fat calories.

Secret 4. Take vitamin E. Vitamin E, and other anti-oxidants, help your body get rid of the free radicals from your digestion that can cause cancer. Vitamin E is available in many forms, but the best natural source is fish or fish oil capsules.

Secret 5. Exercise daily if possible. Exercise helps your body to run normally. Sweating will clear the skin of toxins, and the motion of exercise will help to keep you regular. Your appetite will be improved for the right foods, and you will lose weight. Exercise is discussed many times in this book, so I will only give you one guideline here: get enough exercise of any type you wish to add up to 3 1/2 hours a week, and spread over 3 or 4 days of the week. If you haven't exercised for a while, and that can mean years or weeks, you are probably going to feel lousy the first dozen times you do it. However, the rewards will come every time after that when you feel refreshed, stronger, and more energetic following each period of perspiration and deep breathing.

Deadly Prostate Cancer
Use the Natural Detection Secret

The usual ways of detecting possible cases of prostate cancer are the finger in the rectum examination (or DRG for digital rectal examination) and the fiber-optic rectal examination, but these depend upon either being able to feel the cancer or being able to see it. Since these are both somewhat uncomfortable examinations most men are reluctant to have them regularly, and many cases of prostate cancer are not detected until they reach an advanced stage, and this is the most common cancer in men. Now there is a less well known test which can often detect prostate cancer without the discomfort of the other methods, and it only requires a pin-prick for a small blood sample. It can even detect prostate cancer in cases where the other tests fail, and much earlier in many cases.

The test is called the prostate specific antigen (PSA) exam, and every man over the age of 50 should get it every year or two, as well as younger men if there has been prostate cancer in the family. Men over the age of 60 should have the test every 6 months. The PSA can detect prostate cancer up to four years before it shows up in other tests. A level of 5 or less is normal, and up to 100 can be caused by illnesses other than cancer but should be checked out, and anything higher than 100 can be very serious. When this cancer is found early it can be treated with surgery or radiation, but when it is advanced it usually kills.

Detect and Treat Breast Cancer
What Every Woman Should Know

First, be on the alert—180,000 American women are diagnosed with breast cancer each year, and each year there are 46,000 deaths from breast cancer. You are at a high risk for breast cancer if you have a family history of breast cancer, although most of the new cases each year have no family history of breast cancer. Death is not inevitable with breast cancer, especially if it is caught early, and lumpectomy with chemo therapy and radiation therapy are now just as effective treatments as mastectomy, so you do not necessarily lose your breast if you have breast cancer. However, treatments are not standardized, and the patient is often called upon to make treatment decisions. Even with the best advice your doctor may give you it is still necessary that you know as much as possible when you are faced with a case of breast cancer.

It is important for you to know the risk factors which affect who gets breast cancer. If you decide that you are in a high risk group you can at least be tested more regularly, as well as watch yourself more closely to catch any changes in your breast that might signal a case of cancer.

RISK FACTORS: (a) The known risk factors are a family history of breast cancer, and the closer the family member who has had it the higher your risk. (b) Your age, since after the age of 50 breast cancer rates increase, and 2/3 of the cases are in women over 50. (c) If you have had an early onset of puberty (age 12 rather than age 14), or (d) a late menopause (after age 55), with these having to do with estrogen production in your body. (e) Childbearing after the age of 30, or no children, and these are also related to estrogen production. (f) Women with a history of cancer of the female organs. (g) A diet high in fat, especially saturated fat, and obesity. Diet can also be protective if it is high in beta-carotene, vitamin C, and fiber. (h) A history of over 4 years on oral contraceptives. (i) Drinking more than 2 alcoholic drinks per day. (j) Estrogen replacement therapy is a possible risk factor, but it is not confirmed and there are known good effects from taking this treatment.

EARLY DETECTION: This is virtually the only thing that can save your life with many cancers, and especially with breast cancer. Because the breast is not on the internal part of the body, and may be easily examined, there is no reason for not having early detection if you will take some of the responsibility yourself for breast examinations. There are only two basic forms of examination, and both are painless. The first is a manual examination for lumps or changes in the breast, and it can be done by either a doctor or by yourself. However often you go to a doctor for a breast exam, you should examine yourself at least once a month, and you can do it more often than that if you are worried about breast cancer for any particular reason.

The second method is mammography, which must be done by a doctor, and should be done periodically. Women over 50 should have mammography exams on a regular basis.

TREATMENT: If you are one of those in whom cancer has been found, what are the basic types of treatment you will encounter. The initial treatment is surgical, with the objective of removing the tumor from your body. While mastectomy has been used in most cases, studies are adding considerable support for the equal success of lumpectomy, where only a portion of the breast is removed. In either case, follow-up treatment consists of radiation and chemotherapy. Both of these procedures are carried out to kill any malignant cells that may be in your body, and prevent them from starting new cancers to grow. The rule of thumb is that any breast cancer treated before it has distributed malignant cells through your body is essentially cured. Once distribution has taken place treatment becomes more difficult, and the odds of survival decrease with the stage of the cancer—your doctor should explain all of the details of this with you if you are being treated for breast cancer.

PREVENTION: There are some procedures being developed now which hold out the hope of detecting breast cancer before it has even formed a tumor, and then administering drugs to keep cancers from forming. When this becomes a fact, and it is not possible to say just when it will be possible, most breast cancers will be arrested and prevented and most mastectomies will be avoided.

Foods With Indoles: Proven Cancer Preventers

It has long been known that people eating diets high in certain vegetable foods have much lower cancer rates than those eating normal American diets high in red meats, fats, and sugars. The active ingredients found in these vegetables that fights cancer are indoles.

Foods richest in indoles include broccoli, cauliflower, and cabbage. An added advantage to eating the foods high in indoles is that they also contain other cancer fighters called phenols, and sulfides.

How to Cut Colon Cancer Risk by 50% with Aspirin

Early studies has found that long term use of 1 aspirin a week, 325 mg, can decrease the risk of colon cancer by 50%. This study is still in a very early stage so don't expect anything out of the government for several years about this. In fact because of the cost and time involved, the government may take 5 years or more before they will come out with either a recommendation or a denial of the colon cancer prevention association.

The good news is that you don't have to wait for the government to give its decision before you can take action. Aspirin is cheap and plentiful, and one aspirin a week isn't going to hurt you even if you have a stomach problem.

If there is any problem in taking the aspirin though, there are some alternatives you can use instead. Aspirin is an anti-inflammative which contains no steroids. And when other non-steroidal anti-inflammatives were checked, it was found that both Nuprin and Motrin gave about the same results in cutting colon cancer. However, this doesn't mean you can use any non-steroidal anti-inflammative and expect the same results. When Tylenol (acetaminophen) was tested there was no change in the risk of getting colon cancer.

A good preventive approach would be for you to take one of these anti-inflammatives beginning now, and keep your eyes open for more information in the future. They are thought to work by stopping the cancer cells from reproducing so fast that they damage organs and block up our internal systems. Further knowledge is sure to come out in the next year or two.

Life After Cancer

Especially now that you can usually survive most cancers, it is important to ask how you go about picking up your life after cancer. For one thing having an operation for cancer is not like having your tonsils out, there is a lot longer period needed to recover and a lot more pain. The same goes for straight drug treatments and radiation for cancer, the physical effects on you during treatment keep you from having a normal life and afterwards require a lot of readjustment.

The first person you may think to talk to about readjustment would be your doctor. However, doctors are trained to treat your body and they are usually not too good about helping you to live a normal life afterwards. For this kind of help you are going to have to find yourself a support group.

If you don't have family members or friends close by, or your treatment was very severe, your best bet for a support group is probably one made up of cancer survivors, and under the guidance of a psychologist. The psychologist acts as an advisor and keeps the group members focused on their reason for being there. The members themselves are able to share directly with you, and understand what you have gone through. They can lend you very specific support having to do with your treatment and the readjustments required. At some point you are going to reach the limit of how much good this support group can do you, and how much good you can do it. At that point you need to find a support group which knows you personally, and which is more separated from your disease.

This second support group is going to be made up of your family and friends, even if you only have one or two that you can talk to. If there are no family and friends you will need to join a local social group, and you will find people who want to listen to you and help you, but this is a second choice only. Once you have found this group you must spend time with them doing things, anything, but above all talking about your feelings and listening to their suggestions. Over time, and it may be over years, your need to share all of your feelings in this way will diminish. At that point you will have completed your readjustment and be completely reintegrated into life. But never try to do all of this alone.

The Mineral that Will Reduce Your Risk
of Colon Cancer by 30%

A recent study of cancer patients showed that those with a high intake of calcium had a rate of colon cancer reduced by 30%.

While the exact intake levels have not been determined, it is thought that adequate calcium nutrition inhibits the tumor producing processes of fatty diets. A proper calcium level in the diet combined with controls on dietary fat might even lower your risk of colon cancer by more than 30%.

Prevent Colon Cancer With Exercise: Get the Facts

Colon cancer, because it develops without symptoms until it is well advanced, is easier prevented than cured. Besides changing your diet to cut your risk of colon cancer, you can also get a preventive effect from exercise. A study of 17,000 men by Harvard University, over a 15 year period, found that those men who were at least moderately active had a 50% decrease in cases of colon cancer. While this study did not include women, there is a very good chance that they would benefit to the same degree as the men.

Saccharin or No Saccharin? Decide for Yourself

The most popular artificial sweetener for many years has been saccharin. This was true for many and many years, until the FDA came out with a statement that saccharin caused cancer in laboratory animals, and since that time its use has been somewhat restricted. Nevertheless it is still the major ingredient of "Sweet N' Low,' as well as of many other on-the-shelf sweeteners.

The problem with anything containing saccharin is that it has been proven to cause cancer in laboratory animals, at high doses. Will it also cause cancer in you? Probably not, but nobody knows for sure. When things are studied by our government and are found to cause cancer, they may or may not be banned or controlled. Tobacco has been known to cause cancer in humans for 50 years and nothing much is done at the Federal level to control it, while other things which can cause a few dozen cases of cancer a year are totally banned.

Nevertheless, should you be using something, like saccharin, that is known to cause cancer in animals in the laboratory? Probably not. While a dose 1000 times what you use in a month can cause cancer in animals, you can't be sure that your dose may not cause cancer in you. If it is a problem of weight loss, that is another problem. To cut out the calories of sugar you might just cut out the sugar, but if you want a sweetener what should you use?

The most popular of the non-saccharin artificial sweeteners is aspartame, which is a bit more expensive in the market than saccharin. Nevertheless it might be your best choice for non-cancer causing artificial sweeteners. No tests, so far, have found any cancer-causing effects from using aspartame as a sweetener, and this is good news. So long as you feel that you really need an artificial sweetener, you would do good to use aspartame rather than saccharin.

If you are still a bit in doubt you might consider whether or not you really need an artificial sweetener anyway. Sugar contains 18 calories in a teaspoon. If you use 2 teaspoons in a cup of coffee and worry about the calories you might also consider the calories in a cookie that you sneak in the afternoon. Cookies usually have 50 to 100 calories for each one that you eat. If you eat 3 cookies, depriving yourself of the 4th, then you are getting the calories of about 10 to 15 tablespoons of sugar. If you are the type of person who likes to have 10 cookies over an afternoon you would have to drink about 15 or 20 cups of coffee with 2 teaspoons of sugar in each to get the same calories. Sugar is not the worst calorie food you have in your diet. The best advice is probably to avoid saccharin, for the cancer risk, and use aspartame for artificial sweeteners, or to just use sugar in moderation and not worry about risks other than weight problems.

Stop Cancer Cells
A Spice that Inhibits Cancer Cells

The big problem with cancer is that cancer cells grow in places that interfere with how our bodies work. A Pennsylvania State University has found that the popular spice garlic can inhibit the growth of cancer cells. They have even found that garlic stops cancer-causing chemicals from attacking cells and causing cancer. It has been a mystery as to why countries like Italy do not have higher cancer rates, since they do many of the things that cause cancer in America. One of the answers may be that they use large amounts of garlic in their diets. Garlic is also used in large amounts by people from Vietnam, where cancer rates are also very low. These facts do not prove that garlic will stop cancer from starting, or cure a case of cancer, but they do support what many people have been saying for a long time, that garlic will protect you from cancer.

If you want to increase the amount of garlic you eat, but don't like the odors that are part of it there are some things you can do to help. Garlic capsules are available in health food stores, and should work just fine. Fresh garlic, and raw garlic, have often been recommended, andj8 while they are perfectly good, are not necessary. For low odor ways to put garlic into your diet try aging garlic in wine to reduce the odor and sharpness. Also boiling it will make it sweet, but frying or sauteing it may not help at all. So far as is known it does not matter what form of garlic you eat, the cancer protection effects are good with all forms.

Don't try to cure yourself of cancer with this or any other home method. But taking garlic, if you have cancer or not, will not hurt you, and may very well be a great help. From the Penn State study it would appear that the doctors are coming around to what the natural health foods people have been saying for a long time anyway.

Supplement to Avoid Cancer from X-Rays

X-rays are used to treat many cancers, after all it's one of the standard treatments. But X-rays are also used by dentists on teeth, and by doctor's to look at broken bones, internal injuries, and to diagnose cancer. If you have any long term problem with these types of illnesses, then you may very well have been X-rayed many times. If you also happen to be older than 40 or 50, many of those X-rays were with machines that have now been decided to be too dangerous because of radiation leakage and excess dosages. Now that we have included most of the American population, it is time to tell you what you should take to prevent getting cancer from the X-rays themselves.

Well, not surprisingly doctors have been looking at just the problem of what nutrition is best when you are being given radiation therapy. Now while this can't exactly tell you if the same nutrient will prevent cancer from X-rays as well, that is only because there needs to be large tests of people who have gotten X-rays and taken different supplements, and then to see who gets cancer and who doesn't. So in place of that kind of information what we have is a study of X-ray treatment for cancer, and which nutrient is most effective in preventing further cancers from developing.

The winner in this study was beta-carotene. The beta-carotene was given to mice with cancer, who were then given X-ray therapy. So long as the beta-carotene was maintained, the mice were able to resist getting tumors, and had a normal life span. Even when the mice were taken off of the beta-carotene after a few weeks it was 2/3 of a year before they developed tumors again. Then when the beta-carotene was again given, along with radiation therapy, the tumors disappeared.

So for cancer resistance in the face of X-rays I would recommend that you add beta-carotene to your supplements.

The Cervical Cancer Vitamin C Prevention Diet

Can vitamin C prevent cervical cancer? It is so good for so many other things, why not? Vitamin C is an antioxidant which helps the immune system and attacks infections and invasions of things that make us sick. Well cancer certainly makes us sick, and even though it is the cells of our own bodies attacking us, it acts like some outside infection. As it turns out vitamin C works very well as a cancer preventive vitamin. Studies have found that women who take large quantities of vitamin C prevent 80% of the cancer precursor conditions to cervical cancer from occurring. These precursor conditions are the early changes in the cervical tissues that happen before you develop cervical cancer. By stopping the early changes you prevent the cancer entirely, not just cure it after it has attacked you and caused all of the damage that cancer can do to your body.

If you are now saying that it seems like a good idea for you to go onto a high vitamin C diet, but you need some ideas of the best way to do that, well here are some. For natural foods citrus fruits have always been the best, but some others are very useful too (especially if you have an allergy to citrus). Other than citrus you should eat as much as you can of strawberries, cantaloupe, broccoli, and tomatoes.

To help the effects of the vitamin C you should also take in large amounts of folic acid. Folic acid is found in whole grains, fruits and vegetables.

For a good all around program the American Cancer Society has one which is a proven winner. The ACS diet stresses a high fiber and low fat diet, with fruits and vegetables in every meal. For an extra vitamin boost eat fruits and vegetables in season. And to avoid contamination from pesticides you should use either fruits and vegetables you grow yourself, or those you can get that are certified organic. But even if you can't you are better off eating large amounts of fruits and vegetables, even canned and frozen, than a regular American diet of white flower, sugar, high fat, and high protein.

This is in Your Medicine Cabinet,

and It Can Cut Your Risk of Getting Colon Cancer

by a Full 50%

The common, and inexpensive medication, that you can buy for one penny a day, and which can cut your risk of colon cancer by 50% is aspirin.

It is amazing but true that simply taking one aspirin a day from the age of 45 on can decrease your risk of colon cancer by 50%. There has been a lot of talk lately about aspirin decreasing the risk of heart attack and stroke, and this is because aspirin is an anti-coagulant so that it stops the clots from forming that cause the strokes and heart attacks, but almost none about its affects on cancer. No one knows as yet why aspirin should have this wonderful effect on colon cancer, but maybe it prevents the cancer cells from lodging in the colon and beginning the growth of cancerous nodules. No one knows for sure just what the effect is, but the information so far is that colon cancer, and deaths from colon and rectal cancer both, are cut by up to 50% if the aspirin is taken at least 15 times a month (or every other day).

There is one caution though, if you already have any digestive disorder, like ulcers or hemophilia, you need to check with your doctor before starting any program with aspirin. Since aspirin affects clotting, it may make these kind of conditions worse even though it protects against the other problems.

7 Skin Blemishes, Bumps, and Rashes That Could be Early Warning Signs of Cancer

One of the best ways to protect ourselves against cancer is to watch our own bodies. The more closely we watch the changes in our bodies, the more likely we are to catch cancer at an early stage, when it can be most easily treated, and we can be saved from serious illness and even death. The seven changes in our skin that we may see, and what they mean, are:

1. Waxy brown lumps, which often are seen after the age of 30, are usually harmless when they occur alone, and can be removed without surgery by freezing. However, when there are chronic itchy, areas with dozens of bumps, they may be a sign of internal cancer, and immediate medical care is needed.

2. Spidery blotches are often seen on the face and chest of pregnant women, and are harmless in these cases. When they become numerous, however, they can indicate hepatitis.

3. Butterfly rash is a red rash on the nose and cheeks which is harmless and treated with antibiotics. The dangerous form of this rash is seen in women over 20, covers the cheeks, forehead, nose, and face, and may signal lupus, which is a serious disease which can lead to arthritis and heart and kidney problems.

4. Itchy breast patches are more frequently seen as simple allergic reactions in women with new clothing or new cologne. This is serious when the patches formed are crusty and oozing, and can then indicate a form of breast cancer called Piaget's disease.

5. Flesh-colored growths, known as skin tags, are harmless and are easily removed. However, a rapid increase in such bumps over a few months can indicate diabetes or cancerous polyps.

6. Leg scales, dry and flaky skin on the legs, are easily caused by exposure to wind and sun. But when such scaling becomes brown and covers the body over a long period of time, it can signal Hodgkin's disease, a cancer of the lymph nodes.

7. Below-the-surface bumps are usually just harmless fat deposits or ingrown skin, which are easily removed. However, when such bumps occur over the joints and are hard, they can indicate rheumatoid arthritis, and if somewhere else on the body, they may indicate cancer.

News Flash:

Trace Mineral Cuts Breast Cancer Risk by 72%

Recent studies have found a common trace mineral to cut the lifelong risk of breast cancer from 82% to 10%, for a savings of 72%. The wonderful mineral is selenium, and it is common in many of the foods we eat. It attacks cancer by slowing the growth of tumors, which may give our immune systems a chance to kill off the tumors themselves. In addition to its effect upon breast cancer, it also decreases the risk of heart attack by as much as 66%, men as well as women should make certain that they are not low in their intake of this important trace mineral. Your best defense against disease is a varied diet with abundant fresh fruits and vegetables, and as little fat and sugar as you can manage.

Vitamin Protection from Cancer,

A Simple Combination that Works

While you can often find studies about individual vitamins and minerals that cut cancer risk, you don't often find combinations. It is not that combinations of nutrients are less effective, it is just that they are harder to define since they are more complicated. But since cancer is a complicated disease, it is only logical that combinations at least have the potential of being more effective than any of their individual parts.

With that said, the combination we have here has been recently studied, and found to greatly reduce the risk of cancer. The three nutrients in it are beta carotene, vitamin E, and selenium taken in combination. This is not something that the medical profession believes in, so you will not find support from your doctor, but that also does not mean that it doesn't work. Each of these ingredients has individually been identified by various people as having anti-cancer qualities, so a combination of them should have great promise. So, while established medicine won't support you, you cannot be hurt by these nutrients, and you might just be protected from cancer.

Vitamin Proven to Lower Cervical Cancer Risk by 80%

A recent study has found that one of the B vitamins, folate, were deficient in 80% of the women who developed cervical cancer. It was concluded that folate probably protects women from developing cervical cancer, in every woman who makes certain that she receives an adequate amount in her diet.

If you are one of those who are not sure if there is enough folate in your diet, then you need to take some precautions to make certain you are protected by this wonderful vitamin. In foods, folate is richly found in broccoli, fresh fruit, leafy green vegetables, and legumes. The most pleasant way of getting your folate is to include at least two servings of these foods in your diet every day. If for some reason you are not able to eat enough of these foods on a daily basis, then take a daily multi-vitamin. While a vitamin pill does not supply all of the other benefits found in natural foods, like roughage, it can nevertheless be a very good, and inexpensive, insurance policy for your health.

CELLULITE

Treatments that Work, and Ones that Don't

Cellulite are those little wrinkles and bumps you get on your arms, legs, and body as you get older and more out of shape. They are particularly noticeable on women, but men get them too. The problem with getting rid of cellulite is that it doesn't seem to be attached to any particular muscle, so you don't know what to exercise, or how to diet to get rid of it. It's just little lumps just under the surface of your body, and exercise routines don't seem to do much good.

The real reason that exercise routines don't seem to do much good is that you expect to see improvement in a month, and you should really be looking at 6 months or a year. Weight loss is another necessity, but the main reason you collect fat on a portion of your body is because extra weight gets distributed around depending on whether you are a man or woman. If you have weak, sagging muscles in addition, you will suddenly discover that you have a terrible case of cellulite.

To get rid of cellulite you have to do both, lose weight and exercise. Take a look at Jane Fonda, or one of the other over 50 women dancers and entertainers, they don't have cellulite. The reason they don't is because they keep their weight where it belongs, and they exercise. If they don't have any personal dis-

---

cipline, then they buy some by hiring a personal trainer. If you can't afford a personal trainer, then at least join the "Y".

So long as you keep your body in good tone and keep your weight down where it belongs you will not have any cellulite. But if you let yourself go for a year and gain 20 pounds, and quit exercising, you will have cellulite all over your body.

Before I go I would like to remind you that only exercise and diet will cure cellulite. Body wraps may shrink and tighten your skin for a few hours, but by themselves they will not cure cellulite. Also, sucking the fat out of your body with a machine may help some of the local fat, but it won't tighten your muscles and give you muscle tone. Don't spend your time and your money on these procedures since neither of them, either alone or together, will get rid of cellulite.

CHEST PAIN

Try Safe and Effective EDTA Chelation Therapy
Instead of Surgery, and 94% Effective

EDTA is a protein-like molecule which works to remove metal ions of lead, mercury, and calcium from your body. These metals combine with cholesterol in your blood to form the plaques that block your arteries. It is this blockage that causes you pain, and can cause heart attacks and stroke. Taking EDTA chelation therapy has been effective in bringing relief to 87% of angina patients, and symptoms have not returned over time, and death rates from heart attacks have also been lowered.

Taking this therapy is also attractive because it is relatively inexpensive and is handled as an outpatient procedure, unlike surgical techniques to correct blockage. When nearly 2,000 patients were studied on the effectiveness of this therapy, over 90% reported relief from pain, and the same number showed an increase in ability to increase physical activity. When this problem is corrected through surgery there is a death rate of 5%, and complications another 30%, so using an EDTA therapy program saves lives as well as being extremely effective.

If your own cardiologist is not familiar with this treatment system, don't be too surprised. Most cardiologists are basically surgeons, and EDTA chelation therapy is not taught in medical schools. In fact doctors training for one mode of therapy usually learn very little about any other modes. Surgeons are not effective internists, and they prescribe medications for many things which might best be handled surgically. To find physicians who use this therapy contact the American College for Advancement of Medicine (ACAM), in Laguna Hills, California.

Two Nutrients That Can Relieve Chest Pain

To any of you who have suffered from it, you know that chest pain does not always mean heart attack, but it frequently does mean heart disease. Nevertheless it is possible to live a long and productive life even with heart disease if you take care of yourself and follow your doctor' orders. The problem comes in that even with the doctor's orders, you are often still left with the chest pain, and the chest pain all by itself can make you nearly an invalid.

But now, with the research of Dr. Linus Pauling, a two time winner of the Nobel Prize, comes a prescription for chest pain relief that may be better than traditional heart medication. What Dr. Pauling suggests is that you increase your intake of vitamin C to perhaps 6 grams a day, and that you add lysine to your nutritional program, at 5 grams a day. What this combination does is eliminate many of the factors that are responsible for the repeated attacks of chest pain.

First off, the vitamin C prevents the build-up of a chemical called Lp(a) that forms the plaques that coat our arteries. By simply keeping their numbers down it is less likely that they will start to cause us problems.

Next the lysine goes one step further, it prevents any Lp(a) that we do have from forming plaques, and may even help to reverse the plaque build-up on the artery walls. This last action will actually cure chest pain because you will no longer have any blocked arteries messing up your blood flow.

In a friend of Dr. Pauling's, their chest pain disappeared completely after a few months, and it has been as effective for others as well. Remember though to check with your doctor before you start taking these nutrients since you don't want it to interfere with any medication he is giving you. Also, since he is your doctor ask him to watch for changes, hopefully progress, resulting from your taking these nutrients.

CHILDHOOD EMERGENCIES

First-Aid for Choking in Children

Choking takes place when something gets stuck in the throat. In children it doesn't have to be anything very large, but often times it is something they have picked up off of the floor and just shoved into their mouths, the way small children do. When this happens to a child over 1 year of age, the first procedure to carry out is the Heimlich maneuver. To do this get behind the child and place your hands just below the base of the rib cage, then pull your hands toward you in what is called an abdominal thrust. Very often anything lodged in the wind-pipe will be dislodged and expelled.

If the Heimlich maneuver doesn't work you need to next go to the finger sweep. For the finger sweep you kneel beside the child's head and open his mouth. Then take the hand on the part of the body toward the feet and put it into the child's mouth. Grasp the tongue and lower jaw with that hand and tilt the child's head back to clear the tongue from the back of the throat. Now look into the mouth for anything lodged in the throat. If you see anything put the little finger of the other hand into the mouth, sliding the finger down along the inside of the cheek to the base of the tongue and sweep the object from the throat.

Do the finger sweep only if you can see something in the throat, and be careful not to push the object further into the throat when you do it.

If you want detailed instructions write to the American Academy of Pediatrics for a free brochure on choking prevention and first aid. The address is AAP, Dept. C-Choking Brochure, Box 927, Elk Grove Village, Il. 60009-0927. Be sure to include a self-addressed, stamped envelope.

The First Step to Take in the 6 Most Common Situations

What do you do first if your child is injured? Stop the bleeding, ask where they are hurt, call 911, just what should you do first? This is a practical question that can become critical when you are faced with the problem in the flesh. Of course children are hurt in real situations, and often one that you are a part of.

Just think of car crashes. Many children are hurt every year in car crashes, and most of the time their parents are with them. If a crash happens and your child is hurt you have to do something to help until the professionals arrive. And this is what you have to start planning on today. Of course there are other common causes of accidents to children, and some of these will be given too.

But before we go to the individual situations there are a couple of things you must do first to prepare for the emergencies that might arise. If you don't know CPR, then take a course at your local YMCA and learn it. After all, it's only a day and some of the most common type of accidents children have cause them to stop breathing. Next find the nearest emergency room equipped hospital that take a special interest in children, and even go so far as to pay them a visit. With these two basic preparatory steps you are ready to look at what you should do as a first step when your child is injured and needs emergency treatment.

1. Injury due to falling. The first emergency area we will look at is the one you are most likely to encounter on any given day. Your child may not even tell you about most of the falls he or she has had, but depending on the age of the child and the seriousness of the injury, you will usually hear are a falling down injury sooner or later. If the fall has been serious you will probably hear about it from someone else, first, don't panic. Go to your child, and don't move him. If he is conscious, find out where it hurts to see what might be broken. If he is unconscious then make sure his breathing is good, and give mouth-to-mouth resuscitation if it has stopped. Call 911, and if there has been any injury to the neck or back wait until they arrive to check for spinal injuries (don't move his head either). If he has had a blow on the head, and especially if he was unconscious, he needs to go to a hospital to be checked for a concussion. Concussions can kill since they can leave blood clots in the brain.

Less serious injuries also require emergency treatment. Scrapes, even rather bad ones, usually don't need a doctor's attention. Clean off the area and protect it with an antibacterial cream and a sterile bandage for a day or two. If there is bleeding you need to be much more careful. A bad cut, even if it stops bleeding, may need stitches to prevent scarring. Simple cuts, of course, can be treated at home with just a Band-Aid. If you get any persistent pain in a part of the body, particularly if there is swelling, you may well have a broken bone to deal with and your child must go to the doctor. For most children, injuries due to falls which need professional attention are rather rare, but nearly everyone needs this kind of attention at least once or twice in their lives anyway. Don't be too shocked or surprised if your child requires a doctor's attention for a fall at some time in their childhood.

2. Swimming accidents are next to be considered because they are not only common, but they are usually serious as well. Most swimming accidents involve drowning, but they also include hitting other swimmers in diving, or hitting a board or the side of the pool in diving. If the injury is the result of drowning, this is critical as to how long the child has been underwater, and whether or not he is breathing. If he is not breathing you need to perform CPR, and if you don't know how to do this take a course at the YMCA or YWCA. Parks and recreation departments often have courses, and a fire department will often send out trainers to

non-profit groups. You must also make sure the lungs are clear of water, and this should be part of your CPR training. Once you have gotten the child breathing, it is still necessary that they go to the hospital to check for further injuries.

But suppose the drowning did not go on till the child became unconscious, then what? Well, everyone swallows some water now and then, but they don't drown. If little water has been swallowed, and there has been no unconsciousness, then you can take care of things at home just by keeping the child warm for a while, and in an hour or two there should be no problem. But use your judgment on this. If you do what you can and there is any continued problem in breathing, go to the hospital. Complications can be hidden.

Now for accidents where your child is struck by someone else diving, or has hit a diving board or the side of a pool. You are going to have to use your judgment here too. If there is any unconsciousness, go to a hospital, or call the paramedics. If it is an injury to the back, neck, or head, and there is unconsciousness or obvious physical injury, use the professionals. If there is difficulty breathing, use CPR. And if it is broken arm or leg, then immobilize it as much as possible and either take the child to a hospital or call 911 if there is any bone pushing through the skin, or breaks in more than one area.

3. Choking is a class of emergency all in itself. You don't even have the warning, or time, that you do when you see your child in the water drowning. If your child is choking you have only a very few minutes to act or there will be brain damage or death. All choking is serious, but should not happen to any infant less than 1 year of age. A child under 1 year should never have access to anything they can choke from, and should always be in a supervised environment and under observation. Children over 1 year, however, are usually walking and very active. They will also stick anything small enough into their mouth, and many of those things can result in a choking accident. The first action to take in this case is to use the Heimlich maneuver. It is very easy to do, but on very small children you must be very careful about the amount of force used or the maneuver itself will cause serious damage.

If you are unsure how to do this on your child, then practice before you have an emergency. Get behind the child with your hands on the proper point of the abdomen. Then when you push in on the abdomen there should be an involuntary expulsion of air. Push just hard enough to get the expulsion of air, but not hard enough to cause any discomfort.

4. Poison is another grave emergency, but one which is often difficult to know properly how to respond. Poisons do not all act alike, and an appropriate way of handling a poisoning by one thing can do damage if the poisonous substance was something else. Also many things that can poison children are not labeled as poisons when you buy them, it is just understood that you will not drink bleach, or Drano, or whatever. In these cases the warning about poisoning is often in the small print on the label. But if you have reason to believe that your child ate a poison, the first thing to do is to call a poison control center (the numbers should be in the front of your local telephone book). When you go to the hos-

pital be sure to take the container with you, and know the child's weight. The container is needed so that the proper steps can be taken to counteract the poison, and the weight is needed to know how big a dose of an antidote should be given if that is what is needed. Too much or too little of a poison antidote will be of no use, and can even add to the child's poisoning.

It may be difficult to tell if your child took a poison in the first place. If there is an open container in the area the child had access to, and he is lethargic, or shows other signs of having taken the substance, you have evidence strong enough to justify a visit to an emergency hospital. The other evidence could be pills or powder spilled in the area, or in the child's hands, or of course if anyone says they saw him take it. You can always be wrong, and you usually have some time, but if you delay too long and there is poisoning, there may be nothing that can be done a few hours later. Commit your effort on the side of over-caution if you want to be safe.

5. Fire is just as terrifying to the parent as it is to the child. If your child has his clothing catch fire, the first thing to do is smother it and put it out. You can always practice this to protect your child by telling them that if their clothing catches first they should not run, but should stop, drop to the ground, and then roll until the fire is out. And for your information, running is just likely to fan the flames and result in a bigger fire. If there is no electricity involved, then put it out with water if you have it. But once the fire is out you need to run cool water over the burned area, and you should continue to do this until the area itself is cooled. This may take a while, but it is the only insurance you have that the burning has really stopped.

As a warning, however, do not use ice or ice water on burns because you may do more damage to the skin than was done by the burn. Just stick with the cool water for as long as is needed to cool the area.

When you have gotten the burned area cooled wrap the child in a clean, dry, sheet. Stay away from fuzzy towels or blankets since if the skin is actually charred, the fuzzy material on their surfaces will get into the wound and just have to be cleaned out later. Don't put any ointments on this kind of burn either. Ointments can be used for first or second degree burns where the skin surface is uncharred and unbroken, but not on severe burns where you may injure the skin just in applying the ointment. If you are dealing with a small area that has been burned you can wrap it with a moist, cool, and clean bandage.

Now take the child to the hospital, even if there is no immediate pain. Bad burns often do not show their worst sides until hours, or even a day or two, after happening. With direct exposure to fire there will be blistering, and you never know just how deep the burn penetrated into the body. One of the real dangers of deep burns is the toxins that the body has to deal with during the healing process. There is no way for you to take care of these yourself, so go and get professional help.

6. We will look at the needs in car crashes for our last area of emergency medicine for children. This is not if your child is hit by a car, that is covered under

falls. This is when your child is in a car that is involved in a crash. Even if the child was belted in properly, you still need to check for breathing as a first step, and give CPR if it is needed. If you start to give CPR, then keep it up until help arrives, unless of course the child starts breathing on their own. But never make your declaration of death and give up. So long as you keep oxygen going to the child's body you can have recovery.

Again, watch for spinal cord damage and don't move the head, neck, or back if you can avoid it. If there is fire, then take the chance and move the child clear of the fire. But when you make the move still try to keep all parts of his body in the same position. You can do this by moving a whole seat, if it is loose, or by getting help and supporting all parts of his body while you move him.

In any severe car crash, have your child checked by a physician, even if he has no complaints. Often times internal injuries don't show up for a day or two, and then are fatal. If they were taken care of immediately after a crash, they are more often treatable. Don't make this determination yourself, go to the doctor.

If you can keep all of the emergency procedures at your fingertips, you have the basic knowledge needed to save the life of your child in many of the emergencies they may encounter. In most cases the same actions can be taken for adults as well. But your child is your flesh and blood, and you should make special provisions to care for, and protect, them in the first years of their lives.

NOTES

_____

_____

_____

_____

_____

_____

CHILDHOOD NUTRITION

A Good Diet in Childcare—Don't Bet On It!

You send your child to a licensed pre-school center, and think that they are getting a couple of good meals a day while you are busy at work? Well, don't believe it! A survey of licensed childcare centers in 1992 found that 90% provided meals which were poor in quality, and likely to result in bad nutritional habits as the children grew up.

Meals consisted of foods which were high in fats, low in calories, and inadequate in iron, and vitamins B1 and B2. You would never feed your child a diet like this, but the government accepts these diets are adequate in their licensing system. The result of the poor nutritional state of these children is that they are not able to learn properly in the day care center, and will probably come home very hungry and slightly undernourished.

What can you do about it? Get involved with the day care center you use, don't depend upon the government to ensure that your child is getting good nutrition. This can be done by observing the center at random a couple of times, or at least looking at their diet plan for the month at the start of each month. After all of this you may not be certain as yet that your child is eating what you feel he or she needs. So feed the best diet to your child that you can for the evening meal, and keep healthy snacks around the house. With these precautions you can at least correct any shortcomings that day-care may inflict upon your family.

Free Nutritional Guides for Your Children

It is always news when the professional agencies of our society are willing to give you anything free, and now the American Academy of Pediatrics has 4 free brochures for children from 2 to 6 years of age. The brochures are "Good Nutrition," "Food Hassles," "Cholesterol," and "Healthy Foods." They can be obtained by writing Dept. C, American Academy of Pediatrics, P.O. Box 927, Elk Grove, IL 60009-0927. Above the address put the name of the brochure that you want.

Also available free, from the very popular Weight Watchers organization, is another free guide for children's nutrition. The guide is called "Healthy Diet,

Healthy Kids." To get it ask for it by name, and write to Weight Watchers, Department KB, Box 250, Jericho, New York 11753. Also be sure to include a self-addressed, stamped, business-sized envelope.

Iron Supplements Can Poison Your Child

Children sometimes mistake iron supplements for candy and eat large amounts of the pills. As a result iron pills have become the leading cause of accidental poisoning deaths in children.

The problem with iron pills is that they are colored red and sugar coated. As long as you swallow them without chewing they leave a sweet taste in the mouth that can very easily be mistaken for candy. The number one solution is to keep all iron pills out of the reach of children, but even with this precaution you might forget sometimes. If you have small children in the house try switching to a multi-vitamin source for your iron. The odor and flavor might not be as pleasant, but you could save the life of your child.

Should Milk be in Your Baby's Diet?

Since most of us have been brought up on cow's milk, we also bring our own children up on it too. After all, milk is a perfect food, at least that is what the milk producers, and almost everyone else, says. But how do we really know if milk should be the basic food of our children, and of many adults as well?

The answer is that we don't. We have just been taking other peoples word for it, and then continuing on without paying attention to anyone who questions just how good milk is for us. Now it is becoming clear that milk should not be in everyone's diet, and in infants perhaps it should not be in their diet at all.

Milk, either cow's milk or mother's milk, is designed by nature for the babies of the mothers that produce it. Human mothers' milk is perfect for human babies, and cows' milk is perfect for calves. But humans don't have to grow as fast as calves, or put on weight as fast, and cows' milk has a lot more fat in it than mothers' milk. Actually cows' milk has not only a lot more fat than human babies need, but whole milk has a lot of saturated fat and cholesterol that no humans need. To prevent setting your baby off with a high load of cholesterol in infancy don't use cow's milk in their diet in the first two years. After that stick with low-fat or non-fat milk and leave the whole milk alone except for special uses, but not as a daily part of their diet.

For a baby to start out healthy in life, mother's milk is best. It can be used for several years, but even if a baby only nurses for the first 6 months they will get a big boost in immunity to disease and good health. If nursing isn't practical, or when you stop, go to an iron-fortified infant formula. By the way, cows' milk is too low in iron for human babies too.

Other problems with cows' milk for babies, and small children,is diarrhea from an inability to digest the cows' milk called lactose deficiency. While some doctors think that high use of cows' milk may actually cause this lactose deficiency, once it develops you have to avoid milk products pretty much for the rest of your life.

Juvenile diabetes is another problem which might be linked to infant use of cows' milk. As it turns out there are proteins in cows' milk that are the same as the proteins in our pancreas. If our immune system thinks that the pancreas of children is a protein of milk, we can end up attacking our own bodies and destroying our pancreas with our own immune system. When this happens we get diabetes. This is still being researched, but if it turns out to be true, then we may have to give up feeding our babies cows' milk so that we can stop juvenile diabetes in America.

Another concern with cows' milk is the additives that dairy farmers give to cows to protect them and make them grow rapidly. About 82 drugs are known to be used, and 35 have not even been approved for use in the cows. Now the FDA does test for some of these drugs in batches of milk, but it doesn't test for all of them. So while some of the worst additives are kept out of our market milk, it is always possible that traces of many others are getting to us. While this is not proven, we may be getting antibiotics of many kinds, and growth hormones, in every glass of milk we drink.

A last area of concern for you milk drinkers is the possibility of lactose deficiency. Lactose is a milk sugar, and anyone who cannot digest it properly is going to suffer from diarrhea, bloating, gas, cramping, and nausea. If you drink milk daily and don't have any of these symptoms then you have the ability to digest lactose properly. But if you have some or all of the symptoms regularly, especially right after drinking milk,then you need to take some action. The best, if you can do it, is to give up drinking milk or eating milk products. If you can't do this, or don't want to unless you have to, then stick with chocolate milk since it digests more easily. Eating yogurt before drinking milk can also help by adding the bacteria to your body that you need to digest the lactose. And if you have cheese, get cheese aged 6 months or more since the lactose levels in this aged cheese are much lower than in fresh cheese or milk.

CHRONIC FATIGUE SYNDROME

Doctor's Aren't Sure What's Wrong With You?
The "Mystery Illness"

You have had the flu about once a year, and this year is just the same. After a restless night you awaken with a fever and body ache. You are sure that you have the flu, and take it easy for 3 or 4 days. When you aren't getting any better you go to your doctor for reassurance, and some antibiotic to make sure you don't get any complications. But 2 or 3 weeks, and 2 or 3 more visits to the doctor, and you are still as sick as you were on the first day. What is going on? Why doesn't your doctor cure you or tell you what is making you sick? In either case the doctors aren't helping, so what is wrong with you?

The answer may very well be that you have chronic fatigue syndrome. A debilitating disease that can last for years, and which no doctor can treat rapidly and effectively. They will do their best, once they finally realize what it is, but it is your body that is going to have to heal. There are no microbes to kill, and there is nothing to cut out of you that will make it go away. You don't have a tumor, and you don't have cancer. You have a disease that not only defies diagnosis and treatment, it even defies having a good definition.

Well, to help you a bit in understanding and handling CFS, read the next several entries, and you will at least get some basic information that may get you on the road to diagnosis and effective treatment. Just remember, CFS is just like any other chronic disease, and to get over it is going to take time.

Symptoms of Chronic Fatigue Syndrome

Chronic fatigue syndrome, CFS, has so many symptoms that there is no one symptom that will tell you that you have it. Among the symptoms commonly seen are extreme fatigue, sore throat, swollen lymph nodes, recurring infections, headaches, joint and muscle pains, diarrhea, nausea, fever, and night sweats. There are other symptoms as well, but you should have the picture by now. CFS can have about every non-specific symptom you can think of, and they can all be interpreted as something else.

The problem with telling if you have it is that there is no test to confirm anything you might suspect. Doctor's may tell you that you have it or you don't, but even they are just guessing. Diagnosis is generally made on the basis of symptom, length of illness, and degree of incapacity. But even with this doctor's still have to rule out other possible illnesses before they will give you a diagnosis of CFS.

But what should you look for so that you can tell if you have it? You have already been introduced to some of the symptoms, but other characteristics include a very sudden onset in that you might be fine one day and sick as a dog the next. The only problem is that you don't feel better the day, or the week, after that. You just go on and on being sick. Initially most people just think that they have the flu, or some other common disease. But, as we said before, when the common disease symptoms refuse to go away, and you are extremely fatigued for a long period of time, the diagnosis is most likely CFS. So in deciding if you have it first look for fatigue, then for other symptoms, and finally for how long all of this lasts. The longer it lasts the more likely it is that you have chronic fatigue syndrome.

Treatment for CFS

Before using any natural treatment you need to know two things; first, that there is no standard effective treatment of chronic fatigue syndrome, and second that mainstream doctor's do not believe that natural treatments can have any curative effect on CFS. With that said you may still be interested in trying the most recommended natural treatments, especially since the medical profession offers almost no alternatives. In spite of this, and because of the wide variety of symptoms, doctor's will prescribe a wide range of medications. What I am giving you here are the natural sources of those medications. Of course most doctors don't prescribe natural sources, and if it takes a large amount of a natural source to get a therapeutic dose then eating a serving or two of a particular food will probably not do you any good. Never the less, you deserve to know what the best natural sources are for the medications that doctors are going to prescribe to take care of your symptoms, and to make you feel better. The medications given are from many countries medicines, including both American and Chinese.

Diet, to run your body efficiently, should consist of a well balanced nutritional program. The basic diet is to include both vitamin and mineral supplements, vegetables and complex carbohydrates, little fat, sodium, and refined foods, fresh foods as often as possible, a pattern of small, frequent meals, and a lack of caffeine, alcohol, nicotine, sugar, and refined carbohydrates. You will find this basic diet prescribed for many illnesses, both chronic and acute.

Chinese medicine recommends the use of ginseng (which benefits most of the body functions), and garlic. Many other herbal preparations are also useful, but to find out the right ones you are going to have to go a Chinese herbalist to get a prescription.

American medicine gives us many naturally derived medicines used for CFS. A selection that you might find useful includes shitake mushrooms which are generally beneficial to the immune system (the drug lentinus edodes mycelium or LEM is extracted from them); carob, chocolate, whole grains, raisins, nuts and seeds, in extract, are used from such chronic diseases as herpes (and from which L-lysine is extracted); and vitamin C from many sources which lends its contribution to healing and anti-oxidation.

Since so many potential medicines are used, one or more for each symptom class, most of them are not derived directly from natural products and so there is no diet or supplement plan you can go on that will be able to relieve all of your symptoms. If that is the type of treatment you are looking for go to a Chinese herbalist, an American holistic doctor, or an American homeopathic doctor. If the doctor is good and honest your chances of successful treatment are at least good, and perhaps better than, as if you had been treated by one of the better mainline western doctors.

What Causes CFS?

This is a very tricky question. If we knew exactly what causes it, then we would also know exactly what not to do if we wished to avoid it, as in AIDS. The best available guess is that CFS is an immune system disease, not unlike AIDS, except that it doesn't kill you, and no particular agent is known to be associated with it (like HIV is with AIDS).

Because CFS has so many symptoms, and its sufferers also get so many other infections, it is thought to be simply a case where the immune system has lost its ability to keep everything in balance. It attacks the wrong things, and it protects the wrong things. It doesn't bring anything to a conclusion by killing off invaders to your body. It might even go so far as to protect them and go off and attack your own joints and muscles instead.

One of the best suspects for the cause of CFS is a virus. Because viruses get into our cells they can change the way they work, and one of these changes could be to attack the immune system and send it off on a wild goose chase.

Another strong contender is your genes. The genes you got from your parents may have had a flaw that turns parts of your immune system on and off at different times and produces the symptoms of CFS.

It is also possible that something in your environment can cause CFS. Smoke, chemicals, noise, stress, and other things have all been suggested as causes for this disease. Getting vaccinations with live virus, such as for polio, are a possible cause. And finally getting a yeast infection are considered possible causes.

As you can see, there are so many possible causes of chronic fatigue syndrome that there is nothing that you can focus in on.

Why CFS Can Affect the Heart

Chronic fatigue syndrome may be caused by one of the same hormones that help regulate your heart. The hormone is called cortisol, and is found in your glands and brain. When cortisol levels are high it can cause heart disease, but when they are low they cause fatigue. If this cortisol imbalance is the actual cause of chronic fatigue syndrome, then it should be possible to boost your cortisol level with drugs or nutrition and cure the disease. If you are thinking of this solution though, remember that cortisol also affects the heart, and you don't want to give yourself heart disease in trying to correct a case of chronic fatigue syndrome.

How to Gain Energy, Naturally

To gain energy naturally, even if you may be suffering from chronic fatigue syndrome, requires that you move. Resting in bed might be necessary if you are totally exhausted, but if you are to increase your basic energy level you need to get out and be active.

Besides, look around you. Those people that you see every day don't have any more potential for energy than you do, but they make the effort to go out and garden, or walk, or bike. In any case they use whatever exercise they are able to in order to build their energy levels.

And not only will being active give you more energy, it will also prepare you to better respond when one of those life emergencies happens. And they happen all too often if we are physically unable to respond. Think about your own quality of life, and your ability to respond to the needs of your loved ones the next time you pass on taking a walk so you can sit on the couch for another half hour. It's worth the effort to get up and go.

Fight Chronic Fatigue and Aging at the Same Time

While there are various ways to fight chronic fatigue, there is one which is little known, and which can also fight aging by protecting the cell membrane. The name of the drug is DMAE, and it was studied as early as 1959 for chronic fatigue and depression. The results of this study were excellent, but the drug itself has not come into wide use. One of the reasons for it being ignored for so long is that chronic fatigue was not recognized as a wide spread problem back at that time, and is since something that anyone might run into. DMAE is available in some forms in health food stores, and can be purchased without prescriptions from that source, or may be obtained by prescription. The prescription form of DMAE, from its original producer, is known as DNZ-2, and the producer is Bio-Tech pharmaceutical.

CIRCULATORY DISEASE

Diet Tips to Improve the Circulation

Your blood circulation can be sluggish either because the arteries are so clogged that blood can't get through very rapidly, and when it is you have high blood pressure, or because of certain foods that you eat that thicken the blood. The blood thickeners are also the foods that end up coating the walls of your arteries and giving you circulatory disease. So it doesn't matter what the cause of your poor circulation, you still need a diet that will thin your blood, and keep it from loading up with fats and salts that will slow down its flow.

Foods you need to cut down on, for a healthy circulation, include saturated fats, cholesterol, sugar, and alcohol. The saturated fats and cholesterol will clog the arteries and coat them with cholesterol, the sugar will contribute to diabetes, and alcohol simply slows the action of the system. So cut down on red meats, chicken, plain sugar and baked goods, and alcohol in any form.

Now to really help things out increase your intake of oily fish, raw fruits and vegetables, garlic, onions, oats, avocados, pineapple, ginger, vitamin A, vitamin B6, vitamin C, vitamin E, thiamine and niacin. Besides the food changes, it looks like you need to search around for a good one-a-day vitamin pill that has all of the nutrients you need to increase.

CLOTHING AND HEALTH

Your Necktie can Choke You

Should you wear a necktie or not? That is a question that many men ask, and most of those who work with the public end up wearing them whether they like to or not. But is that the best thing they can do for their professional image?

It' not the best choice if you wear your ties tight up to your neck, the way they are usually worn. Tight neckties have been found to cut off some of the oxygen flow to the brain, and to restrict the carotid arteries that carry blood to the brain. Not unexpectedly this can end up with the necktie wearer having headaches, sweating, and suffering from tension. And don't think that just loosening your necktie can solve all of the problem. If you button your dress shirts up to the top button, and you gain as little as 5 pounds, you may get the same effect as the person who is cinching his necktie just as tight as he can to his neck, and is thereby slowly strangling himself.

What should you do about it ? The solutions are really very simple and logical. If you can stop wearing neckties, and if you can't do that then at least loosen the tie a little bit and unbutton the top button on your shirts. Then you will find that these chances still leave you looking very well, but no one will be able to tell that you are not fully buttoned and tightened. If for some reason these don't work, or can't be done, then at least get some shirts with collars that fit, and get yourself a pre-tied tie that is set to a comfortable level of tightness. While you are at it you need to watch your weight and keep from tightening your dress clothes to the point that you just feel still all day long.

COLDS AND FLUES

A Common and Dangerous Cold Medication to Avoid

When you have a cold, if it is a cold, do not take antihistamines. Antihistamines are found in virtually all cold remedies, even though scientists know that they do nothing to cure the common cold. Antihistamines counteract the affect of histamine, which is released by the body when it is irritated by something we are allergic too, especially in the eyes and nose. The antihistamines stop the irritation and make us feel better, and that is fine. Antihistamines should be used whenever you get hayfever, or any other allergic reaction.

Colds, however, do not release histamines, and antihistamines do not counteract the irritating chemicals the body releases when you have a cold— which are called kinins. But the most important reasons for avoiding antihistamines when you have a cold is that they may cause you harm rather than help you. Look at any cold remedy containing antihistamines and it will tell you not to drive after taking it, that is because antihistamines will make you sleepy. Antihistamines are also dangerous to drivers, or people working around machinery, because they will dilate your pupils and impair your judgment. Taking an antihistamine and working around machinery is like taking a drink and working around machinery—it is a bad idea, and you can have a bad accident.

Colds are caused by viruses, and virus diseases can't be cured. You will get over a cold in a few days without taking anything, and not taking anything is what most doctors also recommend. But if you have allergies, then take the antihistamines and they will help you tremendously, but be careful driving and around machinery.

3 Alternatives to Treat Colds

If you want to do more than just wait out your cold, and are not sure that standard cold remedies are good for you, there is hope in some alternatives that are safer and more natural. Some you may know and some not, but they are all worth a look.

---

1. Vitamin C is the champion alternative cold cure. It has been popularly promoted for many years in health food stores, and even Linus Pauling, the double Nobel Peace Prize winner, has been trying to get people to believe in the curative powers of vitamin C. For colds you need to take about 2,000 milligrams of vitamin C from your first symptoms until the cold has passed. This should make the cold less severe and help you get over it sooner. Pauling, and others, also say that taking high doses when you are well will stop you from getting colds in the first place. Very high doses of vitamin C can be hard on the kidneys, so if you have kidney problems then try one of the other remedies. And don't give these high doses to children, children's' bodies react differently from adults, and they can get overdosed on medicines more easily.

2. Zinc has also been showing up more frequently in the health recommendations for several problems. Studies have shown that using zinc gluconate lozenges will help fight colds. The flavored lozenges are best, but watch out for an upset stomach as that is a problem some people have. Don't give zinc to children, and if you get sick to your stomach stop taking them too.

3. The last of our alternative treatments is an herb which you will get from the health food store. It is called echinacea, and comes as teas or tablets, which are equally good. Echinacea works by getting your immune system working more efficiently. A weak tea can be given to children.

While echinacea is probably the safest of the three treatments, it is the zinc and the vitamin C that are most likely to help with getting rid of your symptoms. A combination can also be used since these are all natural substances that your body needs anyway. Also these are all easier on your body than regular cold remedies that are always being pushed by the drug companies.

In any case rest and eat well in addition to what ever medication you decide to take. At the worst a cold should last no more than a week anyway.

4 Cold Symptoms and What to do About Them

A cold is a rather simple disease, at least so far as symptoms go. The simple and uncomplicated common cold has a cough, a runny nose, a sore throat, and can include fever, headaches, and muscle aches. Any of these last three can be missing, but the first three are usually always there. Because we are so familiar with these symptoms we know we are going to see them more than once each year, and have probably experienced them personally in the last three or six months. Here are a few ideas of what to do to relieve each of the 4 major cold symptom categories.

1. The cough doesn't develop with the first signs of the cold, but once you get it you know it will usually hang around even after all of the other symptoms

have gone their separate ways. A cough has a simple cause though. Simple dryness of the throat is all that it is, and because of that it doesn't need any rare drug for treatment. The medical books recommend linctus, but all linctus is are cough drops. What the medical books don't tell you is that any hard candy will work just as well at relieving a cough as a medicated cough drop. What cough drops do contain that is medical is a cough suppressant, and although they work they also limit the time you can use them exclusively to a couple of days (read the warning on the cough drop box). By sucking on any hard candy, or chewing gum, you will also keep your throat moist and stop the coughing. If you are bothered when you go to bed keep a glass of water near you and sip a little now and then. This can also be used instead of the candy, and works just about as well.

2. A sore throat often comes before the cough, but also goes away faster. You have the sore throat for the same reason that you cough, it gets dry. The dryness can be either from a post nasal drip, or from the expulsion of phlegm. Once it gets dry it gets red and sore. Treatment for sore throat is about the same as for a cough, just suck on hard candies or cough drops. Another helpful treatment is a nice cup of warm soup or tea. The warmth of the liquid seems to help control virus attacks in the throat. For an extra boost use chicken soup, the old Jewish recipe for colds and congestion. It can't hurt, and it will certainly help.

3. Congestion in the nose and the runny nose go hand in hand, and are maybe the most embarrassing part of a cold. If only our noses didn't run we wouldn't feel quite so much like outcasts when we have colds. The best cure for congestion is time, but on the short term a nice steamy bath or shower helps greatly. Remember the steaming inhaler, the steam of a bath works just the same way. You can also take decongestant pills, but these raise the blood pressure and can be dangerous if you have high blood pressure or diabetes. Anyway don't use decongestants for more than 3 days, and don't use antihistamines at all, they don't do any good. Antihistamines work for allergies, and people with allergy attacks who think they have colds and use them for relief have spread the idea that they work for colds too. There is not really good and safe relief from congestion, but in a cold it usually is only bad for a day or two, and then starts to fade.

4. The big three -- fever, headaches, and muscle aches can make a cold ten times worse if you get them. The headaches are part of the congestion problem, but the other two mean that the virus has gotten into your blood stream and your body is bringing out bigger guns to fight it. Fever is often accompanied by a loss of water from the body, and you need to have water with you all of the time if you have a fever. Muscle aches can be relieved with acetaminophen or ibuprofen, and aspirin should not be given to children because of the risk of Reye's syndrome—a possibly fatal disease. Warm baths with sleep and bed rest can often give short term relief. If you have these complications, and that is what they really are, then don't push yourself into working and carrying out a normal routine, but give it a day or two of rest. A little sympathy from your loved ones helps too.

There you have it. All that you have to do is put them into practice for relief. Besides, it will take your mind off of the cold for the 3 or 4 days it will really bother you, and you will be well anyway. Don't ignore your symptoms, treat them, and treat yourself well too.

4 Questions About Colds and Flu that You Should Know

Because anyone may have questions about colds and flu that they don't know until they hear them, there is no guarantee that the questions here will be ones that you want to ask. However, don't make that decision until you at least read the questions. And if you think you already know everything there is to know about colds and flu, then you should read these questions carefully, as well as at least look over the answers. You may be a little surprised, and there may be something here that is useful to you.

1. How do you know if your sore throat tickle is really a strep infection, and should be treated by a doctor? You can't tell for sure by yourself, that takes a throat culture by your doctor, but you can make a guess that is good enough to tell you to go to the doctor or to take care of it yourself. Sore throats are classed at strep, which is caused by a bacterium, or laryngitis or pharyngitis, which are the result of your infection with a cold virus. The laryngitis and pharyngitis are the result of post nasal drips and coughing that constricts the area of the throat. But they usually only last a day or two, and will fade away as your cold does.

But if your sore throat lasts for more than 3 days, is very sore, and you have a fever, then there is at least a good chance that what you have is a strep throat. Strep throats also come on very quickly, in many cases, and the back of the throat will have white dots on it.

But it is still possible to have a strep throat and not have all of these symptoms, so if your sore throat lasts more than 3 days, go see your doctor and have it cultured. He will also give you some antibiotics that should clear it up at that time. If you have a suspicion that you have a strep infection don't just let it go and hope that it cures itself. Untreated strep infections can result in pneumonia, rheumatic fever, and kidney failure.

2. Since a runny nose always accompanies a cold, is there some way to keep it from getting red and sore until you get well? While anyone's nose will get sore and painful if their cold lasts long enough, most of the time we are bothered by this it is largely our own fault. Because your sinuses are infected, and drain constantly for a few days, your nose is always wet and being wiped and blown. All by itself this makes the tissues of your nose tender, but it doesn't make them sore. The soreness comes from using harsh tissues, and from the drying action that you are doing in the repeated wiping. Over a few days you simply wipe off a few layers of skin and all that is left are the raw underlayers. Once you have gotten to that point all that you can do is not touch your nose for a few days and let it heal up. But to prevent the problem in the first place get the softest tissues you can find, and then put a little moisturizer on your nose to keep it from getting com-

pletely dried out. Another trick which will give your nose a little rest is to flush it with some warm water a few times a day. This seems to clear out the sinuses a little higher up than blowing or wiping and will give you a few minutes of piece before you have to face the problem again.

3. You have just gotten over a bad case of the flu, and your cough won't go away, is it possible that you have something else that should be treated? Well yes, it is possible, but don't jump to conclusions. First, it is normal to have a persistent dry cough for even several weeks after having the flu, and there is nothing you can do about that but take cough drops when it gets too bad. But if your cough isn't dry, and you are coughing up yellow or green phlegm, then it is possible that you have either bronchitis or pneumonia, and you need to be treated for either of these. Bronchitis makes you feel very badly, but it is not nearly as serious as pneumonia. In bronchitis you will have a wheezing in your chest that you or someone else with their ear to your lungs can hear. You usually will not have a fever with bronchitis, and will not feel as sick as you will with pneumonia, and you will not have to take time off from work while you get over your bronchitis. But pneumonia is an infection in the lungs, and it can kill you if left untreated. However, with pneumonia you will feel so bad that there will be no question but that you will want treatment. If you suspect that you have either of these conditions go to the doctor, and you will probably be given an X-ray and antibiotics. Most people do not go to the hospital with pneumonia, but you will have to take up to a month or two off of your normal activities and recuperate until your lungs clear.

4. For our last question we want to ask how you can tell if you have a cold or the flu, since so many of the symptoms are the same? You will probably never know which you have had if it is either a severe cold or a mild flu, but in most cases the course of symptoms are very different. Colds come on over a period of 1 to 2 days, the flu over just a few hours. Colds can make you feel tired and weak, and have mild aches and pains, while the flu will leave you exhausted, and with severe aches and pains. Headaches are signs of the flu, but not of colds. Fevers are mild with colds, but can go to 104 degrees with the flu. And the length of a cold is usually pretty close to 1 week, but is usually longer for the flu, and may even last for as long as a month.

Now should you do anything for the flu if you think that you have it? It would not be a bad idea to take good care of yourself if you have the flu. Complications of the flu, but not of colds, include pneumonia, and if you want to limit your period of sickness to no more than a week or two you need to avoid pneumonia.

8 Foods and Drinks that End a Cold or Flu Faster

The worst thing you can do when you are sick with a cold or the flu is to stop eating, or to eat only a limited diet like soup for every meal. Instead you need the best diet you can have because your body uses extra nutrition to fight illness, since you have to attack the infection, get rid of the waste products, and build new tissues for whatever areas of the body are sore or injured. However, because you are sick you may not be able to eat a normal diet, even though you need to have a good diet. Build your diet from the food list below and you will help your body to rid itself of a cold or flu faster and easier than you imagined you could.

1. Soup is especially good food when you are sick. You can put anything into it to make it nutritious. Meat, vegetables, or pureed combinations, and make it to fit your own taste. Soup also works especially well because the extra liquid helps you to swallow, as well as replaces some of the water your body may have lost in sweating.

2. Yogurt and cottage cheese are high in protein and vitamin D. They are also easy to digest, and may be flavored with fruits or eaten plain. Frozen yogurt can also soothe a sore throat and provide a treat at the same time.

3. Potatoes either baked, boiled, steamed, or microwaved are excellent sources of vitamin C, as well as many other vitamins and minerals. If you have little interest in plain potatoes, but want to avoid fats, then try topping the potato with yogurt and you may be surprised enough to put it into your regular diet.

4. Juices work well for vitamins like vitamin C, and can form a very satisfying diet combination. Since you are ill with a cold or flu fresh fruit juices should be mixed with bananas to cut down on some of the acidity. Don't forget to try carrot juice too, and it can also mix with fruit juices.

5. Cooked breakfast cereals, and these can be mixed with extra milk to make them a little thin, are a good source of vitamins and minerals. Using cereals fortified with extra vitamins and minerals may also be wise since your overall diet will probably be cut down.

6. Soft scrambled eggs are a good source of protein, and are easy to digest. Although egg yolks are high in fat, eggs really are a complete food so far as giving us all of the vitamins and minerals we need. If you are concerned about fat use an egg substitute, these are eggs with the yolks removed, but which have all of the protein.

7. Baked custard is another easy way to digest dairy product, high in protein, and it can be picked up in the market in a mix. Its easy to make, and it can provide a nice variation on a limited diet.

8. Protein drinks are a nice fortified food which can be mixed whenever wanted, and even form a complete diet for a couple of days if need be. Try something like Carnation Instant Breakfast, but look at the vitamin and mineral list on

the side of the box, and try a different one if you want some variation or just don't care for the Carnation drink.

How to Avoid the Common Cold

Fortunately common colds do not spring on us out of the night and make us sick, but what they actually do is sneak up on us in the guise of other cold sufferers who we try to avoid. Of course when we are always trying to avoid everyone who has a cold, how come we usually end up with 2 or 3 colds each year anyway?

In the answer to that question lies our means in how to avoid catching the common cold in the first place. Contrary to what we usually think, most colds are probably not caught through someone with a cold sneezing on us. Although being sneezed on can give you a cold, you can also get one by touching something a person with a cold has contaminated and then touching your mouth or eye. And because when there are a lot of people with colds nearly all surfaces like door handles and table tops become contaminated over and over, it gives you many chances to infect yourself.

During the cold season you can be pretty sure that you have been exposed to cold viruses many times whether or not you get a cold yourself. You also may get a cold that is so slight that you don't notice it, and that could happen several times a year more than when you get a cold that makes you feel ill.

To avoid the common cold you cannot get a vaccination though, because there is no vaccination for colds. Too many viruses cause colds, and no vaccine would work. Of course you can continue to avoid other people with colds, although people who are spreading cold viruses around don't have symptoms all of the time so that will only give you limited protection. You could stop touching your face with your hands, except that that is done mostly unconsciously.

So then what can you do? About the best answer is to stay out of public areas as much as possible during the cold season. This means stores, schools, sporting events, and eating areas. If you need to go to them anyway, then do it early in the day after they have been cleaned and disinfected by the employees who work there, and haven't been reinfected by the crowds of the day. Furthermore, in your own home you can disinfect public areas regularly. These include the telephone, doorknobs, and countertops. If someone in the house has a cold then disinfect them every time after the sick one uses them. Otherwise get enough sleep, keep a good diet, and get some exercise to keep your immune system in the best shape possible.

When to Get Your Flu Shot and Why

A flu shot can be one of the best and cheapest form of health protection you can get if you need the protection, but get it at the right time or it may not help to prevent a bad case of the flu. You can always get a flu shot if you seem to be attacked every time it comes around, or if you get especially sick when you get the flu. You should also get a flu shot if you are older than 65 (in general), or if you have any problem with your lungs or breathing (such as emphysema).

But if you decide you need a flu shot when should you get it, or does it matter? As it turns out it does matter. If you get a flu shot after everyone at home or at your job has the flu then it will probably not do you any good because you have already been exposed and your body is doing the best it can. Of course that shot might protect you for next year, but don't bet on it.

Each time the flu comes around it comes in a different form, so last year's shot won't do you much good this year. For this reason wait until October or November to get your shot. That way the doctors will have the right kind of vaccine to protect you, and your body will still have plenty of time to build its immunity before the flu comes around.

CONSTIPATION

Foods That Help You Stay Regular

Some people seem much more prone to getting constipated than others. The problem may be that if you are one of the ones who get repeated bouts of constipation, then it is probably your diet that is causing it. If you eat lunch with someone who is never bothered by constipation it may look very much like the two of you are eating the same mix of foods. But by looking a little closer you may find that your friend has a little more salad, a little lighter main dish, and perhaps more fruit and liquid than you do. While this may not look like much of a difference at first glance, it is actually the basis for a non-constipating diet which will work for anyone who incorporates it into their meals through the day.

As you may have gathered from the food choices in the regular lunch eater, the diet key to staying regular lies in eating enough of the right things, cutting out enough of the wrong things, and then getting as much liquid as you can. The foods that help you stay regular are all high fiber foods, and the foods that are most likely to block you up are all low fiber foods. The main low fiber foods in our diets are meats, foods made from refined flour like white bread and most baked foods, and some of our liquids which have calories but little nutrition.

Now we have already said that you need a lot of liquid in your diet to be regular. If you consider your body to operate much like a steam engine, and that you are best off adding liquid as you use it you are best off, then you will always be on the look out to add liquid to your body through the day. The only problem is that if the liquid you add is anything but water or zero calorie sodas, you are adding calories also. If you add enough calories from your liquids you will not end up wanting your fiber foods, and you will still have a bad digestive system. As a rule of thumb, the more of any calorie containing liquid you want in your diet the fewer the calories that should be found in each serving. One glass of whole milk will be of no harm, but 1/2 gallon of whole milk may give you 1/2 of your daily calories. Make the effort to add as much water, zero calorie, and low calorie liquids as you can in place of full calorie drinks.

Fiber was the other term that keeps popping up. Fiber is basically the part of our food that we don't fully digest as it goes through our bodies. And because we can't digest the silicon coat on plant cells, it is largely the amount of silicon that is in our vegetables and fruits that determines how much roughage we get in our diets. As you can see it doesn't matter whether our fruits and vegetables are raw, cooked, or mixed into a cake just so long as we get a basic 5 or 6 servings a day for needed fiber. Although some fruits and vegetables have more roughage than others, you don't really have to be concerned with how much each of them has just so long as you get the right number of servings and mix up your choices. In terms of vitamins, minerals, and calories however, there are many variations. To minimize calories, and maximize vitamins and minerals it is generally best to have several servings of raw or fresh cooked fruits and vegetables in the diet.

Now as you are adding all of this liquid and fruits and vegetables, what should you be dropping. Start with red meats, and meat in general. You need very little meat each day for protein, and by getting rid of the excess your taste for fruits and vegetables will be stimulated. Now go to anything made with refined flour and cut that out, or at least go to whole grains. Whole grains contain much more fiber and will benefit your digestion. Liquids we have already talked about: cut down on whole milk, alcoholic drinks (which have empty calories), and sweetened sodas. The calories in all of these are empty, especially so since you can get the same nutritional value in skim or low fat milk as you can in whole milk.

There is the basis for a non-constipating diet which will keep you regular and away from the enema.

The Beverage that can Ease Pain in Joints, Fight Constipation, and More

There is only one beverage that accomplishes all of these therapeutic effects, and that is water. The number one reason that you are likely to get constipation is because you have allowed yourself to get dehydrated. Most of us do not drink enough water to keep our bodies functioning at their healthiest. And since your blood and internal organs get first choice of nutrients, if you are low on water its taken from your digestive system. But your digestive system needs large amounts of water to run smoothly. Water is used to process the food, separate out the urine from the blood, and lubricate the intestines as food passes through. If the intestines dry out even a little bit, the waste products in your body can become dry and hard as well. Then you may just stop passing material until it gets to the point that you have to have an enema to get things going again.

The prescription is to drink 8 glasses of water a day, that's 2 quarts, and it can include other liquids as well. You are unlikely to find anyone who drinks as much water as they should, and who has constipation. The other excellent effects of drinking the water that you should is that your skin will smooth out, you will avoid uric acid crystals from forming in your joints and causing you joint pain, and you will be fighting gallstones since you will be flushing the uric acid and calcium out of your system before it builds up to where it can form stones.

CRAMPS

7 Secrets to Relieving Menstrual Cramps

Menstrual cramps can be so light that they are not noticed, or so strong and painful that women have to go to bed during their periods. The level of discomfort and pain that you have as a result of cramps will determine whether or not you need to do something to relieve them. But for many women, doing something is a necessity rather than a choice. If your menstrual cramps are severe enough to make you change your normal activity schedule, then you should probably use one or more of these secrets to help you have a happy and normal life, every day of the month.

Which ones will work best for you really depends upon you and your body. If the reasons for your cramps is medical, then you will probably need a medical treatment. If it is just something that you have once in a while, then hav-

---

ing some things you can pull out and try should be all that you need. The purpose of these secrets is to control the action of the prostaglandin that your body regulates to get you through your monthly cycle. If your prostaglandin level is too high you will have cramps. If it is very high you will have very severe cramps. For your own comfort and care, see which of these you can work into your lifestyle to your best advantage.

1. The menstrual stretch, which can be useful no matter how bad your cramp pain, but which works best if it is not too severe. First lie flat on your back on a firm surface. Then pull your knees up toward your chest, and move your feet in a circular motion. You can use your hands to hold your legs in the right place. Hold this position for a few minutes at a time, and repeat it until the cramping pain lessens. This will stretch out the muscles of your back and uterus, and works real well if you do it just before going to bed, and after getting up. As a less active alternative you can lie flat on your back with your feet elevated a few inches and put a heating pad or hot water bottle on your stomach. If you can relax in this position for a few minutes the cramps will usually go away, and you don't even have to stretch.

2. The diet solution to cramps is just good nutrition advice at any time, but it is especially good if you are having cramps. Whatever your normal diet is, if you make your diet up of vegetables and complex carbohydrates during the time of month when you get your cramps, you may get rid of them. The idea is to keep your blood sugar levels constant, which the carbohydrates and vegetables help do. It also keeps your digestive system working efficiently so that you don't have any constipation problems that could add more cramping. Other actions you can take include cutting out caffeine during this time—that means regular coffee, tea, and colas. And using decaf versions for drinking. On drinking, you should also cut out alcohol at this time since it tends to slow down digestion, and can add to cramping. Anything that you normally eat that takes your body very far from a good balance is going to increase your cramping problems.

3. The stretching solution to cramps has already been discussed, but you can also use any fitness or exercise program to help control pain and discomfort in your menstrual period. Because cramps are the result of the muscles cramping up on you, as the name implies, anything you do that will help you to relax will also help your cramps to be less sever. Exercise works directly by first heating up the muscles, and then allowing them to cool down, and leaving them totally relaxed. If also helps by producing the hormone, endorphin, in the brain which has a very calming effect on your outlook on life. If you like to exercise, or already have an exercise program, then don't stop around your period. Instead do it on a daily basis, with day to day variation, and your body as a whole will be more relaxed and comfortable. Women are no longer expected to be inactive during their periods, but can freely perform most sports and activities. What you can't do at this time is entirely up to you. If you control your cramps using exercise, then exercise is obviously of beneficial use to you at the time of your period.

4. Something that you can do alone, or with someone else, is to get an

abdominal massage whenever you have menstrual cramps. It works perfectly well alone, but if you have a companion the massage can always lead to more intimate things later. Massage is useful because the pain of the cramps is caused by the muscles of the stomach tightening up to the point where it hurts. Since a massage warms and loosens the muscles, it will also decrease the cramps. The best way to get this massage is to lay flat on your back and slowly but firmly massage your abdomen until the pain subsides—this takes about 15 to 20 minutes, but might take longer. The massage will not only get rid of the pain in your stomach, but it will leave you relaxed over your whole body and in much better shape to continue your day's activities.

5. Although you wouldn't think so, there are vitamins that you can take to reduce cramps. Research has found that a daily combination vitamin supplement, with extra B1 and B6 will decrease the strength of the menstrual cycle. If you use 100 milligrams of B1, and 200 milligrams of B6, you will lower the amount of blood which enters the uterus before menstruation, and there will be that much less to leave it, and there will not be as much work for your body to do in order to prepare for the next cycle.

6. One of the things accomplished with a massage is that the muscles of the area massaged get warm as more blood flows through them. To get the same results without the massage you can warm up the muscles directly with a heating pad or hot water bottle. Another way to do it is to take a hot bath and let your stomach soak in the hot water until it cools. This outside heat will also cause more blood to flow through the muscles of the stomach and relieve cramps. There is a time requirement though, you must keep warming the area until the cramps are relieved or this will not work very well for you.

7. Now that we have covered all of the treatments you can do yourself, it is time to look at the medications you can use, and for which you must have a doctor involved. Because cramps are caused by imbalances of body chemicals, it is possible to take additional chemicals to correct or relieve the pain and restore your body's chemical balance.

Prostaglandin has been named as the cause of cramping pain, and the medications are called anti-prostaglandin. You will need to start taking them about 2 days before your period is due, and if you are in pain it will take a couple of hours before the pain goes away. The most popular anti-prostaglandin drugs are Motrin and Anapox, and you will need a prescription to get them.

If your cramps are not too severe, but you would like some relief anyway, there are some over-the-counter medicines that may work. These have lower levels of anti-prostaglandin than the prescription drugs, but are also much cheaper and easier to get. The most popular of these are aspirin, Midol, Pamprin, Advil, and tylenol. While these are certainly worth trying on occasion, if you feel you need stronger drugs or seem to be taking these drugs for too long a time, then talk to your doctor to make sure that there is no other problem.

Causes and Cures of Muscle Cramps

Muscle cramps have several causes, and some have nothing to do with your exercise habits. However, how you exercise is the most common cause. If you exercise only occasionally and don't drink liquids while exercising you can cause your muscles to cramp. Cramping from exercise is caused by a build-up of lactic acid, which is generated by the muscles during exercise, and which takes a while to get neutralized by the body. Drinking water during exercise helps to prevent the lactic acid from causing cramps.

Another major causes of muscle cramps is anything that cuts down on your blood circulation. If you smoke, or have atherosclerosis, or just sit or lie in a position that cuts down on the flow of blood to a part of your body your muscles will cramp. These cramps can usually be helped by just getting up and walking around until they go away. Moving around increases the blood flow through your body and gets rid of the cause of the cramp.

You may also get cramps in the middle of the night, and the cause of these are not very well known. They probably have to do with your eating habits, general health, and physical activity during the day. Although they are very painful they should go right away when you stand and stretch out the muscles. Most of the time you won't have another attack the same night, and they are not something you should worry about.

The last, and most serious, cause of cramps is serious illness. Atherosclerosis, or any disease that narrows the blood vessels and decreases circulation can cause chronic muscle cramps. If you have a lot of cramps, and can't see any reason why you are having them, then you need to be examined by a doctor.

For prevention you need to eat foods that have the nutrients you lose when you exercise. The two nutrients you need the most of are potassium and calcium. Good sources of potassium are bananas, oranges, and potatoes, and for calcium you need milk and dairy products. Otherwise the best thing you can do to prevent cramps is to make sure you don't get dehydrated. So drink plenty of liquids and limit your exercises when the weather is hot.

DEPRESSION

Depression is a terrible and devastating disease that can leave us unable to care for our families, or take care of our daily lives. In its worst form it leaves us unable to carry out any of our own wishes, and is a very dangerous condition to our lives. For this reason we offer some approaches to treating depression which are not well known, but which can cure its clinical effects, and which you should be aware of if you are ever faced with the problems of depression.

Natural Way to End Depression
Four Ways to Talk Yourself Out of it

People who talk to themselves, even out loud in public, may be healthier then those who think this is a sign of mental illness. You are the best person there is to give yourself advice. You know yourself better than anyone else, you have lived with yourself longer, and you have forgiven yourself for mistakes more often than any ever can. Only you know all of your strengths and weaknesses, as well as what your ambitions and needs are. But, if you need a few hints in how to go about talking to yourself constructively, and this need can come up whenever you are having a hard time in life, here are some good ideas.

1. Use the old sayings that so many people make fun of. The sayings about luck is right around the corner, or every cloud has a silver lining, may seem rather corny, but the fact that you can use them without thinking a long time to come up with something useful makes them all the more useful. They also all have a kernel of truth to them. For most anything that happens that is bad, things will get better over time, even if the getting better is just in your accepting what has happened and you are now beginning to live with it. Anything that gives you a little hope is just as important as something that gives you an actual solution to your problems, and anyone with depression needs something to make them feel better about themselves and the world.

2. Be kind to yourself because running yourself down because of a problem is just going to make you feel worse, and add to the problems you already have. Feeling bad about a problem never solved anything. Especially when you are feeling depressed you should never go about telling yourself how bad you are,

or thinking constantly about your problems. If the problem is your job, then look at jobs where you did well, and if it is a personal relationship, then look at the people who love and trust you. Whatever your problems there are always incidents in your life where you have done well, and thinking about them will help you to overcome the problems you have now. A lot of problem solving is just attitude, and those who are more confident solve more problems than those who aren't. Thinking well of yourself is an excellent starting place to solving any problem.

3. Don't try to be a perfectionist, nobody is anyway no matter what they tell you. So many times we think some people are perfect because that is the way they show themselves to us, but by looking a little deeper we can see that nobody is. If you think that your depression is deserved because you are somehow imperfect, then don't. Everyone has failures as well as successes, but it is also true that only those who have successes also have failures. Anytime you try to do anything new in life you risk failure, but failing something new doesn't make you a failure as a person. Anyone who tells you they have never failed, or that they are perfect, is a liar. Don't tell yourself this lie because it won't help you to a happy life. Life can be happy, for the most part, if you accept yourself as someone for whom a failure is nothing compared to the successes you have had, and will continue to have in the future if you keep trying to grow and do new things.

4. Spend some energy looking at your successes. This can be a nice family, a good job, or friends who love you. If you are thinking of your successes you will not be thinking of what it is that is depressing you. Problems and failures cannot fit in the same space as those good things that you have done, and those good experiences you have had. While you may need to return to the problems to solve them, you have already solved many problems in your life, and by looking at them you will gain the strength and confidence to solve your current problems as well. No problem is unsolvable, although some must be accepted and adjusted to be dealt with, but that is success too, and allows you to go on in life to further events that will give you peace and happiness.

Non-Drug Depression Control

There are actually naturally occurring amino acids that can help you get rid of your depression. They work by stimulating your brain to release dopamine, which your body naturally releases to make you feel better, and it is entirely safe. The amino acids do not require medical supervision, and should be available locally. These wonderful nutrients are phenylalanine and L-tyrosine. While they may be a bit difficult to remember, you should have no trouble finding them at a health food store.

People Call It a Miracle
All We Know is it Can End Depression

One of the forms of this disease is called manic depression. This particular form is caused by a chemical imbalance in the brain. People who suffer from this type of depression are subject to behavior varying between uncontrollable outbursts and episodes of hyper-excitement, in which the sufferer just bubbles over with joy. There are three miracle drugs which can treat this condition, and can offer hope for many who do not even know they suffer from such a serious illness. The first is lithium, which has been long used to treat depression, and the other two are Targetol and Depakote, which have been used to treat epilepsy and are now known to act as miracle drugs in the treatment of depression.

DIABETES

4 New Ways to Get Rid of Diabetes

Getting rid of diabetes is not preventing it, it is curing it. Now curing diabetes is always a chancy task. You can "cure" it with diet, but if you fall off of the diet the diabetes will probably come back, and that is how it is with all cures. For whatever reason that your pancreas have stopped working properly, a cure is only good so long as you use it. And there is always the chance that the diabetes will come back even if you cure it once, and follow all of the rules. Diabetes is not even recognizable, unless you regularly monitor your blood sugar, so many people with mild cases of diabetes don't even know they have it. Most of the time such mild cases won't require more than watching, and that is the intent of the 4 ways of getting rid of diabetes that we are going to take a look at here.

1. Fiber has been shown to be effective in getting rid of diabetes. What we are talking about is dietary fiber at high levels. In studies at the University of Kentucky, the effect of a high fiber diet was studied on 20 insulin dependent men. These men were using different levels of insulin, and it was found out that 90% of those using less than 20 units of insulin daily were able to stop taking insulin, they were essentially cured. The next group was taking less than 40 units of insulin, and they were able to cut their insulin needs by 2/3. The third group used over 40 units of insulin, and they had only a slight reduction in their insulin requirements. The less dependent you are upon insulin, the better your chance that a high fiber diet will rid you of diabetes.

2. Chromium, which is the helper to insulin in maintaining blood sugar lev-

---

els. Studies have found that the older we are, as Americans, the more likely we are to have a low chromium diet, and low chromium in our bodies. Without chromium the entire responsibility for processing sugars falls on the insulin, and the pancreas. The theory is that chronic low chromium diets eventually lead to breakdowns in the pancreas, and result in adult onset diabetes. Further, it is felt that maintaining a high chromium diet as we get older will delay or prevent adult onset diabetes. While this doesn't always work, it usually does. To get your chromium, the best sources are brewer's yeast, molasses, and whole grain cereals.

3. Refined sugar has to be minimized in the diet. Studies by the Department of Agriculture found that a diet high in refined sugar, that is as high as the normal American diet, results in an elevation of blood sugar and insulin. Apparently the elevated blood sugar causes the increase in insulin, and in turn puts an increased load on the pancreas. The harder you make your pancreas work, the more likely it is to quit. Diets in which complex carbohydrates were increased, and sugar decreased, experienced no increase in blood sugar or insulin. Refined sugar means honey as well as white sugar. In digestion carbohydrates are converted to sugars as they are digested. But at no time in the history of man has so much refined sugar been in the diet, and it is only natural that this much sugar is going to result in disease.

4. Vitamin B6 is the reliever of diabetic symptoms. Remember the first paragraph, where we said that getting rid of diabetes meant getting rid of the symptoms of diabetes. Well, vitamin B6 will serve to do just that. Doctors at the Thordek Medical Center in Chicago found that the administration of vitamin B6 relieved the symptoms of pain, burning, numbness, and eye problems. If you can relieve these symptoms, and keep them from coming back, you are practically cured.

Those are the 4 secrets to ridding yourself of diabetes. While they may do the job for most of you, they won't do it for all of you. The more advanced your diabetes, the less relief you are going to get. However, that does not mean that these steps won't help to control and relieve the symptoms you have, even if it can't get rid of them completely. Look at these 4 secrets as guides to taking better care of your nutrition. You don't need to be a diabetic to benefit from them either, as they are preventive of diabetes as well as curative of it. Alter your life to save it, and live happier and longer for the trouble.

5 New Ways to Manage or Cure Diabetes

If you have diabetes, managing it is one of the most important jobs you may have to do in order to stay active and healthy. The 14th International Diabetes Federation Congress recently reported some new ways of handling diabetes which can help you to take good care of yourself, and even provide some ways of preventing diabetes in susceptible individuals.

1. A new self-testing method which does not require you to draw blood, and uses only a small hand-held meter. This is still an experimental technique, but promises an end to the constant pin-pricking blood tests that diabetics now do in order to monitor their blood sugar levels. The new meter system works by shining an infrared light through your skin and gives a read-out of the blood sugar level of the blood under the skin. The meter is being developed by Futrex Inc, of Gaithersburg, MD, and does not yet have FDA approval. Inquire from your doctor as to the progress of this instrument, and you may be able to do away with a lot of the monitoring equipment you now have to rely upon to keep your blood sugar level safe.

2. New forms of insulin that can be taken as pills or a nasal spray hold out the promise of doing away with the insulin shot for many people. These are also in the development stage, and are not yet on the market. The insulin pill is being tested in Israel, and has been effective in decreasing blood-glucose levels in 20 diabetes patients for one and a half to two hours. The nasal spray has shown a similar effectiveness, and is being developed in England. While there is no time line on the pills, the nasal spray is expected to be available for use in about three years.

3. Curing diabetes by transplanting human insulin-producing islet cells may be one of the ultimate hopes for the diabetic. This wonderful accomplishment is in a very preliminary stage right now. It has been used on transplant patients who are on immuno-suppressant medication, which would limit its use in a normal population because it isn't safe to have a suppressed immune system— thus leaving you open to infections. A form is under development which wouldn't require immuno-suppression, but those who have already had this treatment have gone for a year without needing insulin. The transplantation is also simple, and only requires an injection into the portal vein in the abdomen, from which they travel to the liver and go to work secreting the insulin that the body needs.

4. Implanting an artificial pancreas is another form of the transplanted islet cell method, which holds out a hope for curing diabetes. This is currently only being tested in dogs, and uses a one-way membrane that prevents the body from attacking the artificial pancreas, but allows its production of insulin to enter the body. The important thing about this technique is that it gets around the immune-suppression problem that was such a barrier to use in the technique above.

5. New tests to measure genetic, metabolic, and immunologic levels in the body and allow us to predict who will get diabetes allows controlling the disease before it develops. Since diabetes is caused by our own bodies immune system attacking the insulin-producing cells of the body, then detecting those who will suffer these attacks before diabetes develops allows the use of immuno-suppressive drugs which will prevent the development of the diabetes. Just so long as the immuno-suppressive drugs are less dangerous than the taking of insulin, this may provide a way of preventing almost everyone from developing diabetes.

6 Step Plan that Can Reverse Diabetes

If you have diabetes, and you have gotten beyond the point where you can control it just with diet, you have probably been told that you would be on medication for the rest of your life. Well that is not necessarily true. A study of this 12 step plan at the Pritikin Longevity Center in Santa Monica found that most diabetics on oral medication only could get off it, and even 36% of those who were insulin dependent could eventually stop all diabetes medication. The secret is that you must follow this plan to have the results, and you must continue the plan after you have gotten the results you are looking for. While this might be a problem, remember that since you are a diabetic you are already making many changes in your life, but this one holds out a good chance for reversing a disease you have always been told is incurable, and something you would have to live with.

The test group had type-II diabetes, where their bodies produced some of the insulin they needed, and this treatment plan works best for those in the earliest stages of the disease. The plan is based on changes in lifestyle, diet, and exercise. It is often said that these are some of the major causes of diabetes, so it only makes sense that they can be used to cure its effects as well. Along with improvement in the diabetes, the subjects also had improvements in their levels of LDL cholesterol (bad cholesterol), triglycerides, and total cholesterol. These are all high risk factors in heart disease, and it is known that diabetes increases these risks anyway, so the plan will also decrease death from heart disease.

This plan is also recommended for you if you have high risk factors for developing diabetes, even if you do not have it at this time. The high risk factors are anyone in your family with diabetes, plus overweight, plus high blood pressure, and thirst which is difficult to satisfy along with excessive urination. If you have more than one of these symptoms you are in serious danger of developing, or having, diabetes at this time. With these things in mind, here is the 6 step plan to help you prevent and reverse diabetes.

1. Start your day with a low dose aspirin tablet. Aspirin is recommended as a daily preventive for anyone over 50 since it is known to lower the risk of heart attacks and strokes. But for diabetics it is recommended for everyone. If you have diabetes, your risk of stroke and heart attack is 3 times the rest of the population, so taking a low dose aspirin will have a much more positive effect than it does for everyone else. For the non-diabetic a daily aspirin lowers this risk by 20%. One thing though, if you have ulcers don't use this aspirin therapy plan. Because aspirin stops clots from forming it will make ulcers worse. Only in high doses over a long time will aspirin actually cause ulcers, so there is no worry in that for a daily low dose.

2. Supplement your diet with vitamin C and vitamin E. These are both antioxidant vitamins and work to protect diabetics against heart disease, and damage to the kidneys, eyes, and nerves. Damage to these areas may be relat-

ed to clotting problems and large changes in the level of blood insulin. You must be protected from these effects of diabetes if you want to be free from their effects. Take a double daily dose of each of these vitamins for maximum effect and minimum risk. Vitamin C is also used by the body in healing, so damage to nerves and eyes that does occur should heal better and more rapidly. Vitamin E helps prevent protein from your body that is circulating in your blood from damaging the eyes and nerves. Damage to these areas leads to poor eyesight and can lead to loss of fingers and toes that do not heal well after being injured.

3. Exercise for 30 minutes to 1 hour every day. There are some very serious considerations in having a daily exercise plan. As a diabetic, especially, you should check with your doctor before beginning regular exercise. Also daily exercise is important for the diabetic, while only every other day is recommended for non-diabetics. Vary your exercise to keep it fresh, and to work different muscle groups. The good effects of taking up this difficult part of the plan are weight loss (which makes diabetes worse), and a decrease in blood sugar level normally. As you build muscle, and exercise, it burns much of the sugar in your body and prevents attacks. A 5 mile walk, spread over a week, will decrease your risk of getting type-II diabetes by 6%. If you have even one risk factor and increase your exercise to 20 miles a week you can lower your risk by another 41% (you would need about 45 minutes of exercise a day for this). The greater your risk the more you need this exercise plan to beat diabetes.

4. Increase the fiber in your diet to 40 grams a day from complex carbohydrate foods. The need for a high fiber diet is its effect in keeping your digestive system working well, and it helps in controlling weight. Using complex carbohydrate foods like whole grain breads and pastas, legumes, oats, and barley helps your body to keep an even blood sugar level because these foods release their sugar slowly into your blood stream. To keep from giving your blood a rapid rise in glucose you need to avoid refined sugar, alcohol, and large amounts of fruit. Sugar is the worst for you and eliminating it would be good for you. Alcohol can be used in small amounts, but should be kept down to 1 or 2 drinks a week, and fruit can be eaten daily, but kept to 2 to 3 servings a day. Don't go on a fruit diet. Also don't go on a high protein diet since high protein meats and eggs have a lot of fat and put a burden on the kidney. The fat adds calories and slows digestion, and kidney problems are one of the major complications of diabetes, so you shouldn't add to their work load with high protein foods.

5. Control the amount of fat in your diet from all sources. For this plan to be effective you must keep the calories in your diet to less than 30% fat. Fat is bad because it is high calorie, twice the calories per once of carbohydrates, and overweight is one of the reasons people develop diabetes. In its early stages diabetes is often controlled by losing weight, something that fat in the diet prevents. Being overweight is also accompanied by other risk factors like high blood pressure, high triglycerides, and high cholesterol, all of which work together to block your arteries. For best results get your diet down to 10% or less fat calories. Also for the fat in your diet, use unsaturated fats from vegetables and fish. They give you the same calories as far as weight loss is concerned, but they won't clog your

arteries and add to heart disease. A final warning is to watch out for the fat free foods in the market. Many of them are high in sugar or salt. Spend a little more care in choosing these and use ones with artificial sweeteners, that are low in salt or sodium free.

6. The final part of the plan, and this is something many diabetics do anyway, is to monitor your blood sugar levels throughout the day. Because of the danger of insulin shock from too much insulin, or diabetic coma, you need to know what your blood sugar level is over the entire day. The ideal is to check your blood sugar before and after exercise and meals, and early and late in the day. The minimum is to check it at the same time each day, and without at least that this plan is not recommended. Following the plan will change the way your body handles sugars, and for your own good you have to know what's going on. You will also need to work with your doctor on this since you should not make decisions on medication without a doctor's opinion. If your doctor advises you not to do it then either get another doctor who will work with you or don't go on the plan. Even more dangerous than your diabetes is going on a treatment plan that your doctor objects to. You may know how you feel, but only a doctor who is treating you will know how your body is reacting to it, and only a doctor can tell you if it is safe to stop taking insulin, or other diabetic treatments that you have been depending on to take care of this problem.

20 Natural Ways to Control Your Diabetes and Lessen Insulin Needs

Diabetes is a complicated disease, and although you can often just take insulin to control it, there are always other things you have to do in your life to stay healthy. To go one step further though, if you can control enough of those other activities in your life that upset your blood sugar balance you can often do away with the insulin altogether, or at least cut down on your dependence. The management methods listed here are for the type II, adult onset, diabetes, and should not be applied to type I, juvenile onset, diabetes. Insulin dependence needs to be controlled because it often leads to complications if carried on long enough. A natural system of control, on the other hand, will keep your body working in pretty much the same manner as it would if you did not have the diabetes.

1. The first is always diet, and some specific hints will be given below. But it is absolutely necessary for you to control what you eat and when you eat it if you want to avoid insulin, and keep your body working as naturally as possible.

2. Weight control, the first dietary need after controlling your sugar intake. Because diabetes affects the circulation of the blood, often resulting in poor circulation to the extremities, losing weight helps to counteract that effect. When you lose weight your blood vessels are not crushed by your weight, and you do

not require as much action by your heart to circulate your blood properly through your body. Also the more overweight you are the more difficult it is for insulin to do its job of regulating blood sugar levels.

3. Exercise every day, and for at least 1/2 hour. Exercise can help you to lose weight, and it can also help you avoid, or reduce, your insulin requirements. Exercise is one thing that most Americans do not do enough of, and if you are a diabetic not exercising can be deadly. The exercise does not have to be very strenuous, at least not every day. But exercise enough to break a sweat and increase your breathing and heart rate. This should take no more than about 30 minutes a day. If you happen to like puttering around your yard, than 1 hour day in yard work and gardening will give you a good basic program of exercise as well.

4. Walking is one of the best low stress exercise you can do, other than gardening and yard work, and it doesn't require any special clothing or equipment. You will also not be alone since you can see walkers in any neighborhood and at any time of day, even in malls. A good walking workout is 5 miles at 3 times per week, which can be done in about an hour of vigorous walking. If you only want to walk for 30 minutes at a time, then do it 6 times a week and you get the same benefit. As in any other exercise you need to walk fast enough and long enough to get up a sweat and increase your breathing. This may not be as pleasurable as just strolling, but if you stroll you will need twice the time to get the same benefit. This schedule of walking will burn 500 calories a week, and will drop your risk of becoming insulin dependent by 6%.

5. Swimming is an alternative for walking, and can work just as well if you like to swim or have trouble walking. To get the same benefit as in walking, or other exercise, you need to work yourself up to 30 minutes of continuous swimming three or more times per week. Of course you can't tell if you are sweating when you swim, but if you are warm in the water you can be pretty sure you are working hard enough. Swimming takes so much energy that usually you start deep breathing as soon as you start moving, so you can't use breathing as a gauge as to how hard you are working. Swimming is strenuous enough that anything that you do that will keep you in motion for at least 30 minutes should give you a proper workout.

6. Something to avoid though is weight lifting. For the diabetic weight lifting can be bad. Because of the tension and strain involved lifting weight raises the blood pressure. High blood pressure is one of the risk factors in complications for diabetes. As a double warning, it also raises the blood sugar level, and that is what you are trying to avoid with diet control and exercise in the first place. Lifting weights is just not aerobic enough to be of help to your diabetes.

7. Break up your meals into light snacks throughout the day. This doesn't mean that you can't go out and have lunch or dinner with someone on occasion, but for yourself, get away from the three square meals a day habit. Food is digested most efficiently when there is only a small amount of it in your stomach. You will also avoid the bloated feeling that comes with large and infrequent meals. Weight loss diets always stress several small meals throughout the day, and for

diabetics it will mean a more constant blood sugar level. Large meals are followed by a gradual rise of the blood sugar to a peak, and then a fall to a very low level to the next meal. This rise and fall is the cause of our hunger and personal energy levels varying so much during the day, and why we like to snack on sweets in between meals to bring our blood sugar back up to where we feel comfortable. For the diabetic it also means that you will need to watch your insulin more closely in-between and right after meals. But if you have a little something every hour or two, then your insulin needs will stay mostly constant throughout the day.

8. On designing your diet, you need to have a high level of complex carbohydrates. Don't be confused though by the term carbohydrate being applied to refined sugar. Sugar is a carbohydrate, but it is a simple carbohydrate and goes straight to your blood stream. Complex carbohydrates are made up of whole grains, fruits, and vegetables, and are transformed slowly into simple carbohydrates during digestion in your body. Refined sugar will make your blood sugar level spike a short time after eating it, but a complex carbohydrate will take time to digest and maintain your blood sugar at a constant level if taken in small meals throughout the day. You need to make up at least 1/2 of your diets in complex carbohydrates, so have a vegetable or piece of fruit for a snack or dessert when you are hungry, and stay away from the cookies and candy bars, at least most of the time. A nice low calorie dish is pasta without meat sauce. Try making a vegetable based spaghetti sauce and you will get loads of complex carbohydrates and avoid the calories of red meat.

9. You should also cut your protein intake. Protein digestion puts a great strain on the kidneys, and too much protein can even result in kidney failure. The normal american diet has 3 to 5 times the amount of protein you actually need to take care of your body's needs, so cutting back won't hurt you at all. The actual need intake is only 12 to 20 percent of your total calories, and many of us get 50 percent or more if we are big meat eaters. While protein is necessary, at least in the United States most of us don't have the problem of protein malnutrition like they do in many 3rd world countries. Save your kidneys and cut your protein.

10. While cutting protein, increase your fiber. You need to have 40 grams or more of fiber in your diet each day. Eating complex carbohydrates will increase your fiber, but eating fresh fruits and vegetables daily will make certain. Some of the best sources of fiber are onions, corn, whole grains, rhubarb, squash, and pretty much all fresh fruits. Most Americans only get about 1/2 of the fiber they should have, so double yours and you should be in the right range. Fiber speeds our food through our digestive tract, and slows the rate of digestion. This keeps your blood sugar more constant, and keeps everything moving the way it is supposed to. If in doubt, add a piece of fruit between each meal.

11. Lower your blood cholesterol level to 150, if its over that. If it is high then aim for 180 as a first step, that's below the definition of high cholesterol, and then work to get it down to 150. A good plan to lower cholesterol is cut down on red meat, eat fresh fruits, vegetables, and exercise. These are all things you need to do to control diabetes so just watch your cholesterol level while you do them.

12. Cut down on fat in the diet. Fat works very much against you if you are diabetic. Even though you can't cut all of the fat out of your diet, even if you are a vegetarian, you still need to get it down to 25 to 50 grams a day for most people. That would be only 225 calories a day from fat, or about what you get in one Big Mac from McDonald's. To get your fat intake this low you will have to cut out most fried foods, red meats, and baked goods. Unless of course they were made specially as a low-fat, or non-fat, way to keep their fat content to a minimum. Other than that you might like the taste of fat in foods, there is no reason for having more than a few grams in anything you eat.

13. As a diabetic, you do not need sugar in your diet. Cut out all sugar, at least so far as you can. The problem is partly calories and partly the problem of having your insulin to handle the sugar when it enters the blood steam. As substitutes use aspertame or saccharin. You may also try fructose and sorbitol, which still have calories, but which are better than sugar. All that eating sugar will do for you is send your blood sugar level soaring to a peak, and then you will fall into a hole. This is exactly what a diabetic needs to avoid. The only way to avoid this type of boom and bust in blood sugar levels is to avoid the sugar to begin with.

14. Get some of the stress out of your life and learn to take it easy once in while. Stress and worry are often solved by Americans eating things bad for them. These are frequently high sugar, high fat, foods which are doubly destructive to you if you are diabetic. While exercise is one of the best ways of keeping your emotions on an even keel, there are some exercises you can do while you drive or work that can help almost as much. One of these techniques is called guided imagery in which you imagine yourself in some pleasant area, like a forest or at the seashore, and recreate the calm emotions you felt there. Progressive relaxation is another handy trick to use when you have a few calm moments. In progressive relaxation you start at the tips of your toes and consciously relax them. Then you just relax each part of your body as you travel up to your head. By the time you get to your head and face you should be completely relaxed, and stress free. For help in carrying these out you can get tapes that will talk you through them.

15. Don't be afraid to talk to yourself. Oftentimes there is no one around to talk to, and you may really need someone to talk to if you are going to keep on a healthy plan and not binge onto a diet buster that could give you an insulin attack. If you express your emotions to yourself, out loud, you will eventually get the same benefit that you would if you had a friend or psychologist to talk to. It does often take longer, but mainly it lets you blow off steam and tell how well you are doing so that you gain confidence in what you are doing. Writing it down is another form of talking to yourself, and may even be better at clearing the air since you can always glance back at it to see how you are progressing.

16. Cut down on, or cut out, the caffeine from your diet. Caffeine raises the blood sugar level. If you are accustomed to having coffee in the morning to wake yourself up, or in the afternoon for a pick-me-up, then you need to start working on a substitute. Most herbal teas do not have caffeine and will still give

you a lift, although taking a 10 minute walk could get your blood flowing a little faster and wake you up and make you more alert just as effectively. Even a cup of English tea, which has caffeine, only has about 1/4 as much as a cup of coffee and can be used as a substitute. You need to stay away from the stimulants that work by changing your blood sugar levels.

17. A good herbal tea which also regulates blood sugar levels is made from blueberry leaves. You need at least a couple of cups a day, one in the morning and one in the evening. Drinking more of this beneficial tea is quite acceptable if you wish to do so, and it takes about 3 months before you get the full effect of the tea. There is also an extract of the blueberry leaf called anthcyanic acid which can be used for the same purpose. It is available at the health food store in your neighborhood, or they can order it if it is not on the shelf.

18. Watch your feet for signs of poor circulation. Poor circulation can result in amputation in extreme cases, and even without that you can be in a lot of pain. Because diabetics tend to have high sugar levels in their blood, a wound on the foot can become infected very rapidly, so also watch for any signs of infection. What would be of little concern to most people can be serious enough to a diabetic to send them to the hospital. The general rule for foot care is to wash and inspect your feet each day, noting scrapes, cuts, and wounds of any sort. Look for signs of infection such as redness, swelling, pus, and pain and treat all of these as serious even if they seem to be minor. Also treat all other breaks in the skin and keep an eye on them.

19. Test your blood for its glucose level throughout the day. It is recommended that you do this 3 to 5 times during the day to watch for changes in blood sugar very closely. A few hours of elevated sugar can leave you in a diabetic coma. And extra insulin, if it gets too high, can leave you in insulin shock. Blood testing is better than urine testing, and what you are really interested in is the level in your blood and not in your urine. The glucose monitors you need for blood testing are available without prescription at the drug store. The needs of diabetics are so well known that there should be no problem in finding just what you need locally.

20. Adapting the old Boy Scout motto, "be prepared," you need to be ready at all times for whatever may happen, or something is going to go wrong. In the case of diabetes you need to be ready to take insulin, or to raise your blood sugar level wherever you are. For the insulin, if you are taking it, you should always carry some with you. For the blood sugar level problem, carry candy, mints, a candy bar, fruit juice, soda, or anything else that can give you an emergency dose of sugar. Besides monitoring your blood sugar level to find out when it is too low, a low blood sugar level will also give you numbness in the mouth, cool moist skin, faintness, and a fluttering in the chest. These signs will tell you to eat some sugar immediately.

Diabetes Breakthrough: Get Rid of Insulin Shots

If you are an insulin dependent diabetic you are probably aware of the attempts to transplant healthy pancreatic islet cells into diabetics to produce insulin naturally. This has been done for several years, but only with very limited success. To get the usually transplant you have to be already on immuno-suppressant drugs to prevent your body from attacking the transplanted cells and destroying them. And because the immuno-suppressant drugs themselves can be dangerous, only people who need them because of transplants usually get them. This leaves out the majority of insulin dependent diabetics from a possibly permanent cure of their problem.

Now there has been a breakthrough in the transplant process, but which looks very promising. A medical team at Washington University has taken islet cells and placed them into plastic fibers which are too small for the immune system cells to get into. The fibers are then taken and put into the pancreas of diabetics where their enclosed cells produce normal insulin. While this looks like a permanent solution to the problem of insulin injections, the fiber transplant method has only been tested on mice so far. Tests on humans should begin this year, or next year. If you are interested into this type of treatment, but don't want to wait 3 or 4 more years until it is generally available, then have your doctor look into the possibility of you becoming one of the test subjects. If he keeps current on his medical literature he should know what you are talking about when you bring up the topic. Also, if he is not interested in it but can't give you good reasons why, he may just not be aware of the procedure and you should ask about seeing someone directly involved with islet cell transplant therapy for diabetes.

Diet Tips for the Diabetic

While we have been giving you some tips on courses of action you can take to control your diabetes, there are also diet steps you need to take as well. Of course your doctor has already advised you on what to eat and what not to eat, but this little capsule of diet tips might give you a few new ideas.

To begin with those foods that you have to limit in your diet, cut down on sugar, animal proteins, saturated fats, salt, alcohol, tea, coffee, colas, and chocolate. You may have heard about all of these before, but if you haven't, take a close look at the list.

Now foods good to eat include whole grain oats, beans, peas, and raw vegetables. Supplements should include vitamin A, vitamin B, vitamin C, vitamin E and chromium. Nutrients which are concentrated in foods you should eat are: whole grain cereals for magnesium, potassium, and vanadium; fish for zinc and essential fatty acids; and various nutrients you need are in meat, egg yolk, beans, peas, fruits, seeds, nuts, and vegetable oils.

How You May be able to Reverse Diabetes in the Future

An over-the-counter compound called vanadyl sulfate is being researched in the laboratory, in animal research, and has been shown to reverse diabetes. This is so new that it isn't recommended for humans yet, and diabetics have to watch what they put into their bodies anyway, but it shows great promise. I wouldn't recommend anyone who is on medication, and insulin is medication, go on their own and start trying to self-medicate. But when you hear of something that can be this important you need to keep your eye on it, and follow up by check-ing with the doctor you go to for diabetes treatment to see if it is still positive, and when it will be available for human use.

Get Off Diabetes Pills With Chelation Therapy

Chelation therapy was studied in Canada as a means of removing metal ions from the blood. The metals that circulate in your blood, if you are diabetic, act as toxins which can cause damage to your body, including the amputation of the limbs. For this reason diabetics are normally given drugs to control these met-als, but they are often eventually unsuccessful. With chelation therapy, which is an intravenous infusion procedure, you remove the metals in an effective manner, and also the need for further drug therapy or the potential of amputation. In the Canadian study 70% of the diabetics studied were totally free of medication with-in an 8 to 13 week period of beginning chelation therapy.

DIAGNOSIS

What to do If Your Doctor Can't Tell You What You Have

You go to a doctor when you are sick because you want him to find out what's wrong with you and fix it. If the doctor can't do this, then you lose valuable time getting no treatment, or getting the wrong treatment. But why can't doctors diagnose you every time you go to them? There are many answers to that ques-tion, and a few are worth remembering so that you will know what to do the next time you want medical help and the doctor isn't giving it.

The first thing is to make sure your doctor listens to all of your symptoms before diagnosing you. Many doctors try to run practices at such a high level of production that they will only give 2 or 3 minutes to each patient. This is acceptable if it is a common illness, but if it is anything that is difficult you will not get proper treatment with this level of attention. So first find a doctor who will give you the time you need.

When you go to a doctor also keep in mind that many illnesses look about the same in their early stages. That includes cancer, colds, stomach aches, and diarrhea. In the first day or two, or even a little longer, you can't tell these apart. But also remember that any illness that keeps up for more than a week should be treated by a doctor. While you may put off going to a doctor longer than that, the longer you wait to treat any serious illness the more likely it is that you will get complications and end up in a hospital. Make up your own mind when to go to a doctor, and don't go at every cough or wait until you can't breathe at all.

But the real problem of getting proper treatment comes up when you have a rare disease. Just because it is rare your doctor may never have seen a case himself. And if the symptoms don't point to the area of the body that is diseased, then you won't even be referred to the right specialist for diagnosis and treatment. This is the area of getting the best treatment that needs the most attention.

The first thing to do for symptoms that have gone on for some time, and which your doctor has not provided relief, is to keep a diary of the symptoms. What is bothering you, when it bothers you, and whether any medications you are taking are doing any good. You take this in with you to your doctor and make sure he reads it over each time. If a doctor says that what you have is just in your mind, and that doesn't help, then go to someone else and look for a physical diagnosis. While you can certainly be ill just from your emotional state, you can also have tiny tumors or slow developing diseases that can give the same effect, and can't be detected unless they are looked for specifically.

If going to doctors and tracking your symptoms isn't getting you anywhere, then you may have to study up on your own problem to find your answer. Every medical school has a medical library that will have the information you need. Even if you have no direct ties, just telling them that you are researching your own medical problems will get you assistance from the librarians. Since a busy doctor can't do this himself, this might be the only way you are going to get relief. Once you have gotten the disease narrowed down as well as you can, take copies of the readings to your doctor, or to a specialist and let them work from there. If your diagnosis is correct, you will soon be getting the proper treatment.

Finally, don't let your doctor or anyone else tell you that you have nothing. If you are ill, and the treatments you get don't cure it, there is a good chance that you aren't being treated for the right illness. Particularly if you don't get better, don't rule out the possibility that you may have a rare illness. If your doctor isn't able to make a complete diagnosis he will usually admit it, and it is time to seek some outside help. Write to the National Organization for Rare Disorders (NORD), at Dept. RD, P.O. Box 8923, New Fairfield, Conn. 06812. Or call: (203) 746-6518. This organization will help refer you to specialists.

The final advice is to never give up. Even if you have a disease that can't be cured, and there are a lot of those, there is always something that can be done for the symptoms. The rule of the medical profession is that even if you can't be cured, you still deserve the best treatment, and relief, for your symptoms. Even incurable diseases can have their progress stopped or slowed, and if you have something that is curable then you deserve to have it cured as rapidly and comfortably as possible.

DIARRHEA

4 Natural Remedies, and a Few Traditional Ones

Diarrhea is one of those mysterious diseases that come on without warning and then take their own good time leaving. Fortunately most cases of diarrhea are over with in a day, although it may seem like a lot longer. There is little you can do about an attack that lasts a day or less, except stay near the restroom, and take the day off. The real danger in diarrhea is when it lasts 2 or 3, or more days. Extended cases of diarrhea not only leave you exhausted and unable to eat, but you will also become dehydrated, and eventually you can have a collapse of your circulation, which would be life threatening. That is why any case of diarrhea that lasts for more than a day should be taken very seriously.

You can always start treatment with some over-the-counter medications, and if they work you will be fine. If they fail you may have no resort except to go to a doctor. But, there are alternative in the natural remedies, and that is what we want to look at here. For 3 natural remedies, and a few less usual ones, read on.

1. The first natural remedy is to increase the amount of fiber in your diet. When you have diarrhea, the effect is that everything comes out in a semi-liquid form. In fact everything in your digestive system is converted to liquid and is expelled. When it is cured the normal rhythm of the intestinal tract is restored, and the problem is to find the best way to restore that normal rhythm. Eating fiber is one of the best ways, and has been chosen as the first. There is always a question as to what is the best way to get the fiber into your system since regular high fiber foods won't digest properly, and are more likely to just become part of the diarrhea problem. That is why anti-diarrhea remedies are frequently combinations of liquefied fiber and a stomach calmative like calcium. But you can also get the same things in natural foods that are easy to digest. For instance carob was given to 230 children with diarrhea and only 3 failed to be cured. Carob works because it is a high fiber food, but you could probably use any other fibrous food that is easy on the stomach. The other one that comes to mind right away are bananas. If you want to use bananas instead of carob, put a banana into a

blender with a cup of milk and make a banana milkshake. Then sip it slowly, and repeat as needed until the diarrhea clears up.

2. The next natural remedy is based on the idea that one of the reasons you have diarrhea is because your intestinal bacteria is messed up. Everyone with a normal digestion has a full crop of bacteria that helps get the process started. When this diarrhea is killed by penicillin or by some intestinal infection, food doesn't begin digesting properly when it enters your stomach. The result is diarrhea, and the diarrhea persists until the stomach and intestines get their normal quota of plants and animals living where they should. Apparently this problem was recognized long ago around the Mediterranean, and it was handled by promoting the use of yogurt. And for as long as anyone can remember yogurt has been a basic part of the Mediterranean diet. In order to test the idea that yogurt really can cure diarrhea, and we hear this from our health food stores all the time too, a group of children suffering from diarrhea were divided into two groups, one of which was given a regular diarrhea remedy, and the other received yogurt. The result was that the group receiving yogurt recovered faster, and to a greater degree, than the group receiving diarrhea medicine. The dose was 1/2 cup at a time, and it was given three times a day for 3 days. While this may be a slow remedy, just remember that it is to be used on serious cases of diarrhea and not on the 24 hour kind of attack.

3. The next natural remedy can be summed up in one word, bran. Bran is the number one intestinal restorer and maintainer. Although many high fiber foods help the intestinal system to behave normally, bran always works. Bran cures diarrhea by thickening the stools, and works just as well on constipation by hardening the hard, dry stools that are part of that problem. Luckily, these days, bran is available in many forms. You can get bran in hot and cold cereal, muffins, bread, and pretty much any baked or vegetable food you can get. You should not only have bran once or twice a day in your diet, you should increase your bran any time that you have an intestinal upset. In fact if you follow this plan you may very well cut out all of the attacks of diarrhea before they ever begin, and not even have the problem of curing them afterwards. Prevention is always a better way of handling an illness than trying to cure the illness after you get it. You can't always cure something you have gotten, but a disease you have never gotten is never going to harm or kill you.

4. The next natural cure comes to us from the British who developed it to treat a special form of diarrhea called "dumping syndrome." This is a problem common to patients who have had intestinal surgery, and is characterized by diarrhea attack with dizziness and gastrointestinal upset. For these patients the condition can be life threatening, and the cure has to be fairly rapid. What the British doctors did was add pectin to a sugar solution given to the patients after their surgery. The result was that all patients had their symptoms lessened or prevented. But what is pectin? Pectin is a fiber found in applies, cherries and bananas, and it helps to absorb water from the colon. While that is pretty simple, since it helps to control a serious form of diarrhea it deserves to be included in the list of natural diarrhea cures. Of course this gets back to the bananas we talked

about a little earlier, as well as the other fruits, but you can also get it in concentrated form from health food stores, or even supermarkets. Pectin doesn't have to be used in very large amounts, the British only used 1/3 of an ounce in their clinical dosages. For you that wouldn't be any more than a teaspoon in a glass of juice or milk, and if it is as effective for you as it was for the British, then only a dose or two should be able to cure your diarrhea.

For the traditional remedies I can't offer any examples of tests that show their effectiveness. All that I can offer is the belief by people somewhere, and sometime that they work. Some of them sound reasonable, and some sound a little strange. If you want to, try some of the ones that sound reasonable, and good luck. So, for your enlightenment and information, here is a short list of traditional cures for the ills of diarrhea: Swiss cheese, brown rice, barley, bananas, and mallow root tea. Some can be found in your market, some in your health food store, and for some you may have to go into the fields and forests and gather your own. Good luck in any case.

DIGESTION

Diet Changes to Calm the Upset Stomach

What upsets our digestion is more often than not what we eat. While we may get a stomach flu for 1 or 2 weeks each year, you have a 1,000 chances each year to cause indigestion by eating something that doesn't agree with your stomach. The result can be pain, that goes away on its own over time, or you may throw up, which is very unpleasant, or diarrhea, which is also not pleasant. Of course you can get all of these plus bloating and burping, and all from a simple meal that you may have even completely enjoyed.

So if you have been suffering bouts of indigestion, what is the best course to follow to get rid of them. For diet, cut back on refined carbohydrates (sugar), alcohol, milk, coffee, tea, chocolate, cola, and fatty and spicy foods. Fatty foods are mainly red meat and fried foods, although it includes donuts as well. Sugar includes the amount you add directly to your food, and the amount in baked goods you may make or buy.

After cutting back on these foods you need to increase your intake of vitamin C and zinc. And there are several teas that are very good for the digestion as well. Good digestion teas include parsley, mint, chamomile, blackberry leaf, and juniper berry. These are all proven teas to calm the stomach and aid digestion.

Natural Way to Improve Your Digestion and Get Rid of "Nervous Stomach"

A nervous stomach is something that everyone gets a few times a year. While you may not throw up, you certainly don't feel very well, and chances are you don't eat very well either when your stomach feels on the verge of coming back on you. So in the way of providing a needed service, here is a suggestion or two by which you can calm your stomach and provide yourself with a happier experience with your digestion.

The most natural way to improve your digestion is by ingesting bran. Most of the time you hear about bran being used to prevent constipation, but it prevents constipation by keeping everything running normally. In one study of 22 patients complaining of nausea, 19 were relieved by taking bran. This should give you an 80% to 90% chance of relief from nausea if you take bran. Of course taking bran on a daily basis may relieve problems of nausea even before they develop.

Now while you were only promised one natural cure for bran, I can't pass up the opportunity to give you a few more, with just a few words about each: Papaya is a tropical fruit which contains a strong enzyme which works to digest protein; Fennel is a local herb that tastes much like licorice, and which relieves many stomach problems when used either as a tea or as a seasoning for other foods; Catnip is familiar to everyone because cats like it, but it is also a good stomach medicine according to Appalachian folk beliefs; Anise also tastes much like licorice and can be used in baked goods for an effective stomach treatment; Mint, such as you get on your plate in many meals, works very well to help digestion, and is also readily available as a tea; Sage, as a tea or condiment, is an old pioneer and American Indian treatment for poor digestion; and Yogurt is used by many peoples in the Near East to cure stomach problems since they are less likely to have fiber in their diets to do the job, but have abundant milk to make the yogurt.

New Study Reveals Foods that Help You Stay Regular

Irregularity is a problem that everyone is bothered by at times, and some people have to suffer with constantly. Eating the right foods, and taking the proper vitamins, can help correct this problem. It is also a good idea for anyone concerned with having a good digestion to pay attention to these ideas.

The best foods to eat and vitamins to take, according to a Tufts University study, are those high in fiber, mainly fruits and vegetables, to drink 8 glasses of water a day, and to make sure you have good intake levels of vitamins A, B, and C, riboflavin, folate, and calcium. If you aren't sure about your diet giving you enough of these foods, take supplements.

DIVORCE

To Avoid Divorce Avoid Psychologists

I f you are getting married, or are married, and spend time reading guides to marriage by marriage counselors and psychologists, you can save your money and time and stop. You would do much better to simply decide if you love your partner, and then overlooking their faults rather than managing them. An Ohio University researcher has found that none of the advice given in the various self-help books on marriage is much good. People get married because they are in love, at least in America, and they stay married for the same reason. No amount of self-help will keep a couple not in love married, and no problems, no matter how serious, will split up a couple that is truly in love.

But is it healthy for you to be in one of these co-dependency relationships? For most people it certainly is. When you have someone close to you it helps you cope with the crises of life, such as deaths, job losses, and moves around the country. If you are alone these events can make you sick, and even kill you. Marriage is one of the best ways of coping with our problem world. Close friends will do the same thing for you, but unless you live with them you cannot get the same support you can from a spouse.

To stay married with all of the bad times our country is having is to be accepting of your partner's problems as well as of their strengths. There is no magic formula. If its snoring or problems holding jobs, love often is sufficient to make the relationship work. And even if everything else is perfect, if there is no love there will be no joy, and neither marriage nor family will make a couple stay together. If you love and accept the one you live with, the relationship will last, and if you or they don't, no advice is going to save it.

DEALING WITH DOCTORS

3 of the Biggest Lies Doctors Tell You

Everyone lies, although we do not like to think of our doctors as also lying. Still, if you want to be charitable, doctors' lies may be more mistakes of giving opinions on things that they don't really know. Too often doctors will give opinions on anything medical whether or not they have actually studied the subject, or bothered to keep up with it. If you ask any doctor a question, they will present themselves as experts, and therein lies the lie, and tell you the absolute truth. A doctor who is honest with himself will also be honest with you, and he will occasionally tell you that he just isn't familiar with the best answer to a medical question that you ask. But don't hold your breath hoping to meet a doctor professionally who is that secure with himself that he can admit that he doesn't know absolutely all that there is to know about every topic in medicine. Now that we understand each other, let's take a look at some of the opinions doctors express that are lies, and very big lies at that.

1. "Most people in America die of natural causes." This lie is based on some idea that the body can't help but get sick, and most of us die of one of these diseases that practically everyone gets anyway. Well don't you believe it. Even today almost every cause of death is known to have events leading up to it that are preventable. Most of our diseases are the direct result of how we live our lives, and if we can find the best possible way to live, although we don't always know as yet, then we can prevent pretty much any disease. The papers today tell us that death rates from heart disease and lung cancer have declined in recent years. This is because people get more exercise and have better diets, and many people have stopped smoking. Keep your eyes and ears open for the best preventive measures you can do to keep yourself healthy, and chances are you will be healthy a lot longer. Some scientists have calculated that the human body should last 150 years before wearing out. The reason that it doesn't is that we do things to ourselves that shorten our lives, and often to the point of losing 2/3 of the lifespan we should enjoy. The more healthy you are the better you will feel and look.

2. "As you get older you will suffer more aches, pains, and illnesses as a natural part of the aging process." Again, there is nothing natural about aches, pains, and illness. Studies have found the body to change in ability by usually less than 1% each year. So at 60 or 70 you should be able to do 80% or 90% of the activities you were able to do at age 50. They talk about the inability of older people to keep up physically with the younger generation, but this is only a half-

---

truth at best. You do accumulate damage to your body as you grow older, but as long as you are active these injuries do not incapacitate you. But if you retire and start to sit around, your old injuries will take over because you aren't keeping the working parts of your body strong enough to take the pressure off of the weaker parts. Why do many people die a year after retiring while those they worked with are still active 10 years later. Often it is because the active ones just stayed active and involved. They didn't let bad habits, or old injuries take over their existence to the point that it killed them. Never accept anyone's statement that you, or they, feel bad because of old age. These infirmities always have a cause, and can always be treated to relieve problems even if not to cure them. We may all die sometime, but we don't all have to die until a lot later in our years than most people think is old.

3. "Because cancer, heart disease, and arthritis are so common in our society, you will probably get one or more of them as you get older." This is a lie based on looking at the statistics of these diseases, not at the lifestyle of the people getting them. If you want to read statistics and scare yourself, just look at crime statistics and you will see that every 3 or 4 years you will be robbed, and in some neighborhoods that's true. But most robberies are very rare, and most of the statistics are accounted for by people who may get robbed several times in a single year. It is much the same as regards the major diseases of the United States. Look around at the older people you know who are in poor health and you will usually find that they have many diseases. If 50 million people in this country share these three diseases, then it may look like 150 million Americans suffer from one of them, and this is wrong. Just remember that only you can prevent arthritis, diabetes, heart attacks, cancer, and premature aging. You do it by the way you live even more so than by your age or the genes you carry. Your life is in your hands, and not some doctors or politicians. Take charge and plan where you want your health to be 5 or 10 years from now, and start working on it.

DOCTORS

5 Questions You Should Answer Yes
About Your Doctor

If your doctor is doing a good job for you then here are 5 questions you should be able to answer yes to. But, you may say, what if I can't answer yes to all of these questions? If you can't answer yes to even one of them, then it might be time to find another doctor, and if you have more than one - no, then find another doctor today.

Remember that there is nothing sacred about a doctor. They are just people who have gone to school and learned enough medicine to get a license to practice. That doesn't make them better people than you, just ones who know more about medicine than you do. Of course they may be terrible people outside of their medical practice, or even inside it. Every profession has people in it who shouldn't be, and you may be a patient the doctor just doesn't care very much about. You could also be one whose problems are really beyond their skill to treat, but they don't want to lose your fees—there is a lot of competition for patient fees and many doctors would rather do a bad job of treating a patient than give up a fat fee. Of course you don't need to know the underlying reason if your doctor is not doing a good job for you. If he is, then go out and find another doctor, the same way you would go out and find another plumber if the one you had been depending on didn't fix things the way you wanted.

Question 1. Does your doctor know you as a person, or just in terms of your medical condition? If you have been seeing this doctor for a year or more he should know something about you other than that you have high blood pressure, or cancer, or a bad skin condition. You do not necessarily have to know any of the details of his life, although that might be good too, but he should know enough about you personally to understand the risks you take with your behavior and how you go about protecting yourself. It should be important to him if you have just gotten a new job, or someone close to you has died. Each of these events is often accompanied by a bout of illness. He should also be interested in your diet, and if you exercise. Exercise can be beneficial, and usually is, but often times exercise is also a source of injury or danger if you have heart disease.

Question 2. Does your doctor counsel you about what you can do to reverse or control a disease that you have? If he doesn't then you are missing out on one of the major advantages of the medical profession. Doctors should know, and usually do, what the major personal risks are that cause disease, and what steps an individual can take that have the best chance of reversing a disease process. For diabetes you should be told about diet and exercise programs you can do so that you can stay off of insulin, if possible. For heart disease, you should be given the same options. Heart medicines are very strong, and will change more of your behavior than the disease itself might. Cancer requires the sufferer to do many more actions than just take anticancer drugs and radiation, yet most doctors seem to stop at that point in giving advice. Your doctor should be knowledgeable, and even anxious in telling you about what you should do to control your disease. You should not have to pry this information out of him either, he should come to you volunteering it for your own good.

Question 3. Does your doctor talk to you about preventive changes you should take in your lifestyle to prevent disease? This is a little trickier to answer. If you don't have a disease, than how can your doctor advise you to do something to prevent it, and if you already have it, then it is too late to prevent it anyway. But the truth be known, if your doctor knows you, your habits, and your family history, then he has a pretty good idea which diseases you are at the highest risk of getting. And as your age or condition indicates to him that your risk of actually getting these diseases is increasing, then he should begin to discuss with you steps you should take for prevention. If you need to lose weight to lower your risk of heart attack, he should not just say that you should lose weight. He should give you some options in terms of diet and exercise, as well as offer you medical support and monitoring during the process. After all, the objective of medical care from the patients viewpoint is to prevent illness as well as to cure it. A good doctor should share this view with you openly.

Question 4. Does your doctor voluntarily inform you of new approaches to treatment and new drugs that can help your medical condition? Now your doctor may not do this for any number of reasons. He may feel that you are on the best possible treatment program that there is, or that your condition is either so delicate or so simple that no other medication or treatment is necessary or useful. And these can be true if your condition is being very well managed, or is very acute. But if you are having any kind of recurrent problem, such cystitis, or the condition you have is getting progressively worse over time, then you should be getting constant updates on new ways to go that might help you more. If you are in this condition and your doctor simply ignores everything else in medicine that is developing, then he may be just too much behind the times to really be of much help to you. You could also suspect him of having stock in a particular drug company, but you could never prove it. The basic truth is, if your doctor never talks about new therapies or procedures that apply to you, then he probably just does not know or understand what they may have to offer. Never assume that nothing changes in the treatment of your problem from year to year. Drugs and therapies change all the time, and any good modern doctor is obligated to stay up with what is going on in his field, and to attempt to bring it to his patients.

Question 5. Does your doctor volunteer do-it-yourself hints and techniques that will cost you little or nothing to carry out, and that will help you stay healthy? Any doctor should come across these pieces of advice in the popular press, except that he should be able to make a better medical evaluation of them, and if they have value he should pass them on to his patients. Even if you read the same items your doctor does, you will not be able to judge their value as well as him, to decide whether or not they are worth the trouble. This also gets back to your doctor having a personal interest in you as a person. If he is interested in you, then he should remember you in his off hours when he runs across something that might help you and his other patients. Even a new doctor should have helpful hints at his fingertips since he is just out of medical school, and should be full of the latest theories and techniques for preventing and curing disease. He can certainly dredge an idea here and there that would help you to maintain your health, or relieve your illness, without charging you a fee every time you use it.

This concludes the 5 questions and some of the reasoning behind asking these type of questions. Your doctor should get to know you, and treat you as a person worthy of respect, if he also wants you to come to him with your life and your money in your hands for medical treatment. If you decide to change doctors because of this little quiz, don't give up, with a little looking you should find just the right person for your needs.

EARACHE

New Method of Handling Ear Problems
Mean Quicker Cures

One of the major problems of getting treatment for severe earache is that the treatment may end up causing you more pain than the earache. For a regular treatment the doctor will look into your ear using a little light, and if that doesn't satisfy him he will stick a little telescope called an endoscope into your ear and look around. This is not a problem so long as the soreness is limited to the outer portion of the ear since the examination hasn't actually damaged anything in itself.

But if the sore area is in the inner ear the doctor will take you into the hospital and make an incision in your eardrum. As a result of this surgery you have a good chance of infection, and even without that you will be off of work for a week healing up. Even so the doctor was not able to look very far into the inner ear up to now.

However, a new micro-surgery technique using the endoscope has changed all of that. In this method a small slit is made in your eardrum in the doctor's office, and the endoscope is sent through it to look around the inner ear. A lot more can be seen, and there is little risk of infection. You will also be able to return to work the same day, and have a much more rapid healing.

This procedure isn't available just yet, but you should always ask about it if you are having problems with earache. It has been developed by the Lahey Clinic in Burlington, Mass., if your doctor wants to know where it comes from. And you could even contact them yourself to see who in your area is using the technique.

ECZEMA

You Probably Cause It, and You Can Probably Cure It

Eczema is a dry, flaky, sore skin which may or may not weep when the scabs come off. Not surprisingly it is not something people sit around and discuss at lunch or dinner. It is ugly and it is painful, but it is not an infectious disease. In fact it is not usually a disease at all, at least no more than a broken arm is a disease. It is certainly an illness, and it needs to be treated if you are to get over it.

Although eczema as a result of disease is seen in some countries from poor diets, most of it in this country is the result of exposing our skin to chemicals around us. The most common type we are liable to see is better known as "dishpan hands." It is known as dishpan hands because housewives, and people working in restaurants, who have their hands in soaps and hot water all day washing dishes end up with red, irritated skin. Once you have gotten this condition started it is impossible to cure unless you get your hands out of the dishwater, and away from the chemicals. The next best solution, in this modern age, is to get an automatic dishwater so that you never have your hands in hot, soapy, water. You can also put on waterproof gloves every time you wash, and that should help a lot even though your hands will continue to sweat.

So let us suppose you have at least stopped the process of continual irritation, and you want to heal up the eczema that you already have, what do you do? Well for one thing you need a medicated cream since your raw sore skin is an open invitation to infections. For that I would suggest an aloe vera medicated lotion. In terms of other measures, vitamin C is often associated with speeding the healing process so I would also increase my intake of vitamin C to between 1 and 3 grams a day. With these measures, and perhaps a few weeks time most eczema on the hands and arms should clear up.

If your eczema was caused by exposure to an industrial chemical on the job you need to see a doctor. Often chemically caused eczema is just an indication that you have come into contact with a highly toxic chemical that can affect your body chemistry. And if possible make it someone other than the industry doctor that you see, after all they have a good reason to tell you that you have nothing to fear.

ELECTRICITY AND HEALTH

Is Your All Electric Life Good for You?

In these modern days it seems very much as if everything that we do is run by electricity. Our kitchens, cars, and entertainment systems are all electronic. We even go to sleep under electric blankets at night and depend upon electric shavers and hair dryers to get us ready for our day in the morning. We rarely question the use of electricity, and outside of getting shocked by our appliances we never question its safety.

There is some information now that our unquestioning faith in electricity may just be somewhat misplaced. Electrical fields have been linked with leukemia and the disruption of cell growth. There is as yet no definite proof that watching television will give you cancer, but the evidence is important enough that you may want to take some precautions even now, just for your own self-protection.

Electric shavers by men, when used for more than 2 1/2 minutes daily, may cause the risk of leukemia to double. To minimize the risk from electric shavers they should not be used on a daily basis, but only when you are too rushed to use a blade razor or are away from home traveling.

The only study so far was done on electric shaver use and leukemia, but some tips on minimizing exposure through other electric sources is also appropriate. Hair dryers should not be used routinely at home, but only professionally and not at chest height. Massager and vibrator use should be minimized. Microwave ovens should be avoided by pregnant women altogether, all others should be at least 3 feet away, never get on their backs or sides, and have the microwave checked periodically for radiation leakage. The TV should be kept several feet from all viewers (a safe distance can be found by using a portable radio—turn it on and back up until static fades). Laser printers, fax machines, and photocopiers should be 4 to 6 feet away from the nearest worker's desk, and should be avoided completely by pregnant women. Electric blankets should not be kept on all night while you sleep, but can be used to warm a bed completely before you retire, and should then be unplugged when you go to bed.

While you needn't get too overexcited about the risk from electrical sources, after all there are many worse sources of exposure around, there is no reason to ignore it either. The doubling of risk for leukemia for shavers may sound very bad, but the government does not even begin to look at risks until it reaches at least that level. You will probably hear something about this from the FDA in the future, but it is more likely that electric razor manufacturers will simply make some design changes and never tell you about them. Nevertheless, keep both your eyes and ears open, and minimize your exposure to the strongest electric fields in your home to protect yourself.

EMERGENCIES

The 19 Things You Should Have in Your Medicine Cabinet
A Handy Checklist

With these 19 items you will be equipped to handle all of the minor medical problems that arise around the home. Go through the checklist and make sure that you have each one of these readily available. If you also have things not on the checklist, you may take them out or keep them as you please. Of course if anyone in the family has a special problem, such as diabetes, then having syringes and insulin in the medicine cabinet may be more important to you than aspirin and Band-Aids, but you will have to make those decisions according to your own needs.

1. Tweezers are a very useful little item to keep available. They are good for splinters, but can also be used to clean a cut or scrape, as well as dead skin off of a healing wound.

2. A magnifying glass is useful for the same reasons. If you get a small piece of glass, or plant sticker, in your finger or foot, a magnifying glass may be indispensable for finding and removing it. No matter how painful or ugly a wound is when something is stuck in it, the pain and swelling usually go away very rapidly once the foreign object is taken out.

3. Thermometers are good for only one thing, but nothing else can take their place. Thermometers are either oral or rectal, and rectal is necessary for very small children. A thermometer can also be placed under the armpit if that is more comfortable, but the body temperature there is about one degree lower than under the tongue. There are also temperature strips which change color according to body temperature, and these are very useful and quite cheap. Also remember that a low temperature is a sign of sickness the same as a high temperature is.

4. Band-Aids, gauze, and tape are the basic tools for closing small wounds to the body. While many cuts and scrapes are best left open to the air, closing them can help keep them clean as well as assist in stopping bleeding. If

you close up a cut for a day or two, then be sure to leave it uncovered for a while so it will dry a bit, and you may find that it will heal much faster then. A handy hint is to cover any dry and cracked skin on the fingers with a Band-Aid for at least a day, and that will probably allow the dry skin to heal. Unless you have bleeding, you usually don't need to put antiseptic under the wrap, and some Band-Aids are antiseptic themselves anyway.

5. Sugar is useful as an antibiotic ointment. This is common table sugar, and works the same as commercial antibiotics in that it kills bacteria and draws fluid from the wound. To use it make it into a paste and apply it over the wounded area. While you can keep some commercial antibiotics handy, you may find that sugar works better than any of the others.

6. Hydrogen peroxide is an excellent substance with which to clean wounds, but it must be fresh. All that you have to do is pour or wipe it over the wounded area, and it won't sting. To make sure it is fresh you will have to put in a new bottle at least a couple of times a year, but hydrogen peroxide is inexpensive so that the main problem is remembering to do it.

7. Solarcaine is good for both sunburns and rashes, but other topical pain relievers will do just as well. To make a choice just see what the active ingredients are and choose whatever pleases you. One of the most common is benedryl, but there are several others from which you may choose and be just as happy with.

8. Aspirin, Tylenol, or Ibuprofen all work well to relieve headaches and minor body pain. These are all called nonsteroidal anti-inflammatories, and it is a good idea to have more than one available. Some have cautions about use for flu, or when you have certain medical conditions (don't use aspirin if you have an ulcer). You will also need children's forms available if there are children in the house.

9. Coffee has a variety of medical uses, other than for drinking, and all connected with its caffeine. Caffeine is useful as a pain reliever, or taken with other medicines it speeds up the rate at which they work (some pain relievers, like Excedrin, contain caffeine for this reason). Coffee is also useful as an enema for migraine headache (but never use hot coffee for this). A small jar of instant coffee is probably all you would need, and it is good over a long period of time.

10. Fish oil capsules are good for headaches and migraines. The fish oil stimulates anti-inflammatory prostaglandins which will improve blood flow, and lower blood pressure, thus relieving the headaches. This is something you are going to have to try to believe; the dose for headache is 4 to 6 capsules. Fish oil is also loaded with vitamin E, which is an anti-oxidant.

11. Ice is extremely useful, but how do you keep it in a medicine cabinet. Ice in the house is best kept in the refrigerator, and on a car trip a cooler of ice is a good precaution, but if you are somewhere where you can't have fresh ice then carry along a couple of ice packs. Ice should be applied to bruises to control swelling, and to the head or back of the neck as a general pain reliever where it

decreases blood flow and lowers the local blood pressure. A trip across the desert in a car which is not air conditioned can also be made comfortable by just having a cooler of ice along for cold drinks and water.

12. Sominex is good as a sleep-aid. This can be a necessary medication when you are sick, under stress, or traveling. Aspirin also works well to relax your body, as does spending a few minutes reading before trying to go to sleep, but keep a medication for this available for those occasions when nothing else works.

13. Echinacea, Goldenseal, and Astragalus are all herbal remedies for colds and flu. These are much used in Europe, though not in the United States. They can be found as a tablet or capsule in health food stores or at an herbalists, and they don't require a prescription. They also are included in many Asian herbal medicines, and you might find them more useful than you think.

14. Garlic capsules are also used for colds and flu, but also to lower blood pressure and cholesterol, and to lower the clotting of blood if you have a problem of circulatory disease. While garlic capsule are made from the garlic oil of the cloves, they do not produce the body order problems you may get from eating garlic cloves. However, if you prefer you can eat garlic cloves instead of taking the capsules, and get the same benefit.

15. Metamucil, or other high fiber digestive aid, is especially useful in the treatment of constipation. Constipation can strike at virtually any time, and you can become incapacitated with it over just a few hours. Constipation is usually caused by some sort of blockage in the digestive tract. The best, natural cure, is abundant liquid in the form of water, and vegetable and fruit fiber. Since meta-mucil contains fiber, it provides you with a natural means of curing constipation. While you can probably cure it with your diet anyway, this is also a natural way which might work a little faster.

16. Vitamin C is also used for irregularity, which seems to work very well in controlling constipation as well as diarrhea. Vitamin C can be gotten in chew-able form, or tablets just to be swallowed. A diet rich in citrus can also supply vit-amin C as well as fiber if you wish.

17. Heat is also very good in many cases, such as chills and fevers, and can be had in a packet with a chemical that heats up when massaged, so that it will be always available. If you are at home, simply heat up a wet towel in the microwave for a couple of minutes, and use that. But anywhere else, a heat pack may be the best thing you can have.

18. Red clover with Cascara Sagarada is also good for constipation. The natural treatments for constipation are abundant and very effective, and there is no reason to worry greatly if this is a problem that you occasionally encounter. Any physical discomfort which persists for more than a few days should be checked out by a doctor.

19. Ace bandages are a relatively cheap and very useful item to have available. They can be used to wrap sore limbs, broken bones, or even stop areas of sever bleeding. Look at the athletes in the news, and how many times

do you see an arm or leg wrapped with tape to prevent further injury as they compete in their sports. A nice firm wrap, which does not cut off blood circulation,is a very good cure for many of the aches and sprains you may get to your limbs. When you have to go about your business with a sore arm or leg, then wrap the area with an ace bandage to prevent further injury, but don't try to act like the professionals at this time and compete in very strenuous sports, do something more relaxed and you will be surprised at the amount of satisfaction you will derive.

Why Hospital Emergency Rooms are Bad for Children

Most of the time when you go to an emergency room it is because you have to. And when you go for your child it is because you are fearing serious injury or death. Because of this it is doubly tragic when the emergency room adds to the danger to your child.

Emergency rooms don't do this because they want to hurt children. They do it out of a lack of proper preparation. Equipment for children must be smaller than the same equipment for adults. Thus, such things as oxygen masks, blood pressure cuffs, defibrillator paddles, and breathing tubes are often stocked in only the adult size. When this life saving equipment is used on a child, the child has less of a chance for survival just because things don't fit as they should.

Short of buying and stocking all of this stuff yourself, which is not a good idea since you don't really know what you need, it is best to go the the emergency rooms in your area and ask how they are equipped to service children who come in with emergency medical conditions. If an emergency room cannot satisfy you that it has equipment in the proper size, then go on to the the next hospital and ask again. If there are more than one or two hospitals in your area then at least one should have what you need. But if none do then start putting pressure on the local emergency rooms with letter writing campaigns and other political action until at least one stocks what you need. Also make sure you go to the best equipped emergency room when you have a medical emergency in your family.

ENDOMETRIOSIS

A Mystery Problem Women Should be Aware Of

Endometriosis is not exactly a problem that you can fix with diet or exercise. In fact doctors are not quite sure how much of a problem it really is, but it is certainly something women should be aware of since it affects only women, and sometimes it can take a serious medical turn.

To begin, the endometrium is the mucous membrane that lines a woman's uterus, and endometriosis is the occurrence of this lining outside of the uterus. Obviously you don't want body tissues growing where they are not supposed to, but does that mean that it is a serious condition?

Actually not always, although some doctors believe that this tissue can turn cancerous. This does not mean that you should be too concerned about cancer if you have endometriosis, but you will have other problems that you need to be concerned with. For one thing this tissue, since it comes from the uterus, behaves just like the uterus as you go through your monthly cycle. That is, every month it bleeds, causes pain, and can cause fibrosis, or growths of tissue outside of the uterus. Non-cancerous fibroid tumors outside of the uterus are not uncommon, and are not especially dangerous. It requires surgery to remove them, and they are usually left in place unless they start to bother a woman, or unless she has a C-section and they can be taken out easily.

If you have been told you have endometriosis you should also know that this tissue can grow in the in the lung as well as in the body around the uterus. If this happens you may get monthly bleeding and pain from your lungs and think that you have cancer or tuberculosis. Of course both of those conditions are much more serious than endometriosis, and a doctor should be much more able to deal with the endometriosis than either cancer or tuberculosis.

What you should always remember is that doctor's are not at all sure what this tissue will do once it starts growing in places where it shouldn't. It can cause you injury, or you may never be aware of it. You might just have a few extra cramps during your period, or it might grow in any area that affects your breathing and has to be removed surgically. Since you never know what it will do, if you are told you have it, just make sure that your doctor keeps an eye on, and don't go for anything radical without having a good reason since treatment can sometimes be more dangerous than the problems they are trying to correct.

ENERGY

4 Tonic Teas to Pep You Up

While the majority of people use caffeine drinks like sodas or coffee as pick-me-ups, you can also use herbal teas for the same purpose, and avoid the caffeine. The problem with the caffeine is that you can actually overdose on it to the point where you get the shakes and an accelerated heart beat. For some medical conditions you are restricted from having caffeine, but you will still need your energy. For those of you who are looking for an energy booster, and would like to get away from the usual caffeine sources, here are 4 tonic teas that will do the job.

1. The first of the tonic teas is peppermint (Mentha piperita), which has been chosen because you can already find it in so many foods at the market. Peppermint teas are also easy to find, and you probably already have some in your home. Besides making a refreshing cup of tea, peppermint is excellent for the stomach. Before or after a meal, or in between, peppermint will help you to feel better by promoting digestion, eliminating heartburn, and curing any common stomach upset. This will get you on the right road to more energy and more activity.

2. The next tea is raspberry (Rubus idaeus), which has several interesting qualities. It is good as a diarrhea cure, but also works well as a treatment for sores in the mouth and bleeding gums. For women though, raspberry has special powers. It has been used for many years for anything having to do with pregnancy helping babies come to term and for good deliveries, It is also considered a good general women's' tonic.

3. Now that we have taken care of the digestive system and women, this next tea is for the nervous system. It is made from oat straw (Avena sativa), and is most useful for any;one undergoing stress and emotional strain. If you are trying to stop any addictive habit such as smoking, this tea will cut down on some of the anxiousness that you are feeling whenever you miss your normal smoke, or other activity. Give it a try for this or any condition that gives you frayed nerves. If you tend to have a high-strung and nervous personality this may be just the thing for you to put you in a more mellow mood.

4. The final tonic tea is something that you would not normally think of as a source of tea. Stinging nettles (Urtica didoca) will not sting you as a tea, but can supply help to the kidneys and a control for allergies. Nettles are useful in many things having to do with your body, and can help you overcome asthma, high blood pressure, arthritis, and eczema in children. Even though it was left for the last, stinging nettles is one of the best herbal teas you can use for many

things. You can always go out and gather the nettles yourself, but if you don't want to your best bet is a health food store since the local supermarket isn't likely to carry something like this. Good luck and good health.

Burn Fat for More Energy, Here's How

Studies have recently shown that taking potassium-magnesium aspartate increases physical endurance, and energy, by up to 50%. This over-the-counter nutrient has the ability to increase the body's rate of fat burning to supply energy. Of course this also adds to the replacement of body fat with muscle tissue, and increases general health. With the difficulty of weight loss, it is wise to take advantage of anything that you can to keep your weight in an ideal range. And when you can do it at the same time that you build muscle, you are already halfway down the road to fitness that you want to be on.

EXERCISE

3 Tips to Safe Exercise

Every time you go out to have some exercise there is a small risk that the exercise will cause a heart attack. The risk is about 1/10,000 of dying from at this time, but only about 1/1,000 of having some kind of an irregularity with your heart beat. In either case you don't want to put yourself at risk unnecessarily.

Luckily there are ways that you can cut down even that small risk, and they are worth taking because the benefits of exercise lower your overall risk of heart attacks and cardiac problems to 1/2 to 1/10 of what they would be if you don't exercise. To lower your risk is mainly to go through the following 3 steps whenever you exercise. You will have to decide exactly how to carry them out, but here are the general guidelines.

1. Before you do any kind of exercise take some time to get a good warm up. The warm up is going to loosen up your muscles and get your blood flowing a little faster through your body. That way you won't have to strain quite so much when you actually start to exercise so your heart rate won't have to increase so rapidly, and you will be less likely to get an injury that will stop your exercise plan. A 5 or 10 minute period of stretching arm and body movements, with maybe a 5 minute walk included will do the trick and get you ready to go.

2. During your activity don't overdo it. Don't try to do your best every time you go out, once a week or every two weeks will let you know if you are making progress in your maximum abilities. But that doesn't really matter since all that your body really knows is that your muscles are getting some work. By planning a series of different kinds of exercise through the week, at different levels of difficulty, you will know in advance that some days will be harder than others and on some you can just take it easy and get good and comfortable without getting sore.

3. After exercise take some time to cool down properly. Cooling down after a run usually means walking around a bit until you feel your body start to cool and relax. If you are biking or swimming cooling down might be stretching and deep breathing before you go in to change. You will be able to get a good estimate of how your exercise for the day measured up to your level of fitness a few hours later, or the next day at the latest, if you are stiff and sore. If there is no soreness then you could have done more, but if you are in some real pain than you know that you were close to an injury point. For safety in exercising try to keep your level of effort to the point that you are never extremely sore the following day. A little stiffness is normal and no problem, but that is also the reason that you do not want to do very strenuous exercises 2 days in a row. It's also more interesting to do many physical activities, and it gives you more skills as well.

4 Secrets to Prevent Skin Problems When You Exercise

We usually think that everyone who exercises has nice, healthy, and clean skin. But when we begin our regular exercise program we have all sorts of acne problems and little rashes which makes our skin look worse than before. You should know that these problems are not unusual. If you haven't worked out regularly for a while, and have just started then your skin isn't used to the extra work it is going to be doing in heavy periods of sweating. When you exercise your skin sweats heavily. When it sweats the pores open and swell shut the openings to the oil glands that we have all over our bodies. This trapped oil causes the acne, and if the sweat doesn't evaporate right away, or isn't washed off right afterwards, it will also irritate the skin and cause a rash. This gives a pretty good picture of what the problem is, but not of what the solution should be. First, the problem will only last a few weeks, or maybe a month or two. After that your skin will get used to taking care of the extra work during exercise and will take on a very healthy look without any extra work from you. But in the meantime you should use the 4 secrets we have here to keep your skin looking well, and yourself looking healthy.

1. Before you go out to exercise remove any make-up or personal care products from your face and body. For women this usually means make-up, but for both men and women it can include hair treatment like moose or hair spray. All of these kind of things will break down when you sweat heavily, clog your pores, and irritate your skin to cause rashes. No one expects you not to sweat or

have messy hair while you are exercising. You will feel a lot better afterwards freshly made-up, and you will have to do this anyway, even if you don't remove the make-up beforehand.

2. When you have completed your exercise the most important thing you can do is to shower immediately. If you are still perspiring while you shower anything on your skin will wash right off, and nothing will get into your pore or onto your skin that could irritate it. Besides just rinsing it off is also a good idea to use a soft washcloth or sponge to clean your skin surface. You don't want to rub very hard, but a nice rubdown at this time will take off any dead skin or oils on your skin and help keep it healthy.

3. If there is a problem with showering then you have a real risk that you are going to have a skin rash or acne within a few hours. In this case at least wash up those areas you can get at easily. These should include your face, neck and back and you can use water alone if that is all that is handy. Pat yourself dry, and have a shower later in the day whenever you are able. It is not a good idea to do this every time that you exercise, but it is a lot better than not cleaning up at all.

4. Clothing can also be a problem. Don't let the ads of people sitting around in their workout clothes after exercising make you believe that this is a good idea. This clothing, including leotards, will have trapped everything on your body, and will undoubtedly lead to skin problems if you do it very often. Change to clean clothing, and don't re-use the exercise cloths without washing them out first. If your exercise clothing is tight, like leotards and bicycling jerseys, and you have skin problems then change to different fabrics and wear something a little looser for your workouts.

6 Week Plan to Get In Shape for those Over 40

If you are over 40 and lead a good and normal American life then you are probably out of shape, most Americans over 40 are. The problem with being over 40 and out of shape is that your age not only catches up to you, but it goes right on and gallops right on past. The reason why some people are young at 50, 60, and 70 is often a result of the effort they have taken to care for their health, and to keep in shape throughout their lives. But if you are over 40 and haven't kept in shape your whole life, don't give up hope. If you go about it just right it is still possible to get in shape without killing yourself or getting too hurt by it that you give up before it does you any good. All that being over 40 and out of shape means is that it is going to take you a while to get in shape. If you start tomorrow you will feel better 6 weeks from now, so give it a try.

Week 1, 2, 3: this is a program that you are going to build up slowly, so all that you have to do in the first weeks is take a 15 minute walk three days each week. The walk can be fast or slow, it doesn't matter, and it also doesn't matter if you do it in circles in your own living room. Just do it and you will get things moving.

Week 4: you have now had at least 9 walks to make sure you can move, and you should know by now if there are any aches or pains that you can't handle. If everything is still go, then increase your walks this week to 20 minutes each.

Week 5: your beginning to get things moving now, and it is time to increase each walk by another 5 minutes—25 minutes each day. Continue to walk at least 3 days this week.

Week 6, plus: this week we get to our full basic time-on-task for walking. Add 5 more minutes and make it 30 minutes at a time, and 3 times this week. It is also now time to set a distance goal of 2 miles for each of the exercises. You will need to do the 2 miles each time, and if it takes you more than 30 minutes to do it, that's ok. As you go along after this gradually speed up your walks until you can do the 2 miles in 30 minutes. This will assure you a full aerobic, walking, workout three times a week. If you feel good and are getting bored with the walking it is now time to start varying your exercise plan: alternate walking with jogging, hiking, swimming, cycling, and so forth so that you do two or three different exercises each week for the total three exercise sessions each week.

CAUTIONS: Now that you have decided that you are going to start an exercise program and get all of the good benefits you hear about, it is time to take some care to make sure you should do it—after all you're over 40 and out of shape, and you are going to do something that can strain your heart. So here are three cautions to follow.

1. See your doctor. This is to make sure your heart and circulatory system are in good shape. If your doctor says no to this plan for any reason, then ask him what you should do to get exercise. Any doctor who examines you for cardiac problems should be able to give you alternatives that can be done safely. It is a good bet though that even if you have a problem your doctor will not discourage you from this walking exercise plan, but will only tell you to come in for checkups, and maybe give you some medication.

2. Don't overdo it when you are just starting out. You have taken a long time to get this out of shape, and it should not be a problem to take some time to get back into shape. If it takes you 12 weeks to get up to 30 minutes a day instead of 6 weeks, so what. At least you have done it. If you exercise your body it will respond, and you will know it.

3. While you may not feel like it at first, or even for several weeks, aim for 3 sessions of exercise of 30 minutes each. If you can do this your level of health and fitness will increase vastly in a short time, and you will find yourself with more energy, a better appetite, and sleeping better than you have in years. Take whatever time you need to get to this level, but get to it and keep it as a minimum level of activity to stay in peak physical shape for the rest of your life.

8 Step Plan to a Good Exercise Program

There are some general rules to exercising, no matter what type of exercise you like to do, to make sure that you will get the most benefit from your effort. What you want to do is have a good time exercising, keep from getting hurt, and take care of any physical problems in the best way possible. These 8 steps can be followed to get all of these benefits, and can be used with any exercise program.

Step 1. The old saying about exercise being no good unless it is painful needs to be killed. No pain no gain is more likely to give you pain than it is to give you gain. When your body starts giving you pain it may mean more than that it is just tired. You can have pulled muscles and irritated achilles tendons. Any time that you get into an extremely painful situation while exercising take a break. If the pain stays with you after you have stopped and rested then see a doctor. You get as much benefit from a run where you spend half of the time walking as you do from one where you run constantly, and more if you avoid injuring yourself. An injury that prevents you from exercising for a month is much worse for your exercise program than a lighter exercise that doesn't cause you an injury in the first place. Also if you exercise regularly you will eventually be able to do the more strenuous exercises without the pain, but give it as much time as needed and don't try to follow a rigid schedule,

Step 2. If you have any interest in exercising in hot weather you need to rethink what you are trying to do. The temperature that you exercise in does not make your exercise better or worse, but it can endanger your health. Exercise on a very hot day can lead to dehydration and heat stroke. At the very least you will get very overheated and can have heat prostration. Your body has to have a certain amount of liquid in it to keep your cells from collapsing, and if you exercise on very hot days you loose water so fast that you risk a complete collapse—and that can be life-threatening. Anytime that you exercise make sure that you have had a sufficient amount of water first, although don't drink real heavily just before you go out. If the weather is extremely hot in the middle of the day, then exercise early in the morning or late in the afternoon. A jog under the stars or a tennis game near sunrise will be a lot more fun, and do you just as much good, as the same thing at high noon.

Step 3. Never go out for your exercise completely cold. Always take some time for stretching and warm-up exercises or you risk injury to your muscles. Warming up does some of the same things that you want your exercise to do, except that it does it at a slower rate so that you are not breathing hard. When you warm up you stretch out the muscles you are going to use, and you may take some short jogs or runs to get everything else loose. Warming up has the added advantage of letting you know if you have any injuries. If you pulled a muscle a day or two before but thought nothing of it, and you still feel it in your warm up, then you can watch that area of your body and make sure that you don't re-injure

---

the area or cause it to get worse. Exercising without a warm-up is likely to end up causing you an injury whether or not you were hurt before. If you warm up each time you go out to do anything physical, and everything seems to work the same, then you can be pretty certain that it will work just fine and you will get what you want out of any workout, fun and good physical health.

Step 4. You have now finished your exercise, so what should you do now? What you should do now is take a few minutes and cool down to prevent your muscles from stiffening. When you exercise your muscles get more blood and oxygen going to them, but when you stop if all of that nutrient is stopped too suddenly your muscles may cool so fast they they can still be injured, and this is part of the reason that horses who have run hard are cooled down before being put away. You are a lot more important than any horse, and when you exercise you need at least as much consideration. Not only can your muscles cool so rapidly that they are easily injured, but they can cramp and spasm into little knots that are extremely painful. This often happens if you are exercising much more heavily than you have in the past. A good cool down exercise is something very close to what you do to warm up in the first place. If you have been running, then run much more slowly or walk for 5 minutes. Whatever you do don't stop moving until your body feels more comfortable: heavy sweating has slowed, heavy breathing has stopped, and you have no quivering or feeling of collapse in your muscles.

Step 5. If you have gone through steps 1 through 4, and have still had an injury, then steps 5 through 8 are for you. These steps will go through the best way to get over your injury so that you can get back to your exercise program, and feel healthy again. The first of the steps you must take to get over an exercise injury is to rest it. If it is a pulled muscle, then don't do anything that is going to put much of a strain on it. These injuries will probably all be in the sore muscle area, but you might even get a strained achilles tendon. You will need to rest the sore area whatever it is so that it can have a chance to heal, and so that you don't injure it again. Taking some time off of a particular exercise is good advice, since you can always find something else. If you have been a runner, then take up aerobics, or if you have been a swimmer, then do some tennis. It doesn't really matter very much just so long as you get out and use your body. Once your sore areas have completely recovered you can go back to doing what it is that you really love. And since you have not sat around doing nothing all that time you will get back to your old form much quicker than you would have otherwise.

Step 6. In the process of resting the damaged part of your body it is also a good idea to cool it down with some ice. In fact cooling down any injured part of your body should be your first priority. Resting is a long term thing, and can take anywhere from a day to several months, but cooling should take place right away and should take no more than a few hours. The reason you want to cool down injured areas is that when you are injured your body pumps blood into the area and can even make it worse. Cooling slows the blood flow, and the swelling, and prevents this natural reaction from causing further injury. Think of it as putting that part of your body to sleep so that it can have a chance to heal up without having any more strain put on it. Often times it is the strain of the body reacting to the injury more than the injury itself that causes the damage. So cooling can be very useful in curing the injuries of exercise.

Step 7. Going along with the last advice of cooling the area is this one. When you have been injured put a compress on it. A compress is just a firm wrapping, like an Ace bandage, that restricts swelling and gives the area some support. Think of all of those professional athletes you see running around with bandaged elbows and knees, they are using the same idea to control their injuries so that they can continue playing. While they do it so that they can make money, you should do it so that you can continue to go out and continue to give yourself a good body. The compress acts a lot like the ice, it keeps blood from going to the injured area, but it also helps in a different way, it adds strength to damaged muscles. Damaged muscles are weak and sore because they are damaged, and anything that you can do to stop further injuries from happening will help you to heal faster. The compress is nothing more than a support for a sore muscle just like a splint is a support for a broken bone, and both help the damaged area to heal as fast as possible.

Step 8. The last step, and this doesn't seem like any really important act, is to elevate the injured part of your body. Like all of the last 3 steps this is meant to cut down on the amount of swelling that you have. Because swelling makes it harder for blood to enter an injured area, because it is harder for blood to flow uphill, your injured body will not swell as much. Cutting down on the swell will also result in less pain, and should make you feel better all around. Just think how good it feels to get your feet up at the end of the day, when all that they are is tired, and figure that this effect will be multiplied when the arm or leg you are elevating is really hurt.

This completes the steps to better exercise, but don't be discouraged if they do not seem like steps. The first 4 should be done by everyone whenever they exercise. The last 4 should be done by anyone who has an injury as a result of their exercise. If you wonder where these last 4 steps come from, look in any exercise book in the index under R.I.C.E., and you will find the best standard information for getting over exercise injuries. RICE has been used for a long time because it it easy to remember, and it works. The importance of the steps is that they need to be kept in mind by everyone who exercises, whether they are hurt or not.

A Key to Happiness and Healthy Living

When you are asked you usually say that you exercise to control weight for your health. The next time you might consider saying that you exercise to be a happier person. Studies have found that chemicals are released in the brain during exercise that make you happier and more contented. These chemicals are entirely natural, and do not harm you. They are part of your normal body chemistry, but are normally released rarely and at only certain times. With exercise you can get their full benefit at any time. They also do not affect any of the other benefits of exercise such as weight loss or physical conditioning. To get the maximum benefit exercise at least three times a week, and a vigorous walk can be just as good as any other exercise. This is also a handy way to help you overcome stress or depression from any cause. The next time you have any emotional discomfort take a half hour walk and you will feel better. Do this every time you feel stress and you will be able to cope more effectively with all of the problems that arise in the course of your life.

Checklist for Putting Together
Your Own Program of Exercise

Exercise plans come in many shapes and sizes, some hard and some easy. But what you want is an exercise plan that is right for you, and to get it you are going to have to do it yourself. While you can go to a professional trainer and have them design you one, you know yourself better than anyone else is going to. Your exercise plan should be based on how hard you want to work, what your history of exercise is, what your goals are, and how much dedication you have. You may also have a time line that you want to be on, and it may be either flexible or firm, and depending upon what you want to do, it can change from one to the other from week to week. You are more understanding of these needs and aspirations you have than any trainer can ever be. So follow the 8 items as you check your way down to a perfect plan for you.

1. If you are just starting out after a year or more of inactivity, or you are over 50, before you begin on your new exercise program get an exercise stress test. This will tell you if you can take the stress of the exercise you are planning, and what kind of condition your heart is in. It is vitally important to know that you are not putting yourself at risk for a heart attack before you change your way of life. If you wonder about those reports of people dying just after getting one of these tests and beginning to exercise, it is just that no test is perfect and occasionally one does get through. But you can protect yourself much better if you do this before your plan, since it will catch just about everything.

2. Now that you know you are safe as far as your heart goes, it is time to set your goals. These are goals in time, in weight loss, and in fitness that you want to accomplish. You want to do these reasonably since everyone's body reacts different to exercise. It is also good to keep your goals rather loose. If you haven't exercised before and you decide that you are going to run 5 miles at less than 10 minutes a mile in 3 months, you are not going to make it. In fact those are not the right type of goals to set anyway for exercise, those are goals for competition. More realistic goals are that you would be getting 30 minutes of aerobic exercise 6 times a week within 1 month. If you are interested in performance,

than set easy goals first, say 2 miles in under 30 minutes in 3 months, and 3 miles under 3 minutes in 1 year. If you don't want to run, then set goals in any exercise you are going to use. If it's weight loss, don't set it at more than 1/2 pound a week or it won't work either. Keep your goals simple and reasonable and they will help you to see your own progress. Also don't be afraid to revise them every few months, especially once you have reached them.

3. Now set your exercise schedule. While this may have been part of your goals, it also may not have been. What you have to do is to find the number of hours you are going to need to carry out your exercises, and the equipment you are going to need to do it, if any. It is usually hours more than equipment that determines the exercise schedule you will have. If you have not been exercising, then one of the biggest problems to overcome, before you begin, is where you will find the time to do it. You also probably wonder at all the people you see biking and jogging around the neighborhood while you are busy working and doing errands. The truth of it is that they have made exercise a priority in their lives ahead of some of the errands they have to do anyway, and exercising gets their body moving and their energy level up to the point at which they pretty well get everything done anyway. Remember that exercise can take as little as 1/2 hour out of your day to do, and don't tell me that you don't spend that long watching the news, after reading it in the paper, or watching some television show that you don't really like anyway just to pass the evening. How much better it is for you to spend that time taking yourself out of a chair and walking or jogging. If you are into something that takes longer, say 2 hours at a time, then you may only do that once or twice a week, with a couple of additional times limited to the 1/2 hour walk or jog.

4. But don't just walk, or jog, or bike, vary your exercise from day to day. While all of your exercises should be something that you enjoy doing, don't try to do the same thing every single time you go out. Not only will you get bored, but you can also develop injuries. There is no one exercise that exercises all of the muscle groups in your body equally, and often times muscles will be ignored all together. Listen to any professional athlete at the start of the season, or when they are recovering from an injury, and you will find that they always talk about their time in the weight room, golfing, jogging, or doing some exercise other than the one they are paid for. They do this because it trains more of the muscles and because it is not as boring as doing the same thing every single day. The exercise professional call it cross training, and I guarantee that you will find exercise more rewarding and more interesting when you vary the exercises you do from day to day and week to week.

5. Whenever you go out to take some exercise, first take some time to warm up properly and fully. The warm up may seem like wasted time, but it is the preparation that you go through in order to prevent injuries and have a more enjoyable experience. The warm up can also tell you if you already have an injury, and muscle pulls are often not felt until the next time you go out and put a real strain on a muscle. The standard warm up program usually starts with some stretching and bending, not rapidly at first, but slowly to limber up the muscles.

Cold muscles will tear more easily than warm ones. Then when you have spend 2 or 3 minutes at that you can do a few which are more strenuous, such as pushups or deep bends. Give it about 5 minutes at a minimum. When you begin your exercise don't start off at full speed, always take the first 15 minutes on the slow side to get everything working well. By then your blood flow will be better, your heart rate will increase, your breathing should deepen, and you should begin to break into a light sweat. From that point on you can exercise, run or walk, whatever, at whatever level you feel most comfortable. If you never feel comfortable going beyond the beginning stage, you just need to give it some time, and eventually you will feel like increasing your pace and the difficulty of your workout just to give yourself a challenge.

6. Cooling down properly is just as important as warming up properly. Cooling down does not mean sitting in the shade with a cold drink in your hand, what it means is that you keep moving until your breathing slows to normal and you are no longer gasping for breath, if you got to that point in the first place. This usually requires from 15 minutes to 30 minutes, but you can do some of it puttering around home after your breathing is normal. Your goal in cooling down is to get your pulse rate into a normal range, at which point you will fully have cooled down. To cool down properly you should also find out what your resting heart rate is. To do this just take a count of your heart rate after you have been sitting down for at least 30 minutes, at rest. This will be your minimum active heart rate, and will be higher than your heart rate when you are asleep, but higher than when you are up and walking around. If after you have finished your exercise you are in the habit of relaxing for 30 minutes or more, then take your heart rate and find out how soon it returns to its resting level. As you exercise you will find that your resting heart rate will decrease. Where the normal heart rate for American adults is between 60 and 80, those who exercise often get theirs into the 50's, and professional athletes are known to go into the 20's. You will see your heart rate drop as you exercise, and you will periodically have to measure where your true cool off point is located.

7. Now when we talked about stretching to warm up, we did not mean that you should go out and do as many of these stretching exercises as possible, because they can hurt you too. It has been known for a long time that doing sit-ups, especially if done incorrectly, can damage and weaken your lower back. The weakest points in the human body are the lower back and the knees, and it is easiest to injure those two areas. Using deep knee bends, in many repetitions, will result in injured knees and not in strong legs. Repetitions, just like repeating the same exercise every day, can end up in causing muscle as well as joint injuries. It is much better to use exercises that stretch the muscles to different lengths over a longer period of time than to rely upon ones that simply do the same thing over and over. Repetitive stretches will also ignore muscles which are not used in the particular exercise being used. Then, no matter how good the exercise you are doing, there will always be much of your body that you are not exercising at all.

8. Finally, as you are in the process of doing all of these things to give yourself a good exercise program, you also need to keep records. You need a

record of your progress from week to week, and the efforts you are going through to get your exercise. This will give you a true measure of how much you are improving, and it will allow you to appreciate even the most modest gains, and get encouragement from them. Records will also tell you the times when you do not keep up your program, and what the effects are upon you and your body. But what should you put into the records? The basic record should be of your primary goal. If it is weight loss, then you need to weigh yourself several times a week, or at least once a week at the same day and time, and record it. If you are interested in your time walking or jogging some distance, then record that. It is also a good idea to record what you do each week to see that you are doing enough of the right kinds of exercise as you go along.

And that's the plan to set up your exercise program. Now this is just an outline, so you can apply it to any type of exercise and for any purpose. Of course the quicker you get started the quicker you will get results. But any exercise you go on will have the benefits of strengthening your immune system and lowering your heart rate, and both of these are important to staying healthy and disease free.

Don't Like Going to a Club to Exercise
You Don't Have To

Keeping on a regular exercise program is such a problem. There is always something better to do, and at some times of the year the weather is either too hot or too cold. There is also the problem of vacations, or sick children or a sick spouse. Is it any wonder that most of the people who sign up at exercise centers, and pay their money, rarely if ever go and use the equipment.

Of course if you do not go to one of these places how are you expected to lose weight and stay in shape? The answer lies in doing your exercises at home. A Stanford University study found that those who worked out at home got just the same benefits as those who went to an exercise club, and that the results they achieved were more long lasting.

The results were just as good, of course, because those tested did the same exercises, or at least exercised at the same level. Your body doesn't care where you exercise just so long as you get the time and effort into it. This is a good argument for buying an exercise tape, or tuning into one of those exercise shows that are on every morning, and working out along with the celebrity.

But why should the results from home workouts last longer than the results gained by paying your fees and going to a club? The answer again lies in the time you spend and the effort you put into your exercise plan. In home workouts there is no cost past the initial outlay for equipment, and you don't have to go anywhere to do the exercises since you are doing them where you are most of the time. What was believed to be a contributing factor in this study was the monthly follow-up phone call the researchers made to each of the home exercise group each month, the anticipation of this phone call was enough to keep people exercising from month to month, and this at the time when many of the club people had interrupted schedules or quit for some reason. If you want the same benefit, but don't have a researcher to hound you, then look for encouragement from friends or relatives, and you can save yourself trips to the gym and monthly dues to use someone else's equipment.

How to Make Your Exercise Program Work for You

If you are in an exercise program but aren't getting the results you want, or feel you deserve for how hard you work, then changes are due. The first thing you have to do is see how good the exercise program is itself. Is it regular? Do you have realistic goals? Is the difficulty level right for you?

A negative answer to any of these could be the reason things are just not happening the way they should. Regularity means that you exercise an average of about every other day—3 or 4 times a week. Exercise less than that will not do you much good, and exercise more than that won't give you any recovery time. Goals are more personal and harder to define. If your goal is to lose weight, then set a reasonable weekly goal, say of one pound per week, and go for it. Whatever your goals set enough small steps into them that you can see your progress. If your goals are too far away it might explain why you never seem to be getting near them. Difficulty level is a little easier to settle. If you are left exhausted and sore after every workout it is too hard for you at this time—back off a bit. The same goes if you get injured often and it interrupts your exercise schedule. As far as difficulty, just remember that lighter workout more often will do you a lot more good than a break in your program every couple of weeks because your body is too beaten up to go out for some exercise.

Like to Exercise Early
Watch Out for Back Injuries

If you are one of those people who like to get in an early morning exercise, before going to work, then you have to be cautious about possible back injuries. You need to know that while you sleep at night the discs in your back expand with fluid. This makes them tighter and more tense. So if your exercise program has a great deal of bending and stretching of the spine you risk a back injury that will keep you out of your program for anywhere from a few days to several weeks. To protect yourself from this kind of injury wait at least an hour after getting up before you go out for that early morning exercise that you like to take so much. Remember that any exercise that leaves you disabled will cost you a lot more of your ability than easing off a few minutes a day to allow your back to adjust itself to the daily strain that you are going to put on it.

Sore Muscles
2 Vitamins Can Make the Difference

At work out you must suffer from sore muscles at times, and the harder you work out the more chance you have of getting a serious muscle injury. These injuries are caused by asking our muscles to do too much too fast, and a bad one can take week to heal. With a couple of vitamins you can reduce significantly mostof those types of injuries, and allow athletes and anyone else who works hard physically to work longer and do more without injury. The 2 vitamins are vitamin C and vitamin E. They were tested in Australia, and it was found that athletes who were taking supplements of these vitamins trained longer and harder, recovered afterwards more rapidly, and were injured less often. If you are active physically this is a good pair to include in your diet for a better workout, and better performance.

EYE PROBLEMS

93% of the Nearsighted May Be Able To
Do Away With Glasses

Have you ever wished that you could get rid of your glasses, and be able to see just as well as all of those people you see running around without anything hanging from their nose in front of their face? Well I think we all have if we have been wearing glasses. Besides the way they look, they are expensive, they get broken all the time, you need new ones every few years no matter what you do, and they are just a big nuisance much of the time.

Well, if you are nearsighted there is a very good chance that you can get rid of your glasses if you are ready, willing, and able to have an operation. The operation is called a radial keratotomy, and it consists of the doctors making tiny cuts on the cornea of your eyes with a laser. This is a much safer operation than one in which a knife is used on you, and you are usually able to go home the same day that you have the operation.

Of course not every nearsighted person can have the operation, although 93% can. The problem is that some nearsighted people have other problems with their eyes that can't be corrected by this operation .

But assuming you are ready and willing to have the operation, are you also able. Normally insurance won't pay for it, since its classed as an elective operation of something that can be corrected with glasses. The cost per eye, so I understand, is about $1500. You should shop around though because there may be bargains out there, and you may even have an insurance plan that will do it.

The laser cuts are made with a computer aiming the laser, so there is no chance of a doctors hand slipping. And because of the expense some people even go to Russia for it, where they do several thousand operations a year in an automated hospital which is dedicated just to doing this particular procedure.

So if you hate your glasses, have a little money, and nearsightedness is your only problem, then getting rid of your glasses is a decision which is entirely up to you.

Nutrients to Fight-Back Age Related Blindness

Blindness at any age tends to be related to the quality of your nutrition. The better your nutritional state the less likely it is that you will be threatened with blindness. The other concern is that as people get older they often lose their appetites. The result is a regular pattern of malnutrition in the aged, and that in turn contributes to a general deterioration in health and development of disease. The attack on eyesight is just one aspect of the nutritionally based deterioration of health that older people experience. But because it is nutritionally based it is also at least partially curable by increasing vision related nutrients in the diet.

Vitamin A is the carrot vitamin, and the one most indispensable for making sure that your eyesight stays in good shape. A chemical in your eye called rhodopsin is broken down in seeing, and vitamin A is necessary for your eye to rebuild its rhodopsin and keep your vision operating normally. Vitamin A can be gotten in carrots or as a supplement.

Zinc is necessary in addition to vitamin A since zinc ensures that the blood supply in the eye stays at an optimal level. Patients with night blindness have been cured by receiving supplemental zinc. It has also been found that giving patients vitamin A, who were deficient in zinc, did not have their vision improved.

B vitamins have also been recently implicated in maintaining vision. B vitamins apparently are necessary for the health of the optic nerve. They are available as supplements, or in green and yellow vegetables.

Part of the function of the eye produces destructive oxidants that may also damage the vision. Vitamin E, as an antioxidant, counters the destruction effects of retinal oxidation. While vitamin E does not stop this process, it is seen as being protective against damage.

Going back to the B vitamins we find that one in particular, B2 (riboflavin), counters the development of cataracts. Cataracts are also one of the chief reasons for blindness among the aged, if they can be stopped, then the number of older blind will be largely decreased. Vitamin C is also involved in this anti-cataract effect, and is found in the highest concentration in the body in the eye fluid. This very high concentration of vitamin C occurs naturally, and for a reason. Vitamin C also has anti-oxidant property and serves the same purose as vitmin E.

There you have it, a basic list of nutritional elements which are important to the eye. While keeping their levels in a high nutritional level may not be a guarantee against blindness, you can be fairly certain that having a low concentration, or malnutrition, in any one or more of them will contribute to the development of blindness. To protect yourself from deterioration of vision, get these nutrients through your diet, or by supplement, every day.

See Specks CrossingYour Eye WhenYou Read, You Have Floaters

The first thing you should know is that most of the time floaters are not something that needs to be treated. The second is that floaters are usually no more than little specks that float around in the liquid of your eye. The reason they don't need to be treated most of the time is that they usually settle toward the bottom of the eye over time all by themselves, and when they do you probably won't even notice them anymore. The way to deal with the common floaters is to cut down on the intensity of the light you work or read in. It is the bright lights on paper that makes them more noticeable, but it doesn't mean that there is anything serious.

The time to worry about floaters is when they come on very suddenly, and you also notice flashes of light. While the flashes of light don't happen every time, a sudden onset of floaters can indicate serious conditions like retinal detachment. It it important that this condition be treated as soon as possible since retinal detachment can result in blindness. On the other hand, don't worry about a floater or two over your lifetime, since most people will experience the same thing and no treatment is required or recommended.

Sore, Irritated Eyes?
A Home Remedy that Gives Fast Relief

When do you usually get sore and irritated eyes, on smoggy days, or when you have been reading for a long time, or perhaps after a long work day and a drive home? Whenever your eyes get that tired and uncomfortable you need quick relief, and you need something you can do at home.

Now many people, when faced with tired, red eyes will turn to over the counter eye drops which promise to cut out the redness and get rid of the problem. In general these drops do what they say they will. They are largely liquid with something in them to cut the blood flow to the eyes that makes them look red. The problem with these medications, and they are medications even though you don't need a prescription, is that your eyes can become allergic to the chemicals they contain if you use them very often. If your eyes become allergic, then the drops will cause the irritation to get worse rather than cut it out. So I do not recommend these drops, except once in a great while in an emergency situation.

For a daily solution to the problem, I have a much safer method which can be counted on 100% of the time, at least if there is no infection or damage to your eyes. This solution is water! And to begin the solution wash your face thoroughly with water, but no soap, and especially around the eyes, and then dry with a soft towel. This will remove facial oils, and make-up if you are wearing it, which might be the cause of your eye irritation. Then take a wash cloth and get it damp with cool water, not cold or icy and certainly not hot or warm. Fold the wash cloth once or twice, lean your head back, and place it over your closed eyes. After about 5 minutes rinse the wash cloth, fold it, and place it again on your eyes. Do this exercise for 15 or 20 minutes. By then all of the irritation should be out of your eyes, and you should then dry your eyes completely, and keep your hands away from them.

Many times just the washing of the eyes with water will remove all feeling of irritation, and if that is true you are cured at that point. You do not use warm water as a compress because that will just increase the blood flow to your eyes and increase any existing irritation. You do not use cold or icy water on your eyes because cold can damage the eye itself. Remember that your eye is a liquid filled marble, and you do not want to freeze it, all that you want to do is cut down the blood flow for a few minutes, and a cool cloth will do that. The idea is to use the least extreme, and most gentle treatment you can to cure your minor physical problems. And that is especially true when it comes to minor problems concerning your eyes.

2 Vitamins to Cut Your Risk of Cataracts by 50% or More

The common vitamins C and E were shown in one study to cut the risk of cataracts by at least 50%. While we don't know exactly why these vitamins are so effective, they are known to both attack the free radicals in our bodies that cause so much disease, and they concentrate in the eye. It is worthwhile to make sure that your diet is high in both of these vitamins, and remember that cataracts attack 15% of Americans over age 65.

FATIGUE

A Simple Nutrient to Cure Fatigue and Increase Performance

Studies in Sweden have shown that the addition of two simple nutrients to a good basic diet could relieve fatigue and increase athletic performance in athletes. The nutrients are potassium and magnesium aspartate, and they are available in a combined tablet form which can supply 500 mg of each. It was found that six of these tablets a day increased performance by 50%, when taken before an exercise stress test.

Routine use has also been found to be effective against fatigue for nonathletes, as well as protecting against heart disease, diabetes, and high blood pressure. This nutrient combination may well end problems of ordinary fatigue for you, and leave you feeling better and healthier than you have in years.

9 Rare and not so Rare Causes of Fatigue

Are you always tired, or does it just seem like you are always tired? If you think you are tired most of the time then you are, and you have to take some steps to deal with it or you could be tired for years. But before we can do anything about getting over our fatigue we have to understand what might be causing it. And if it is not the problem of just overwork and lack of sleep, then you may have a medical cause, and that is what we want to talk about here in these 8 little discussions.

1. The first of our rare, and not so rare, causes of fatigue is low blood pressure. If all that you have ever worried about is high blood pressure, then you have a new worry, and it just might be the cause of your fatigue. How do you tell if you probably have low blood pressure, just lie down or sit down for a few minutes, and then stand up suddenly. If you get dizzy for more than 2 or 3 minutes, and you are chronically tired, then there is a good chance that low blood pressure is causing your condition.

2. Now that we have gotten you to start thinking of your blood as a possible cause of fatigue, you can also think of something in your blood that can also cause it. That something is iron. This is something that women are more prone to than men because women lose blood each month during their menstrual cycle, and this can lead to temporary iron deficiency anemia. Even a very slight drop in your iron level can result in feeling tired. The usual advice for iron deficiency is to take iron supplements, and to eat iron rich foods. But you shouldn't do this blindly even if you are certain that you have iron deficiency. Studies in Finland have indicated that high iron levels may promote heart attacks, and that low iron levels may protect you from heart attacks. This makes iron deficiency too dangerous to deal with on your own, and if you have it you should consult your doctor for treatment.

3. There is also a cause of fatigue that will affect you only during a part of the year, and it is called SAD, and it will make you sad as well. The full name is "seasonal affective disorder," and it doesn't just cause fatigue. The fatigue is actually caused by depression due to too little sunlight. In other words you just feel bad, and tired, because it is dark outside so much of the time. A good step in getting over this is to go outside as much as you can in the middle of the day. If you live in an area that is overcast much of the time in the winter, you can use a light-box device that exposes you to light several times brighter than the sun. And if you can manage it, a vacation is more fun and will relieve your winter depression and fatigue at the same time.

4. The next possible cause of your fatigue is something that some one else is going to have to tell you about. It is called sleep apnea, and what that means is not breathing while you are asleep. If you are watching some one sleep whom you think may have this sleep apnea, here is what to look for; snoring which stops, followed by silence and gasping, then normal breathing and perhaps a resumption of the snoring. The period of silence occurs when the breathing stops, and of course the gasping takes place when the sleeper is trying to gain their breath. If you have sleep apnea you may wake up tired each morning and never know why unless someone tells you about your sleeping pattern. If you think that you have sleep apnea, don't ignore it. Sleep apnea is associated with high blood pressure, heart attacks, heart failure, and stroke. But if you do need treatment, doctors are fully aware of sleep apnea and can treat it.

5. While everyone has heard of diabetes, most people don't know that type II diabetes can cause fatigue. In type II diabetes the pancreas produces insulin, but your body isn't able to use it. No one knows how type II diabetes

causes fatigue, but it is common with it. To get a diagnosis you will have to go to a doctor for a glucose tolerance test, or a fasting blood sugar. Treatment for type II diabetes is with exercise, diet, and medication, but you probably won't be on insulin. Ignoring it can lead to heart disease and stroke.

6. It is also possible that you get a high level of fatigue an hour or two after eating. Most of the time you might think that this is part of your normal digestion, where your blood is being diverted to your stomach to help you digest your food. But the real cause may be something which is somewhat more of a problem, and that is what is called reactive hypoglycemia. Don't be afraid of the word though, since all that is means is that your blood sugar has fallen to a lower than normal level because of the meal you've eaten. The other symptoms of this condition are headaches and general irritability, but it isn't a very serious condition by itself. Treatment is also not too complicated since all that you are usually required to do is eat more, and smaller, meals through the day, and cut out alcohol, sugar and caffeine from your diet. Because this is also associated with stress, it also helps if you learn stress management, exercise regularly, and pick up some relaxation tips.

7. Now here is a pattern of fatigue that can reveal a disease that is hard to diagnose: if you wake up each morning feeling so tired that you don't think you slept at all, and develop stiff, aching, and painful muscles over time then you may have a disease called fibromyalgia. All that this name means is that your muscles hurt, and that is also all that doctors know about its cause as well. Fibromyalgia affects 3 to 6 million Americans, and most of whom are women of childbearing age. Besides fatigue, it is characterized by widespread muscular pain, headaches, and numbness and tingling in the hands and feet. That is also pretty much how it is diagnosed: a doctor will put pressure on different points all over the muscles of your body, and if many of them are painful, you probably have fibromyalgia. Treatment is complicated; you may be given antidepressants to help you sleep, but also stretching, moderate aerobic exercise, heat applications, and massage can also be useful. With proper attention to this disease, its sufferers can lead pretty much normal lives. But if you think you have this you are going to have to see a specialist for the best diagnosis and treatment. The specialists who treat fibromyalgia are psychiatrists and rheumatologists, or specialists in rheumatic diseases.

8. Are you tired all of the time? Have you gained weight, have dry and itchy skin, constipation, muscle cramps, heavy periods if you are a woman, feel cold all of the time? If you do then you may have thyroid disease. Of course you don't have to have all of these symptoms to have thyroid disease, but you will have some of them. In fact about 3 to 4 million Americans are already known to have this disease. The problem with this disease of hypothyroidism is that it affects many functions of the body, and you can never be sure if the seemingly unrelated set of symptoms you have indicate a thyroid problem, or if you have 2 or 3 other diseases that have nothing to do with your thyroid. But let us say that you have hypothyroidism, and that you have gotten yourself diagnosed by a doctor, what happens next? Next you will be a given medication for it called thyrox-

in, which replaces the thyroid hormone that your body is supposed to be producing. Thyroxin treatment is a life long process, since thyroids do not get cured and return to normal function. When you take thyroxin you have to be monitored very carefully since taking too little can result in heart trouble, insomnia, palpitations, osteoporosis, and arthritis. But taking too much can also cause a continuation of your thyroid disease symptoms, as well as cause high cholesterol and contribute to heart disease.

9. Now suppose that you feel fine just so long as you don't try to do anything, but that as soon as you have any exertion you feel completely tired out. This could indicate that you have chronic fatigue syndrome, or CFS. Now CFS affects quite a few people, although we don't really know how many in the United States. The real problem with CFS is that it can go on for months, and keep you from leading a normal life. But other symptoms, to help your diagnosis, are chills and fever, sore throat, aching muscles and joints, weakness in the muscles, and sleeping problems. The cause is thought to be a virus, but none has been found yet. The usual way of diagnosing CFS is by a blood test called 2'-5'A, and a pattern of extreme fatigue that lasts for 6 months or more and reduces your ability to carry on your life. If you are diagnosed, treatment can also take a while. Treatment consists of anti-inflammatory drugs to relieve sore muscles and pains, and antidepressants to help you sleep better. Otherwise it just takes time to get over it.

Now you have some hints as to what you may have if you have been living with chronic fatigue and can't seem to get over it. But remember that I have only said may. We have looked at 9 things that can cause your fatigue, but there may be more. If fatigue has been plaguing you then see a doctor who you know and trust, as well as who knows you and has your best interests at heart. Oftentimes getting well is as much a matter of who treats you as much as of what you are being treated for, or of how you are being treated for your problem.

What to Eat to Charge Your Batteries

Feeling tired and want a snack to give you a boost? Or do you feel tired often, and want to have a boost all of the time? In either case a little food, or a change in the foods you eat, may be just the thing to get you over that sluggish part of the day. But what should you eat when you are nodding at work in the afternoon, or in mid-morning?

To begin with make sure that you eat something at least every 4 or 5 hours through the day. When you go longer than that between meals your blood sugar level falls and that is when you begin to feel tired and sleepy. And for something that will wake you up have some cheese, yogurt, or tuna. These are all high protein foods, and will not make you even more sleepy than you already are.

Next, stay away from the candy bars, and other sweets, that all of the television ads say you can get instant relief from. For one thing the relief you get from them is not going to last very long, since the sugar goes directly into your blood, and for another thing after a little while your blood sugar will fall to an even lower lever and you will feel an even greater need to eat.

Now to cure the fatigue, other than eating frequently, make sure that you get a balanced diet. Fatigue and irritability can be the result any time you are short changing yourself on one of your required nutrients. So in your diet you must be sure to include vitamin fortified foods, fresh fruits and vegetables, and at the very least some 1-a-day supplemental vitamins.

And finally, for foods to help you rest eat carbohydrates. Not a big meal of them, but a snack of crackers, popcorn, or a couple of pieces of toast. Digestion will help your body to release tryptophan, which is a natural chemical that will help to relax you.

If you have done all of this and you still aren't comfortable and relaxed, then take a 30 minute walk. The walk will both warm up your muscles and relax your body and your mind. Within a few minutes of taking the walk and going to bed you should be asleep.

But say you are at work and trying to get through the afternoon, and have also done all of the diet tricks you can think of, but you are still tired and irritable, what can you do? Take 5 minutes and stretch, go to the bathroom and wash your face, or go to the water cooler and get a drink of water. These little actions can activate your brain and get the blood in your muscles moving again. The only other thing is that you might have to repeat this routine every 30 minutes to get through an especially difficult afternoon, but even that is preferable to falling asleep on the job, or of becoming too hungry to work just because you haven't had anything for 3 or 4 hours.

Setting Yourself Up for a Good Night's Sleep

Have trouble sleeping, or wake up 2 or 3 times during the night? If you have these types of problems then it's time to take some steps to give yourself a better nights sleep. But what can you do? You certainly don't want to start taking sleeping pills, not when you may have to do it every night. No, it's better if you can do something natural, and the truth is that you can do several things that are natural, and one or more of them may work. Anyway, here are a few ideas that you need to look at.

The first thing to do is make sure that you are tired when you go to bed. For instance, if you have a habit of taking naps during the day, and can't fall asleep at night, then you are simply not tired enough when you try to get your night's sleep. Cut out the daytime naps and you will automatically start sleeping longer.

Now if you are simply not getting enough exercise during the day to feel tired at night, then you have to become more active. You have to tire your body out, and relax it, so that when you go to bed your body and mind will be ready to rest. Good exercise for this, if you don't have anything you like to do now that is active, is to take late afternoon walks of 30 minutes or an hour. This will do the job by warming your muscles, and by tiring you out.

You must also begin dedicating your bed to sleep, and get rid of the toys and job related items you may have there. By this I mean that many people have typewriters and computers in their bedrooms so they can get a little work done before they go to bed. Then when they go to bed they continue to think of their bedrooms as areas to do business in and they never get fully relaxed. Keep your area of rest and relaxation separate from your areas of work and business.

Now get the climate of your bedroom so that it is completely comfortable for you. You want the room cool, but not cold, and you want the mattress firm, but not hard. If you have special needs you may want a hard or soft mattress, and you may want a very warm or cold room, but for most people aim for the middle ground.

Now get yourself ready to rest by reading something enjoyable, or listening to music. Also perhaps have a massage, or a nice warm bath. All of these things will put you into what is called an alpha state, which is a condition in which your mind and body are at rest and you can slip into a comfortable and restful sleep.

Set yourself a routine time to get up and go to bed. When you are changing your time of retiring from day to day your body never really learns when it is time to rest. And make no mistake about it, just like we learn everything else we also learn to go to bed and get up at certain times of the day and night.

But if you go to bed at your usual time and are just lying there awake, don't torture yourself. Take some more time to put yourself into a relaxed condition. Read some more, or watch some television. Don't do anything too active, but put yourself into an activity that you know will leave you relaxed.

Diet is also important in getting a good night's sleep. If you have hunger pains when you go to bed you may just sit there wanting something to eat. If you have eaten too much during the evening, you may just feel bloated and unable to relax and get to sleep. In either case you are not going to sleep very well. So if you are hungry then have a little snack, and if you are too full, then take a walk and cut down on your diet the next day.

If you have trouble sleeping cut out all drinking of either alcohol or coffee in the evening. People who feel a drink relaxes them should know that it also disturbs sleep patterns. The same goes for coffee, although it is usually those who drink it in the evening as well as in the morning. Remember that coffee is used in the morning because the caffeine speeds up the heart and wakes you up by giving your brain more oxygen. You don't want this at night because you can't sleep well if your heart is racing and your mind is stimulated by an oxygen load.

There you have a nice little collection of tips for improving your night's sleep. It is now up to you to carry them out. Of course if your insomnia persists in spite of everything you can do for it you need to see your doctor. It might be time for medication or other professional help. But don't give up before you try, in most cases you will be able to cure yourself just by changing your habits.

FEELING GOOD

5 Tips to a More Satisfying Life

Many times you may be just uncomfortable with life. If your job isn't quite right, you have a few personal problems, and your health needs improving, you could actually be suffering from the inability to take charge of your life more than you are from those things which seem to be your biggest problems. In spite of what anyone or anything does to you, you are actually in charge of most of the activities you go through every day. But unfortunately most of the time you probably just don't take the time to appreciate your self, and to make the conscious decisions that would let you know that your life is being run by you, yourself. While you have to actually make the decisions, these tips will give you a little guidance as to where you can start. Even if you give just one or two a try, you will find that your life is much better than you thought, and that you really do feel good about your self.

1. Cut out some of your life's complications, and simplify things for yourself. This is a hint that you may be trying to do too much with your hours and your days. Don't wash the dishes every day, or mow the lawn every week, or take the kids out every weekend. You can be sure that you have overcommitted yourself in life if every minute of every day seems to be occupied with doing things you need to do, but not with those things you want to do. As a way of giving this a try, pick something out which you impose on your self, but which others do not seem to notice you do, and stop it. Even if the task still has to be done, you can be pretty sure it doesn't have to be done with the dedication that you were putting into it.

2. Take some time out for your mind. If you carry out the first step, and cut something out of your daily or weekly schedule, you will have a little more time. If you don't just fill it up with another task, but give yourself a rest there is no telling what you may be thinking. In fact you will actually be able to think things over and make some plans, or read a book, or do something really important that you want to do. It could also mean taking a walk or a little exercise, or taking a nap because you have been too busy for that for a long time. The idea is that you, and your thoughts, are just as important as at least some of those other things that keep you busy every day.

3 Simplify your diet, so that it is not a burden to follow, and so that it accomplishes what you want. This can mean many things, such as don't plan to cook a big meal every day, or don't count every calorie, or don't try to balance every single thing you eat. A good diet can still be a simple diet, and it should not consume your interests. Of course if your diet is already simple, which it is for a few people, then you can relax and enjoy it. But if it occupies anything more than a couple of hours a week in planning, then you are spending too much of your time on diet.

4. Give newness to your family and friends. Life, and love, are precious, and appreciating those around you is just as important as appreciating yourself. In appreciating them you don't have to serve them, but try to do something together, either for fun or to accomplish a task. Because you have loved ones, you have the opportunity to share with them those things in life that needs to be done.

5. Enjoy the moment. Perhaps you can't enjoy every minute of every day, but there are minutes in every day that you can enjoy. Your mind and your memory make it possible for you to enjoy what pleases you at any time you wish. You may need to make an effort at first, but by enjoying your moments each day you will be building your own satisfaction with life, and feeling better about yourself every day. Eventually you will see that you have more to cherish in life than life has problems to give you. Every one can find enjoyment in their lives, since they are not tied to accomplishments or money, but just to how you react to those things that come your way.

6 Natural Secrets to Feeling Good

Since you control how you feel for the most part, by your actions you can either make yourself feel good or feel bad. Often times you do things that are supposed to make you feel good, but end up making you feel bad, sore, and sick. These are some of the secrets we are going to look at. For the moment we will ignore the actions you might carry out that you know are bad for you, but you do them anyway because they make you feel good at the time (you know that we're talking about smoking, drinking, taking drugs, and just taking chances in general). But for now let's concentrate on what we are doing to ourselves in trying to make the transition to a healthy and perfect person, and why we are often hurting ourselves instead.

Secret 1. Stop over-exercising, because exercise doesn't have to be painful to be helpful. You get the benefits of exercise, and this means the heart and weight control benefits, by frequently exercising to the point of sweating and breathing hard. Now while you can do this through very vigorous exercises like jogging and mountain climbing, you can also get the same benefits by walking an equal amount of time at a 3-4 mile an hour rate. The slower you go the longer you should walk, but otherwise you will get the same lift as your muscles warm and your brain releases endorphins. Now if you really like to have a hard exercise, but you are often in pain doing it, and afterwards as well, then start pacing yourself. Have a hard exercise once a week, but then have lower impact exercises 2-4 more times a week. You will find that you are no longer sore and in pain, but that you feel as well or better than you did with the other program.

Secret 2. Learn to love fish and canola oil. What you want to do is get away from saturated fats and cholesterol as much as possible. Fish contains Omega-3 fatty acids that reduce fat levels in the blood, and canola oil is the lowest saturated fat oil on the market. Red meats, and even chicken, contain large amounts of saturated fat and cholesterol. You can't continue to eat these foods on any regular basis and keep your levels down. You could of course become a vegetarian, and everyone should be a vegetarian a few days a week anyway, but that isn't necessary. If you limit your servings of red meat to 3-4 ounces, no more than 3 or 4 times a week, and substitute fish and vegetables for the other meals you will get rid of most of the fats you don't want anyway.

Secret 3. Increase the fiber in your diet. Fiber has been shown to aid digestion, prevent constipation, and protects against colon cancer by keeping your digestive system working efficiently. If also helps in weight control because if lowers the calories absorbed from the foods we eat, as well as making foods move through us more rapidly. Good sources of fiber are potatoes, whole grains in any form (bread, muffins, or cereal), bran, vegetables, and fruits. Foods to avoid are meats, refined flower and sugar, and excess alcoholic drinks. For a treat try putting an ear of corn, in the husk, into your microwave oven for 5 minutes. This will give you a quick meal which is high in fiber, and can replace foods you want to avoid.

Secret 4. Use supplemental vitamins and minerals. You don't have to use supplements for your whole diet, although 1-a-day type might be a little insurance, but if you are not getting enough of any particular vitamin or mineral in your diet then start taking supplements. Remember that the governments recommended daily allowances for basic nutrients are insufficient for many things, even if you are healthy, and are too low for many if you have any special needs. The government sets minimum needs just high enough to prevent deficiency diseases, but that doesn't mean that your body has all of the nutrient that it needs. Diseases that take a long time to develop may be related to nutrient levels that do not cause immediate disease, but which still lead to deterioration of the body. Remember that the government level for vitamin C is only 60 milligrams per day, while medical research puts it as high as 3,000 milligrams a day. Just because a food has 100% of the minimum daily requirement of a nutrient, it may still lack the amount you need to stay healthy.

Secret 5. Learn to breathe deeply. Sounds simple enough, but many people go for years without exercising their bodies enough to take a deep breath. If you are one of these, then you should know that you are doing harm to yourself, and that is one of the reasons you do not feel as good as you should. Deep breathing puts oxygen into the blood, relieves stress, cuts feelings of fatigue, boosts your personal energy level, and helps your body to function more efficiently. Now while you can just stand in one place and take some deep breaths, this isn't good enough. You have to get out and move, and a vigorous walk is sufficient, and you have to move fast enough and long enough to increase your breathing and keep it deep for several minutes. Usually a 1/2 hour walk at a good walk will do the job. Any other exercise can also be used that gets your heart moving and your breathing going.

Secret 6. And this is a real secret, don't diet. To feel good, lose weight, and be healthy, you don't have to starve yourself. You will lose weight on a diet, but when you go off the diet you usually gain it all back plus some. What you need to do is redesign your eating habits so that you are eating the right foods. This will automatically cut out a lot of fats and calories from your diet, and you might even begin to lose some weight at this point. But you can't ignore the other half of the method. You have to get out and get some exercise, and you have to do it nearly every day. It doesn't have to strain every muscle in your body, and it shouldn't, but it should be regular and give you at least 3 hours of workout spread over 5 or 6 days every week. If you have the time, then do 2 or 3 times that amount. The 3 hours a week will benefit you, and it is just a survival rate. As you do more exercise you will feel like doing even more, and so on. As strange as it seems, inactivity is actually more painful than activity, and all that it takes is time.

8 Ways to Stop Negative Feelings
from Spoiling Your Day

To feel good sometimes you first have to stop feeling bad, and many times you feel bad because you are thinking negatively. Negative thoughts come up in the question of: is the glass half full or half empty? Those who see it as half full are positive thinkers, and those who see it as half empty are negative thinkers. If you are always seeing everything from the negative side, then there is no way that you are ever going to be happy. But all is not lost, if you read through our 8 ways to handle negative thoughts, you should be able to take care of any potentially negative situations that you come up against.

1. First we will deal with motivation by answering this question: which do you think is healthier, being a pessimist or being an optimist? Give up? Being a pessimist is less healthy than being positive, and it just means that you are negative about practically everything. Pessimists tend to get depressed more, since they always feel that the worst possible outcome is going to happen no matter what they do, and that also depresses the immune system. Because of that pessimists also get sick more often, and when they get sick they get sicker than optimists. On the other hand optimists have healthier immune systems, and will do more to take care of themselves if they do get sick since they expect to get well.

Optimists, since they have a better outlook on life, try harder to exercise, eat right, stop smoking, control drinking, and to have better and more satisfying relationships, all of which add to being healthier persons.

2. The next question has to do with the type of people you spend your time with, and whether they can influence your outlook on life: do you believe that the state of happiness or unhappiness of your companions can be passed over to you? The answer is that they can. Moods and outlooks on life can be caught from your companions, friends, and family just the same as a cold or the flu. This is fairly easy to prove, just think about the last time you were in a very sad situation, perhaps a funeral. It doesn't matter much if you knew the person well or not, you begin to feel sad and unhappy that they have died, and sympathetic to those most sad in attendance. Now think of a very happy situation, say walking around in Disneyland or some other amusement park, it is very hard to feel depressed when all those around you are in such a generally happy mood. If you are having problems with depression and unhappiness, then get in a happy crowd. If you don't have a happy crowd to get into, then rent some comedies and watch them, as well as read a joke book. Anything just to put yourself in a pleasant frame of mind, and you will soon find your whole outlook on life has improved. Happy people have just as many real world problems as you do, but they can handle much better just because they tend to have a good outlook on life, and spend time with others who feel the same way.

3. This question has to do with how you see other people and how you see yourself: do you see a difference between aggressiveness and assertiveness? If you have trouble finding the difference then you may have a clue as to your own unhappiness. Aggressiveness is an attempt to control others primarily through attitude and behavior. Overly aggressive people are viewed negatively by others because most of us do not want to be controlled by those we often feel has no right to exercise the power that they use. Assertiveness is related to aggressiveness only in that one person may be seen as exercising both behaviors at the same time. But assertiveness is actually a refusal to accept the power or opinions of others without being able to express your own feelings and thoughts. Assertive people will clash with aggressive people, but will generally get along very well with other assertive people. Aggressive people will fight most strongly against other aggressive people, and can never get along with them. If you are aggressive you will be truly disliked by others, but if you are only assertive then you should be able to get along with anyone who will allow you to participate in decision making processes.

4. This question has more to do with how we see others, and how we may think we should conduct ourselves to have warm and satisfying relationships: do you feel that going out of your way to make a good and positive impression on everyone you meet results in better and more satisfying personal relationships? Now we all know this type of person, he may be our best friend, or our boss, or just our neighbor, but are his relationships better because of this? These impressionables seem to get a good break in life, often, and to make friends easily, but does that translate into being a better and healthier person? Actually it does not.

The effort to make a good impression on everyone usually overlays a rather low level of personal confidence, as well as a lot of unresolved stress as to how to respond to others so as to show their true selves. In other words, the person who wants everyone as a friend is likely to be someone who has trouble relating to others as real individuals, and of differentiating real commitments in social relationships from superficial back-slapping exchanges such as politicians familiarly use to gain votes. You are better off, and more trustworthy if you give yourself and others time to get to know each other before making a commitment to friendship with anyone, and that goes for both men and women.

5. This next question has to do with your own attitude toward cleaning up your emotions: do you believe that blowing up and venting your anger will make you feel better? If you think so, then you are wrong. If you do give way to your anger you are just responding to your feelings, but it doesn't get rid of the pain you may feel. Look at anger as a chemical reaction in your body. Those chemicals are going to take time to go away when you get really angry, and the best way to get your body chemistry back the way it should be is to increase your activity level. This produces endorphins in the brain that will give you a feeling of peace and serenity. If your anger is especially intense it may take several days of walks and other exercise to get rid of it.

6. Now how to deal with those really close to you when a possible competitor comes around: if you get jealous of others should you show it? The answer is no, showing jealousy is more likely to make your relationship disintegrate than become stronger. Jealousy is a sign of insecurity and that what you really want to do is to control the person you say you love. To be jealous every time someone you think is better looking or more intelligent comes into a room simply shows that you do not believe in yourself, and others, no matter how much you say you love them, are going to distance themselves from you if it happens all of the time.

7. Now about things, and who has them: do you feel that envy is a sign that others have things you respect and wish to have for yourself? In this case this is true. You only envy what you want to possess, and that goes for accomplishments, property, money, or self esteem. You should never treat envy as a destructive force just because it does not make you feel good. Envy can be constructive if it tells you that you need to change the direction of your life so that you have a chance of obtaining those things that you feel envious of.

8. On maleness we want to find out how you feel you should consider others in order to show your true sexuality: is it true that a real man, testosterone rich male, is more likely to express himself as tolerant of the sexual threats of others than a male who is less assertive? Actually no, the stronger a male feels the need to follow a strong sex role model the more likely he is to express jealousy and a lack of self assurance in the modern world. If you are this way then reform, and if your companion acts this way, then you will never be on an equal footing with him in your dealings with the world.

For a Long Healthy Life Find Some Friends

You can't go it alone, either in life or in health. Good health, like a happy life requires that you have close family and friends around you every day. Those polls about single men and women really say the same thing, only they confuse you more than inform you. Both single men and women have more trouble with their health when they are alone, only single women have an easier time getting close to their friends, and men don't let their guard down fully except with their families.

The best companions for a healthy life are close family members and good friends. If none of your family is living close to you, or if you are not on good terms with them, then you need good friends. Actually you have got to have good friends if you want to live healthily and happily.

You have to have people close to you to be healthy because joy, grief and setbacks in life have to be expressed to others around us. No culture anywhere isolates anyone except to kill them. If someone is cut out of the fellowship of others, then they are invited to go away and die, and no one would know. Unfortunately the same thing happens when we cut ourselves off from family and friends.

People who are alone are sick more often and die sooner. They also are sick and depressed more often than a person who has someone close to them who they can express their feeling to. Just think of it, a girlfriend (or boyfriend) has just left you and you have no one to talk to. Your feelings are hurt, and all that you can think of to do is abuse yourself with drink or food. Do you think that this will make you healthier, that's doubtful. More likely you will trigger something off in your body that will make you really sick before you will be able to adjust to the loss and find someone else.

Consider the same thing when you have someone around you who you like and trust. What do you do? You go and talk to them about it over and over until you get bored with it. In the meantime you are looking around yourself and eventually you find that there are others lovers out there, and you can survive. When it is a death the loss is much more permanent, but you can still find that there is a reason for living—whether it is to help yourself or to help others. The point is that any time something happens and you don't have anyone to confide in, then you end up holding in the pain, and the pain causes your body to changes in ways that are going to make you sick, and may even kill you.

FERTILITY

Turning Back the Clock
for Successful Pregnancies

Women over the age of 40 lose more pregnancies to miscarriage than do younger women. In fact every woman over this age knows she is taking a chance with her baby's life when she gets pregnant. Nevertheless, many women in this older age group would very much like to have children, and have long needed a means of doing so which would cut their risks of losing the baby.

The one method that has been developed so far that turns back the clock is in vitro fertilization, or IVF. A USC study of 65 women between the ages of 45 and 55 was able to achieve 32 pregnancies with only 5 miscarriages. These were women who could no longer produce fertilizable eggs, and donated eggs from fertile women were used. The sperm was from the women's husbands, and of course the women themselves supplied the uterus.

The results were exciting because the donated eggs produced babies more often then when the older women's' own eggs were used, and the numbers of successful pregnancies were more like those of women years younger than the test group. The conclusion reached by the researchers was that if you are an older woman and want to have a successful IVF baby, you increase your chances significantly by using eggs from a younger fertile woman. The effect of using sperm from a younger man was not tested.

FEVER

When is a Fever Not a Fever?

When ever you have a fever you are sick—or are you? Sometimes your body temperature can vary by a degree or two from its normal 98.6 degrees, and not mean that you are ill. Even without doing anything else, or having any illness, your body temperature will be lower in the morning by maybe a degree. As people get older their body temperature will go down to perhaps 95 degrees, but be perfectly normal for them. Also if you are exercising, or if a women is ovulating, the body temperature will rise a degree or two. So body temperature fluctuations which are small, and without other symptoms, can be safely counted at normal situations which do not require medication.

But just how much variation can you put up with in your temperature before you can say you are sick? A little more than you probably think. A University of Maryland study of 148 men and women found a normal temperature range of 96 degrees to 100.8 degrees. The average was 98.2 degrees, but the most common measured temperature was 98 degrees. This means that you can have a temperature of 100 degrees and not be sick at all, or one as low as 96 degrees with the same conclusion. It also means that you can feel hot and flushed, or cool and chilled, sometimes and it means nothing. Your body will do everything it can to maintain the temperature of your brain and vital internal organs, and that includes sacrificing the external circulation that you measure. That is why you get a range of temperatures with thermometers, your body is either trying to get rid of extra internal heat, or trying to conserve the internal heat to bring up the temperature inside your body by a degree or two.

One area that you need to watch out for though is that of night sweats. If you seem to only sweat, and run a temperature, at night, but feel normal in the daytime, it can never the less be a sign of serious disease. Any time you develop a pattern of night sweats which lasts for more than a week you should see your doctor for a screening. If he is a good doctor he will take your concern seriously, and give you a proper screening to see if anything is wrong. Night sweats do not always mean that you have something serious, but many times that is the only way your body will show you that something is wrong and must be dealt with.

FOOD POISONING

81 Million Americans Suffer Each Year
What to Watch Out For

How many times have you had food poisoning over the last two or three years, one, two, ten? You can have food poisoning many times without even knowing it because most of the time you won't get sick enough to go to the doctor or the hospital—of course those cases are put in the statistics, but probably not those of you or your family. Food poisoning is so common that about one out of every three Americans will get sick with it each year.

How can you avoid food poisoning? You can't completely, but you can cut down the chance that you will get it if you watch out for certain foods and pay attention to what you eat. The food poisoning that causes most of the cases comes from <u>chickens</u>, <u>eggs</u>, and <u>beef</u>. These cause a lot of poisoning because they are very good for the common organisms that cause food poisoning to grow on—salmonella bacteria. Anytime you eat any of these foods make sure they are fresh, and that they have been well cooked if you want the best insurance that they will not make you sick.

If you like raw <u>milk</u> then you are always taking a chance, and you can't avoid it completely. Find a raw milk supplier you trust and stay with them, at least you will know who to blame if you do get sick.

<u>Pork</u> carries a parasite called trichinosis, which is a little worm. In spite of all of the meat inspections and controls in this country, American pork still has trichinosis, and any time you eat pork which is not well cooked you run the risk of getting a live dose of this worm. An extra special warning on pork is that a few people in the United States die of trichinosis poisoning each year, so don't fool around with raw pork at any time. Also wash your hands after anytime you handle raw pork or chicken because you can get poisoned this way too.

Finally, watch your <u>canned goods</u>. Everyone has canned foods in their house that have sat around for years, and at some time or another you may decide to eat. Anytime you take a canned good out to open, and this includes new ones as well as old ones, if the top is pushed out it is bad—don't use it. Also if you open a can and hear a little rush of gas, although you sometimes get this in newly canned foods too. If you even think something might be spoiled, then smell it before you eat it since bad canned goods usually smell strangely as well. These precautions also include any canned foods that have become rusty.

Why be so careful around canned foods? The gas you hear, or that pouches out the can tops, comes from gas producing bacteria—the most common of which is botulism. Even a small dose of botulism can kill or cause permanent disablement. With a little care you won't be one of the 81 million sufferers of food poisoning in the United States this year, or in any year.

10 Causes and Symptoms of Food Poisoning

If you have food poisoning and would like to know why, this list will give you a handy guide to finding the cause so you can decide what to do about it. The list starts with the most common and goes to the least common, and gives some easy tips to see where you got your dose. The basic way of telling if you have food poisoning is if you get an upset stomach after eating, along with the added threat of vomiting and diarrhea. But different causes add different symptoms to the list, and can call for different treatments to suffer the attacks in most comfortable manner.

1. Salmonella: this will attack you from 6 hours to 3 days after a meal. It is probably the most common cause of food poisoning, but is usually the least

serious, except in babies, small children, and people who are ill or poorly nourished. The symptoms are nausea, vomiting, diarrhea, cramps, fever, and headache, and it usually lasts no more than a day or two.

2. Staphylococcus: attack is from 1/2 hour to about 8 hours after a meal, and it is the second most common cause of food poisoning. While it can be much more serious than salmonella poisoning, it is not usually so. The usual symptoms are vomiting and diarrhea, and occasionally there is weakness and dizziness.

3. Hepatitis A: the attack is from 15 to 50 days after eating, so you may never know where you got it. It is pretty common, and can be very serious for some people. The symptoms are fever, nausea, abdominal pain, loss of appetite, and after 3 to 10 days you may turn yellow with jaundice and have dark urine.

4. Campylobacter: the attack takes place 2 to 10 days after eating. This form of food poisoning can cause some scary symptoms so you should probably get it checked out by a doctor if you see them. Symptoms are the usual muscle pain, nausea, vomiting, fever and cramps, but occasionally also a bloody diarrhea that might be mistaken for cancer if you don't expect it.

5. Clostridium perfringens: this is a common cause of food poisoning that attacks you 9 to 15 hours after eating. The symptoms are common, consisting of diarrhea and cramps, and will probably be mistaken for something else, but that is not important since they will probably stop before any medication you take could be of help.

6. Norwalk virus: while you don't run across this name every day, it is a common source of food poisoning. It attacks 1 to 2 days after eating, and the symptoms are the usual nausea, vomiting, and diarrhea, but with the added risk of headache.

7. Scombroid poisoning: this is a rather uncommon source of food poisoning, but you should have an easy time of deciding whether or not this is what is making you sick. The attack happens anywhere from 5 minutes to one hour after eating, and has symptoms we haven't seen before. Along with the abdominal pain, vomiting, and diarrhea seen in other causes, this one also has facial flushing, headache, dizziness, a burning sensation in the throat, and hives. If these symptoms come on right after eating you can be pretty certain that you have food poisoning and not some form of heat rash or measles.

8. Botulism: this is certainly one of the most serious forms of food poisoning since a drop or two of botulism can kill a person, but it is rare and that is good. Symptoms develop from 12 to 48 hours after eating, but it can take up to 8 days before a person knows they are sick. The symptoms are pretty much like the other causes of food poisoning; abdominal pain, diarrhea, vomiting, and nausea, but there will also be double vision, and difficulty speaking, breathing and swallowing. If you have been in a group where any member comes down with these symptoms go to the doctor immediately, because once you have developed all of the symptoms it will be much more difficult to treat you.

9. Listeria: this is also a rare form of food poisoning, but one which can

be very serious in some people. The attack comes on from 2 to 4 weeks after eating, and the basic symptoms are just flu-like with fever and chills. The real danger is if very sick people get it, or newborn children, or pregnant women. Listeria can cause spontaneous abortions and stillbirths to women, as well as death to those other people who are not too well.

10. Trichinosis: luckily this is also rare, but can be very serious if you get a heavy dose. Symptoms come on in 1 to 2 days after eating, and consist of fever, edema, and muscle pain. Trichinosis comes almost entirely from under-cooked pork, in the American diet, and all pork must be assumed to be infected even though only a small amount actually is. The fact is that even though there are controls and inspections for meat everywhere in our country, pork still has trichinosis. Other sources of trichinosis are game animals like bear and deer, so hunters also have to be careful about eating or handling any game they may kill. Trichinosis kills a few people in our country each year, and it is because they are not careful how they handle their food, or eat meats which are undercooked.

How to Avoid
The 7 Most Common Types of Food Poisoning

Food poisoning is not rare, in fact it is so common that 65% of raw meat and poultry are known to carry salmonella and campylobacter, which are both common causes of illness. With the expectation that you will come into contact with foods that can make you sick nearly every day, what precautions can you take so that you won't be getting food poisoning all of the time? Here are the major food classes that make people sick, and what you can do to make them safe.

1. Raw meat, poultry, eggs, raw dairy products, fish, and untreated water; basically cook everything thoroughly. Always wash your hands and the surfaces you work on after food preparation since a dirty kitchen area can contaminate other foods hours later, and to be especially safe never eat unpasturized dairy foods or drink untreated water. Water doesn't have to look cloudy or smell bad to carry bacteria or pesticides.

2. Cooked meat and poultry; never let these foods sit around at room temperature for hours before serving. Keep them above 140 degrees until served, and if you do let them cool then refrigerate and reheat thoroughly before serving. Hard boiled eggs can pick up bacteria through their shells, and if they are are not completely cooked in boiling they may keep the salmonella that most of them are contaminated with when they are laid.

3. Raw shellfish, and any foods handled by people who have handled raw meat or milk products; raw shellfish is best avoided since you cannot tell when it

is carrying bacteria. Also shellfish can harbor things like DDT and lead because it feeds on the bottom of the ocean, so it is best not to go out and gather your own shellfish even if you are going to cook it. Commercial shellfish is collected in clean areas and is inspected for poisons. Also don't eat anything prepared by dirty food handlers, there is no way of cleaning it after it has been prepared and then contaminated. It is better to skip part of a meal than end up sick for 2 or 3 because you were hungry or were trying to be polite.

4. <u>Mackerel, tuna, and bonito</u>; these favorite game fish are often found in the fish market, and fishermen frequently bring home more than they can use and give some away to neighbors. Only eat these fish if you are sure they are fresh, if they have a peppery taste there is something wrong and you should stop eating it.

5. <u>Spoiled canned goods and honey</u>; these are all foods that can carry botulism, which can kill. Even fresh honey is known to have a trace of botulism. While it will not hurt an adult, infants have been made sick by honey, and occasionally have died from it. Canned goods are another story, no one should eat anything that has been improperly canned, comes out of a damaged or rusted can, or from a can that has developed gas so that the top pushes out. Botulism is a gas producing organism, so if a can has gas in it, it is a good bet that it has botulism too.

6. <u>Raw milk, cheese made from raw milk, and processed meats</u>; these are especially dangerous to pregnant women. Raw milk can carry salmonella or typhoid fever, and cheese made from raw milk can have the same things. Recently there were several deaths from contaminated cheese, and it was not even claimed that the cheese was made from raw milk, but cheeses and milks we think are safe could be one of the main causes of food poisoning each year.

7. <u>Pork</u>; pork gets its own category because it is the only thing in the supermarket that carries trichinosis, and anyone who eats undercooked pork is going to get to know this little worm much too well. To be safe always cook pork and pork products, like sausage, thoroughly—and to a temperature of 160 degrees.

What To Do for a Poison Free Picnic

Many cases of food poisoning start in the picnic basket. Picnic food is often precooked, and then taken unrefrigerated to the picnic site, where it may sit a few more hours before being eaten. It is the unrefrigerated, raw or precooked, food that is most likely to make you sick. A few hours of normal temperatures are enough for many foods that left our homes safe to eat to become poison packages that will make you sick for days. Picnic foods should always leave the home in a cooler, and should be kept cool until the food is eaten or cooked to be eaten.

If the car is hot then take the cooler out and set it in the shade, or at least put the cooler in the passenger area of the car rather than the trunk because the passenger area at least has some ventilation and will be a little cooler.

If you do bring raw meats, poultry, or fish on a picnic put it in a separate cooler from other foods. Most of these fresh meats and things carry contaminates that must be killed in cooking, even if they have been frozen since purchase. They also tend to have juices that can run onto, and contaminate, other foods that are otherwise clean. When you prepare these raw foods you can also pick up contamination on your hands or cooking utensils, so keep food preparation areas separate, and wash up everything afterwards, as well as your hands before handling or serving any food.

Mayonnaise is feared by so many people as a picnic poisoner that you may be surprised to learn that you have nothing to fear from mayonnaise. Mayonnaise is made from eggs, which is a perfect place to grow bacteria, but it is also made very acidic so that bacteria cannot grow. Mayonnaise in potato salad will help to keep the eggs in it from growing organisms that will make you sick. So, while you have nothing to fear from mayonnaise itself, it is still a good idea to keep the things it is mixed into chilled since mayonnaise does not guarantee that nothing poisonous can grow in anything it is used in.

Finally, if you have left over prepared foods, meats, chicken, potato salad, beans, whatever, put them back into a cooler as soon as possible after the meal, or some of the picnickers may be visited by the food poison princess after the picnic rather than during it. Some of these foods, and you can't tell which in advance, can become poisonous in just a couple of hours if left unrefrigerated. Put everything that was freshly prepared back into coolers, and keep them refrigerated until they are eaten.

FOOT PROBLEMS

The Common Way to Relieve Foot Pain
That Doctors Overlook

Your feet have been hurting and all that you can stand is to soak them, and put them up at night. You've given up what little activity you were doing on the weekend because you just can't stand to get up and walk around on those painful feet after a hard day at work. So what does your doctor tell you? Pretty much nothing, since you are already doing the basic therapy that you will get most of the time for painful feet, although your doctor might also tell you to take aspirin, or some other pain reliever.

But what has your doctor overlooked? The main thing he has overlooked is that your tired and painful feet are probably the result of poor circulation, and have nothing to do with disease or damage to your feet. Of course if you keep treating them long enough like they were objects of disease, pretty soon they will not want to work at all, and then your feet will really be in the condition that you think they are now.

While you might really get a problem that will cause your feet to be painful, like planter's warts, most of the time it is just poor circulation. Don't think that just because your heart is beating your circulation is just fine in all parts of your body. Our bodies work to make sure that the circulation to our internal organs is constant and in good shape, but the circulation to our hands, arms, legs, and feet might get cut off in the process.

Why do you think that your feet get cold on a cold winter day? It is because your body has cut the blood flow to your feet in order to keep the temperature of your brain nice and warm. Your feet are expendable since you can live without them, and that is also the reason that you can get frostbitten feet, but never a frostbitten brain.

But, back to your painful feet. Most of the time your feet hurt because you have been standing around on them all day cutting off their circulation. To get them healthy again you need to go out and take a walk or a jog. That is all it takes, and I will bet that you don't hear that very often from your doctor. Actually, any exercise is good, but you have to do exercise that gets your heart beating faster and your blood moving through all parts of your body. While I won't bother giving you a run down of all the good things that a 1/2 hour walk each day will do for you, just note that in most cases it will take care of your painful feet.

Type of Shoes to Prevent Corns, Bunions, and Hammertoes

Most of the problems you may have with your feet are caused by the type of shoes you wear. If you wear shoes that are too small you are going to have a problem with hammertoes or corns. The ends of your feet are pushed up against the top of your shoes. The distortion of your feet will also cause bunions because they will not lie comfortably flat in the shoe.

All of these problems come from buying shoes made in Asia, but which carry American sizes. An American made size 6-B might equal an Asian made size 6-D. Instead of going into a shoe store and buying something that has your size written on it, you need to fit your feet to the type of shoes being sold. A study at the University of Southern California has found that 90% of American women have this habit of wearing shoes that are too small, and that 76% have foot problems from it, so you are not alone.

To solve your foot problems start wearing the more comfortable athletic shoes if you can. If that isn't possible, then at least buy soft leathers and low heals, and always have your shoes fitted or try them on for a few minutes when you buy them.

GALLSTONES

Dangerous New Surgery for Gallbladder Removal that Can Increase Your Chance of Serious Injury

If you haven't had surgery in the past few years you might be very surprised at the microsurgery revolution that has taken place. Microsurgery has been done on knees, hearts, and brains, and now it is being done on the gallbladder. And don't get me wrong, microsurgery has many advantages over the old techniques. The same repairs are done, but the damage to your body is less, and you are able to return to normal activity much sooner. At least that is true when it is done right. But when it is done wrong, it can be just as devastating as any other botched operation.

And that is where we come in looking at a new surgical technique for gallbladder removal. They call the surgery minimal access surgery, and the gallbladder is removed through a cut that is less than one inch long. The official name of the surgery is laparoscopic cholescystectomy, and in it the surgeons make four holes in your abdomen. They then put in little tubes which are used to light the area that they are operating on, and which contain the surgical tools they need. They even have a little television camera on one of them, and the television picture they get is what tells them where to operate.

The problem comes when surgeons are just starting to use this procedure. When they go in to remove the gallbladder they have to cut what is called a bile duct, which attaches to the gallbladder. However, near the bile duct is another one which is connected to the liver, and which they do not want to cut. This is the cystic duct, and if it is cut or damaged by accident you can die. Other complications include pain and infection, and it is these last two that you are more likely to have. However, the two ducts look very much alike, and damage to your cystic duct is not something to be taken lightly.

The doctors who usually have this kind of accident, cutting or nicking the cystic duct, are the ones who are just starting to use the procedure. After a doctor has performed 25, or 100, of these operations he no longer has any problem in deciding what must be cut and what must be let alone.

So how do you protect yourself from this kind of accident? Find yourself a surgeon who has done as many of these as possible. Never entrust yourself to a surgeon who is in his first 2, or 10, or 20, laparoscopic cholecystectomys. This will minimize the risk you have that you will be one of your doctor's early mistakes. Of course you can never remove all of the risk of accidents like this, but finding the best experienced, and most successful surgeon you can will be a huge step in the right direction.

NOTES

_____

_____

_____

_____

_____

_____

_____

GOUT

Isn't Gout Extinct?
Then Why Have I Got It?

Actually gout is just one of those diseases that were popular in some of the older movies. As a disease gout is doing very well in inflicting pain on people in the 90's every day. Gout is a very real disease, if you don't have it, it can attack almost anyone, although most victims are between the ages of 40 and 60. While gout can be inherited, it can also be caused by overeating, drinking alcohol, dieting, and joint injury or surgery.

Of course knowing what can bring on an attack of gout doesn't tell you what actually causes it, and the cause is something we produce in our own bodies. Uric acid, which is produced and should be eliminated from our bodies, if it isn't eliminated it can build up in the joints and cause gout. The uric acid comes from our body's breakdown of such foods as coffee and chicken which contain purines. When this uric acid doesn't leave our body as it should it can crystallize in the joints and cause reddening, swelling and tenderness. The big toe is often one of the first places gout will develop because circulation through that part of your body isn't as good as through other parts, but you can get it in any joint.

Once you get an attack you need to get it treated or you can get more attacks, and even permanent damage to the joint. Treatment is a problem because there is no real cure. For this reason you have got to use prevention if you have a history of gout either personally or in your family. The best preventive methods in those cases are to avoid alcohol, cut down on fatty foods, and cut down on such foods as chicken that contain purines and raise uric acid levels.

Treatment that is available includes medication and a proper diet. Medication can be had for pain and inflammation, but that is about all that you can expect so far as effective treatment for this condition.

Simple Plan that Get the Gout Causers Out of Your Diet

The basic cause of gout is a build-up of uric acid crystals in your joints. The uric acid comes from the proteins you eat, and is one of the digestive products your body produces. If you want to get rid of gout you have to get rid of some

---

of the protein, to cut down the amount of uric acid in your body, and eat some foods that will help your body to get well.

First, to cut down on the protein, cut way back on the amount you eat of red meat, organ meats, fish, shellfish, asparagus, cauliflower, mushrooms, spinach, beans and peas. Some of these are not high protein foods, but they do contribute to the acid crystals in your blood.

Now increase the amount you eat of fiber, green leafy vegetables, celery, and parsley. To get more vitamins, since you are losing a lot by cutting out all of the protein foods and some vegetables, take vitamin C, magnesium, zinc, raw vegetables, fruit and vegetable juices. From your back yard, or a health food store, you can use dandelion root or leaf, and nettle tea.

GRIEF

Steps to Dealing With Grief

Grief is the loss of a loved one, family or friend. We often grieve over pets or the loss of personal property, like our home, and the process of getting through and getting over it is the same. Dealing with grief does not mean forgetting what we have lost, it is just what we have to go through so that we can go back to living in the world. Grieving is a process that takes time, as much as a year if someone close to you has died, but as little as a few days or weeks for more distant friends or relatives. Following these 9 steps will give you a plan to follow to help you survive your grief, and a guide when you just don't know what to do next to get through the day. Grief often makes it impossible for us to think clearly until we start to emerge from under its cloud.

1. Anticipating grief can be a very important step in surviving it as a whole person. If someone close to you is expected to die soon, you can be supportive of them, as well as a companion in carrying out their wishes. This is very important because the first expression of grief that you are likely to experience is the sense that you should have done something for the person who has just died: you should have been nicer to them, or visited them more often, or given them some little gift that they have long wanted. The inability to do that after they have gone produces an overwhelming guilt many times, that runs through the whole grieving process.

The other side of anticipating grief is to dispel the fear you may have at the impending loss of someone. You may fear the loss of their companionship, or death itself and the closeness to it that someones death brings you, or that you will be unable to cope with the world afterwards. By making some plans as to how to handle the loss

---

and what to do afterwards can bring both them and you peace of mind.

If the person who is dying is very old, or has been very ill, the anticipation of death often does not seem so frightening. However, you should still plan because a personal loss always leaves a hole in your life.

2. Share your anticipation with someone close to you. This can be a close friend, spouse, or children in some cases. You want to do this sharing with others who are going to be directly affected, and have them help you to plan your part in the loss and what you are going to do afterwards. Without sharing these important people you may have the entire responsibility thrust upon you, or you may be cut out of any part in taking care of things afterwards.

If the loss will be of someone to whom you have direct responsibilities, then talk over disposal of the body and distribution of the property. If there is a will, then when and where should it be read, and who should be executor if no one is named in the will. Don't try to do these things alone because it will just end up with problems and emotional upset. Even close relatives who have become distant will usually unite if a parent, brother, or sister is dying. The loss of a home often results in a close relative offering help which is unavailable otherwise. Get everyone closely involved into the discussion if you can. And if you can't, then at least get one close family member to cooperate with you to go over all of the details of what has to be done and how, in order to adjust physically to the loss.

3. Prepare yourself to grieve in advance. Losses come in many shapes and sizes, and they all require some of the same processes to get over them, and grieving is just the process of getting over a loss. While getting over the death of a close friend or relative is much more serious than getting over the loss of a raise, they do bring up some of the same emotions. The common emotions that we feel in grieving are rage, anger, guilt, impatience, and finally acceptance of the loss.

By consciously learning how to deal with these emotions in less serious situations we can learn how to deal with them in the most serious ones. And because minor losses are so much of the daily life of people, you can constantly practice how to handle major losses.

This works best if you are anticipating a loss, but it can also be helpful even if you do not think anyone close to you will die or have a major tragedy. Loss, and grief, are just proportional to what we lose and how we lose it. Unfortunately too many times we are overcome by our losses and unable to handle them at all, but that is usually because we never think of what we should be doing when losses occur, and they do to everyone.

If you can't handle a minor loss on your own, then you should not expect to handle a major one without help. But if you can take care of things without going into dangerous depressions every time some bad happens to you, then you will probably be fine if there is a major catastrophe in your life.

In spite of the violence in America, most people still die as a result of diseases. And most deaths by disease do not happen without some sort of warning.

People usually die because they are sick, or have not taken care of their bodies, and are at a risk of death at any time. Because most of us have a family member or friend who is in this kind of a threatened condition, we should always be aware that death can occur around us at any time, and that it could be of someone we care about.

In spite of that it is still good to remember that even though someone we know may die at any time, they will probably not die when we think they will. Death is unpredictable most of the time. So plan and prepare, but don't look at everyone you know, even if they are seriously ill, as if you think they will die tomorrow.

4. The stages of dying have been discussed in several books, and they can give you guidelines to how your feelings are going to run when you do have a loss. These stages are the result of the chemistry of your body, and they do not have anything to do with whether or not you are a good person, or have prepared for the loss of someone close to you. Humans, and probably animals as well, react to loss by going through feelings that have nothing to do with our intelligence, wealth, or fame. It doesn't matter who we are, we are going to feel these feelings, and have to deal with them. If you don't know what they are and run into them, as everyone does, then you may be overwhelmed and end up in a dangerous state of depression yourself. If you do at least know what they are, then even as you are going through them you will at least know how what you are feeling fits into the stages of getting through a close personal loss.

The stage of dying, and of grief, are denial, anger, bargaining, depression, and acceptance. These 5 stages are felt by people who are told they are dying, and also by those who experience a loss. Denial is just the unwillingness to believe that our life, or of our loved ones, is over. Anger is a defense, the same as what we feel when we are attacked, except that it cannot overcome the loss. Bargaining is a logical process of trying to buy our way out of the loss we know we are going to have to face. Depression is the realization that we cannot bargain our way out, and is really just a complete physical and emotional collapse. Acceptance is the emergence from depression, and is the final step to recovery and adjustment. How well, and how soon, you come through these stages depends upon how well you can follow the other steps of the grief process that are given here. No matter what you do you will still go through the 5 steps, only you can go through them more quickly and in better shape if you prepare yourself well, and do the most you can in advance.

5. Don't be afraid, or ashamed, of how you feel. The feelings you are having, and you are going to have, are what everyone feels. Your feelings are part of your humanity. They have to do with your ability to love and relate to others, and are nothing to be ashamed of. If you did not go through the emotional states of grieving, and dying, you would not be able to adjust to your loss, or to going on without the support of the one who has died.

Accepting your feelings as real and appropriate means that you will not be afraid to discuss them with persons close to you, or to fully express how you feel at any given time. At funerals these feelings often come out as inappropriate laughter, but that is just the result of being in the most stressful situation you can be in when someone close to you has died. Laughing at a funeral you are part of is not a sign of disrespect, but a sign of how deeply you feel and how much you want to fulfill your role in laying that person to rest.

To express your feelings it is probably best if you can talk freely and openly about them as you wish. If that is a problem, you are still going to have the feelings, and the need to resolve them. If there is no one else to talk to, than talk to yourself. Write them down, put them on a tape recorder, or just go to a mountain top and yell out how unfair and evil it is that your loved one has died. This is an absolute necessary part of grieving, and should not be looked on as weakness or indifference to loss, but as a supreme expression of grief on the road to self-adjustment to loss.

6. If you feel like crying, then do it. Crying is an open expression of grief, or pain, or happiness, or sorrow for everyone at some time. Crying is a complete surrender of yourself to emotional expression. When you are crying you are signaling to everyone else how badly you feel, and everyone will accept it as a deep sign of affection and respect for someone who has died.

When you have finished your crying, and it can go on for a few minutes or several days, you will feel clean and cleansed of the greatest depths of your grief. You will still remember and still grieve, and you may cry again, but you will have given yourself over fully to the process of getting through the grief.

Crying is one of those things humans do, that is like the purring that cats do, we know what it expresses but we don't really know why it is done. Perhaps it is just a pure expression of your emotional state. Crying happens more for most of us in situations of love or tenderness than of grief, but it always expresses the same thing. It shows that we have accepted the emotions we have, and that there are no words or thoughts that can solve our feeling better than giving over to them in a period of crying.

7. Go to your social support system for strength. It really doesn't matter very much what these people do, you need them around you in times of grief. Social support networks are the family members and friends who we depend upon to express ourselves. A distant family member or a friend we had not seen in 10 years is not of much use as a support for your emotions. But everyone you have come to depend upon in times of both joy and grief will give you the support you need when the situation is most desperate to you.

Social support systems are usually made up of people you see every day, or at least very often. They are the ones you trust when you have a real problem, and those to whom you turn when you have a real triumph. The expression of joy in your support system is just as the sympathy you get in times of grief. Joy and triumph will usually bring resentment in strangers, but feelings of congratulations and acceptance in friends and family. Those who will pull for you in any crisis will certainly try to help you in any way that you need in times of trial.

To make use of your social support system at a time of grief, just get them around you. Spend time with them, whether or not you can express your grief openly, but be in their presence anyway. These people will not reject you if you show anger over a loss, nor will they go to your depths of depression when you have given up hope that one who has died will come back to you. They will just be there, and by their presence they will lend you their strength without condemning you for needing it. Everyone needs others at some time in their lives, and especially at times of grief and personal loss.

8. Eat right to overcome grief. Too much caffeine, or too much alcohol, when you are in the process of grieving will just add to how bad you feel rather than help you get over it. Grief is also an appetite killer, but it does not stop the processes your body uses to keep you alive and healthy. An extended period of grieving, with a poor appetite, can leave you with malnutrition that can add to your own physical problems, and an even greater state of depression.

You do not necessarily have to eat the same way you do normally, but when you are grieving you still need to make certain that you have a nutritious and well balanced diet. It would be best if someone else looked after your eating habits in such a time. But those people around you who would be best able to do so are also going to be grieving, and will be busy looking after their own diets.

Take a few minutes out and plan a good diet for yourself. Not a heavy diet and not a light one, but one which is well balanced and which will be good for you. Diets can always be changed, but having a poor diet at a time of grief can only add to the time you will feel bad, and the length of time before you can really begin to take command of your life again.

9. Rest sufficiently so that you are not exhausted all of the time, but not so much that you spend all of your time in bed. Years ago a grieving woman was expected to go to her bed and be waited on for weeks, when she would have recovered. Now there is nobody to wait on us, and it is our own responsibility whether or not, or how well, we recover from the tragedies that overcome us.

If you do not feel like sleeping at your normal bedtime, don't resort to sleeping pills or you will just end up drugged and dependent for a long time. Instead do something, anything, to take your mind off of your grief, and rest. Read or watch television, or maybe lie in bed and talk to someone close to you. If you have trouble resting for a full night because of your grief than lie down for a couple of hours at a time several times a day. Don't try to push your body even if there is much to do as a result of someone dying. Everything takes time, and taking care of the affairs of a missing relative can take months to resolve.

Rest is more than just sleeping, so don't worry if you don't seem to sleep very much for a while. At least relax and give up the duties of the day for a time. If nothing seems to work, and you really feel that you need a sleeping aid, then talk to your doctor before you start depending upon one. If you are under the care of a doctor, he can monitor you and take you off of it when you no longer have the need.

Above all remember that grief takes time to get over, and no one gets over the grief of a close, loved one in just a few days. If you are grieving deeply then give yourself at least a year before looking into getting professional help. A group support system may help sooner, but a social support system made up of close friends and relatives is better, In any case don't try to do it alone. You are a social person, and you must have those around you whom you trust and who love you to get through the trauma of grief.

GUM DISEASE

A Natural Way of Curing Gum Disease With No Side Effects

Gum disease is caused by the build-up of bacteria on the teeth. It is now known that there is a natural ingredient in the Aloe vera plant that can kill this disease-causing bacteria, and has no side effects. This extract is still being studied, but you should ask your dentist if it is available. The beauty of this treatment is that it is applied by simply squirting it on the teeth.

If you still need a way of handling gum disease at home, you can simply eat a piece of cheddar cheese after meals. This type of cheese is able to neutralize the acids in your mouth that cause gum disease.

2 Ways to Prevent, or Get Rid of Gum Disease

Gum disease is very insidious, it just sneaks up on us and we aren't even aware of it until our gums start bleeding, or our teeth start falling out. Of course by then it may be too late to save all of your teeth, and gum disease can let a lot of other more serious disease get started. Now we start getting warnings about gum disease as soon as we start going to the dentist. But it seems that most Americans don't bother listening to their dentists since 75% of the people over age 35 have disease gums, and by age 60, 40% of us have lost teeth as a result of gum disease.

Now if you weren't aware that the numbers were so large, that is probably only because no one is going to come up to you and say, "hey, I just lost a molar because my gums are rotten." That just isn't done, and you are more likely to hear about their hernia operation than tooth loss because they hadn't bothered brushing their teeth for a few years.

Of course that is no excuse for you not to take care of your teeth. The dentist ways of preventing gum disease are brush your teeth after every meal, floss once a day, see your dentist twice a year, and avoid sweets. While this will prevent much gum disease, it ignores the nutritional aspects of prevention. Healthy gums come from a healthy diet, and your healthy diet must contain those nutrients that the gums need especially. Did you know, for instance, that the skin in your mouth, including your gums, is some of the fastest growing skin in your body. That means that the gums need the nutrients required to grow and replace themselves at a much higher level than areas of the body that grow very slowly, and therefore only need repair nutrients.

There are 3 vitamins that are especially concerned with healthy gums and teeth. The first is calcium (remember that the teeth are mainly calcium and that they are embedded in bone that is also largely calcium). Women of childbearing age are especially susceptible to low calcium levels since a growing fetus will take its calcium needs from its mother. And after menopause calcium is taken from a woman's bones and teeth because of her loss of estrogen.

The second necessary nutrient for healthy teeth and gums is vitamin D, the sunshine vitamin. Vitamin D is necessary for the body to use the calcium it receives. The best sources of vitamin D are either through exposure of the skin to the sun, as a bone meal supplement, or in milk where it has been added to complement the calcium.

The third vital nutrient, and why it is vital is not well known, is the B vitamin folate. Folate helps to control gum disease after you have gotten it, and it is a good supplement if foods high in folate are not on your regular menu. While you are at it you might as well add vitamin C, since high doses of vitamin C are also helpful in healing.

That is the basic list of nutrients to complement the dentists list of preventive actions you need to take to prevent gum disease, or to cure it after you have gotten it.

HAIR PROBLEMS

Dull Gray Hair

Here's How to Make it Shine

If you have gray hair you can color it or leave it natural. But how do you go about giving it a nice, healthy shine so that it looks its best? Gray hair loses its shine because the scalp is also losing its oils while the hair is turning gray. Consequently the hair no longer has enough oil to shine and look nice.

A simple solution, with ingredients out of your kitchen, is to use a puree of peeled avocado and one teaspoon of warm olive oil. The hair should be wet, and the puree mixture applied and left on the hair for one-half hour. Then the hair should be washed and conditioned as usual. The oily combination of olive oil and avocado will smooth the hair and enable it to reflect light.

While this is a good natural method, which also allows the hair to absorb some oils from the mixture, you may also want to try a commercial hair oil. Although these have largely fallen out of favor with many people, anytime that your have a problem with dry hair for any reason, you can at least add something which will externally replace the oil your hair should be getting from your scalp. This might also be something that you will want to talk to your dermatologist about, especially if you do not know why your hair is dry. Remember that coloring, perming, and treating your hair will also result in a dry hair problem, for which you may want to use the avocado and olive oil treatment.

HALITOSIS

How to Sweeten Your Breath With Your Diet

The big villains in bad breath are sugar, coffee, and cow's milk. First consider sugar and you will see that it promotes the growth of bacteria in your mouth, which leads to tooth decay, and then to bad breath. Coffee doesn't have to grow anything, all that you have to do is sit next to someone who has been drinking coffee all morning in a closed space and let them breathe on you to see how bad it can get. Cow's milk might be a good source of calcium, but it can sour your mouth and add plaque to your teeth, making a very good start on a bad breath day.

But let us say that you cut down on all of those and things still aren't quite as sweet as you would like, what can you do now? Well its simple, just increase your diet in green leafy vegetables, and add parsley (which will take care of garlic and onion in your diet).

Even if you can't clear it up completely in a short time, you can at least disguise it somewhat with fennel (smells like licorice), dill, caraway seeds, and anise seeds. Of course you should try some straight licorice or ginger to change your mouth odor.

HAYFEVER

6 Ignored Secrets to Controlling Your Hayfever

It is called hayfever because you get it in the spring and summer when the hay is growing and ripening, and it can keep you from enjoying either your spring or your summer every year. While hayfever is really just allergies, it can give you all of the symptoms of a cold or the flu. You can have a runny nose, headaches, bodyache, prickly skin, fever, and violent sneezing. Your eyes may run to the point that you can't see well enough to drive your car, and it happens every year. The problem with allergies is that they can be caused by so many things, and you can get new ones all of the time. An allergy doctor can find out which ones you have right now and help to desensitize you to them, but for new ones you have to go through the whole process again. But what you want are some suggestions of what you can do to deal with your hayfever right now, not after some doctor has worked with you for a year or two. And in that spirit, here are 5 secrets to controlling your hayfever that are ignored too much of the time.

Secret 1. Don't try to freeze your allergies. You need to keep your air conditioner at 68 or 70 degrees, and not cold enough to make ice. Doctors have found that rooms that are very cold simply make allergies worse, while those at a more moderate setting help to relieve the problems of hayfever. Why? The answer is really quite simple, very cold air cannot hold very much moisture. Therefore, very cold air is very dry, and it dries out your sinuses. When your sinuses are dry they have no protection between them and the things you are allergic to. Moist noses have a coating of water and mucous which protects the tissues from a direct attack by aggravating pollens and molds.

Secret 2. Shower whenever you think that you have gotten a good dose of pollen, or other things you are allergic to. This can happen because the wind was blowing, or you were cutting the lawn, doing yard work, or cleaning your house (if you are allergic to house dust), and before you do anything else you need to get that stuff off of you. You can take all of the anti-allergen medicine you want, but if you are still covered with the stuff that is making you sneeze, you will continue to sneeze anyway. Like everything else that has to do with our bodies, if you get more of something you are allergic to on your skin, you are going to react. And when you get rid of it, or get a medicine to counteract it, the symptoms will go away. The first step in any treatment for hayfever is to remove everything from your body and clothing that causes the hayfever. Once you have done that you are ready to go on with more medical treatments, such as your doctor might recommend.

Secret 3. While you are at it, and even if you don't shower, at least wash your hair. Think of your hair as a big air filter. Any time the air blows through it, it is going to leave behind some of the solid stuff it is carrying. This includes pollens, molds, chemicals, dust, cells off of bodies you don't want to know about, and anything else that can get picked up and carried on the wind. After mowing your lawn you may have so much of this allergenic stuff in your hair that it will keep your eyes and nose running, and you sneezing, until you get around to washing your hair. Most of us, when we are outside, do not cover our heads. Because of the filter effect of our hair we can be carrying around an ounce or two of something that a pinch of which would send us into sneezing fits. But you get the idea, wash your hair more than once a day if you are bothered at all by hayfever, and the more violent the hayfever, the more frequently you should make sure that your hair, body, and clothes are clean and free of contaminating substances.

Secret 4. Consider it a day when you have a lot of hayfever, and you jump into your car and turn on the air conditioner to get some relief. However, instead of getting relief all that you get for a few minutes is watery eyes, and a lot of coughing and sneezing, and then it all clears up. What is going on here? Is the coughing and sneezing just what you have to go through to get rid of the pollens and molds that are attacking you, or is there something else? Actually there is something else, your air conditioner may have its own load of molds that it blows into your face when you first turn it on, and which in a few minutes is flushed out so that you really do get relief. If you have bad allergies it is really best not to fool around, take some precautions. When you get in your car to drive with the air conditioner on, roll down your windows and let it run for 5 minutes before you button everything up. That will take care of the flushing action, and get molds out and pollens out of your car. Where do the molds come from, why right from the air conditioner itself. Your air conditioner will trap molds and moisture, and give the molds a good place to grow in between uses so that all that you get when you first turn yours on is a big dose of mold. Now, while the flushing method is the cheap and quick way of getting rid of these pollens, you can also have the air conditioner decontaminated for about $75 by the factory dealer. It's up to you how you want to handle the problem, but don't just sit in your airconditioner stream every day and cough, sneeze, and choke, until it all clears up on its own.

Secret 5. But now let's suppose that you are bothered by hayfever, and that you are also tired of being locked up in your house for 4 or 5 months of the year, what can you do? The most direct action you can take is to give yourself a dose of anti-allergen medicine before you go out, and then go out and have a normal life. You may wonder what a dose of antihistamine is going to do for you when you have no symptoms, but the answer is it will prevent the early symptoms from getting you at all. Allergies have to start somewhere, and if they can't start, they can't bother you. Some patients have reported that this prevention type treatment has resulted in their being able to discontinue any allergy medication after a period of time. While your degree of sensitivity will have a big impact upon how important this kind of treatment is, it is only reasonable that taking a medication before you are attacked by something that will make you sick will only help you resist the attack. The medication will either boost your immune system, or it will desensitize your body to the allergic attack. Consequently, you should have no allergic attack, or a very much lessened one. In either case you are far ahead of the game for the price of a dose of your allergy medication.

Secret 6. This is a secret that you are not likely to have run across anywhere else. Allergies or pollens or other substances might also show up as itchiness in the mouth. This is very strange, but it also may not be quite what you think. When you are attacked by an allergy, say in a pollen, it may make you especially sensitive to the fruit of other plants that have some characteristic in common with it. For instance, if you are allergic to grass pollens, then you may very well get an itchy mouth feeling when you eat melons, oranges, peas, or tomatoes. It might even be a problem to swallow them normally when you have this dual allergy attack. Okay, so you have an itchy mouth during the summer, when your allergies are bothering you, what can you do about it? Actually the immediate problem is very easily solved, just eat canned or cooked fruits instead of fresh ones. Only the fresh foods will cause the itchy mouth problem, and never the canned or cooked type. Probably the fresh foods have either some of the pollens on the skin of the fruit, that you then also eat, or there are oils in the skin or the fruit when they are fresh that boil away when they are cooked. In either case, if you shift to prepared foods any time that you experience one of these itchy mouth attacks, you can avoid any further problem with that particular food, and continue to enjoy it to your heart's content.

HEADACHES

Clothes that Can Cause Headaches and Tiredness

It seems rather silly to think that your clothes could cause such things as headaches and tiredness, but its true if they have been cleaned with certain kinds of resins to keep them wrinkle-free. These resins can contain formaldehyde, which the clothing will give off in the form of a gas as long as you have them. You won't notice any effects immediately, but after a few months, if you wear them daily, you will start to develop headaches. If you breath in enough formaldehyde you can also develop tiredness, coughing, watery eyes, and breathing problems. While these problems may not threaten your life, they can leave you feeling chronically ill, and untreatable.

The only way to avoid formaldehyde poisoning from your clothing is to avoid the clothing that contains formaldehyde. Natural fibers are generally not treated with formaldehyde, and should be worn by anyone who has any of these symptoms over a period of time. Also do not buy clothing made of fabrics which call themselves "easy care," or "no iron." You usually find these on cotton clothing, and it can mean that they were treated with formaldehyde. While the easy care type of clothing may be more convenient for you to use, it isn't worth the pain if it is also making you sick.

The Vitamin to Avoid if You are Taking Aspirin

Aspirin is still the most popular headache medicine taken. But whether you are taking aspirin for headaches, bodyache, or to prevent heart attacks you should not take vitamin C at the same time. Studies have found that large doses of vitamin C and aspirin taken together are very irritating to the stomach and can lead to ulcers. If you have a history of stomach problems you need to be especially careful, and if you notice any upset when taking aspirin and vitamin C, then it may be that this is the cause. For best protection to your stomach, if you are taking both and want to continue, is to take them at different times of day. It is also good if you do not take them on an empty stomach. If you have aspirin in the morning for protection against heart attack, then wait till lunch or dinner to take your vitamin C. And if you need aspirin in the evening for bodyache or headache, then skip the vitamin C until the next morning. No difficulties were found with natural sources of vitamin C like orange juice or grapefruit, and you might consider using these as alternatives to vitamin tablets.

HEALING

How to Heal Faster from
Cuts, Scrapes, Bruises, and Surgery

What I want to give you here are a few ideas on healing in general. There are always things you can do for each type of injury—cuts, scrapes, bruises, and surgery. But what we want to focus on are some ideas that can help you heal faster no matter what you are healing from.

When your body is injured and is in the process of healing, it uses protein to make new cells and blood, and you need to have an adequate amount of protein in your diet. To promote healing of all kinds you will never go wrong if you increase your vitamin C to 2 or 3 grams a day. While the protein is available for cell building, and vitamin C speeds up the healing process, you also need the other building blocks of healing, and vitamin A is one of these. Vitamin A increases the rate at which cells are built. While you are at it you should also include a supplement of zinc, which is necessary for cell growth, and vitamin E, which helps keep wounds from becoming infected. That is the basic tool kit which works for all types of wounds and cuts, and although you may see parts of it in many places in this book, you need this specific combination to heal.

But because most of our wounds and injuries are on the outside of our bodies, you might as well include a good topical lotion to help those areas heal. The best that I can think of is aloe vera, which you can get in plant form and grow yourself. You can also get it now in everything to medical lotions to shampoo, and it's generally very inexpensive. In any case, whenever you have a cut or scrape put some aloe vera on it along with whatever you usually use.

HEALTH CARE

Free Health Care
Where to Look to Find It

Where first not to look, don't go to your doctor and ask where you can get his services for free. Doctors are not going to undercut their own business by getting you free care. They are more likely to refer you to another doctor who will either refer someone else back to them, or to someone who will split fees in some manner. But why would they want you to have free care. And if you aren't one of their patients and come to them for this advice, they won't even see you to begin with.

What you need to do is to write to: Information USA, FREE HEALTH CARE, P.O. Box E, Kensington, MD 20895. This is a pamphlet which gives you a list of mostly unknown government programs which provide free health care. Programs are listed in every state, so no matter where you are you shouldn't be too far from the help you need at a cost you can afford.

HEALTH INSURANCE

Cut Your Rates by Nearly 50% With these Tips

Everyone's health insurance rates are way too high, but by making a few good decisions you can cut the amount you pay by at least 50%, and perhaps even more. Here are 4 good ideas that can help you save on the amount you pay for health insurance, and give you the coverage you need.

1. Sign up for insurance through a professional organization. This makes use of the group insurance rates and avoids the problem of being a single person or a single family trying to buy insurance from a company. This is open to anyone who is a member of a professional organization, or anyone who can join one, and is a great way to spread your risk over the other members of the organization. There is a caution though, check the deductible in the group rates and make sure that it won't threaten any savings you are getting.

2. Join an HMO to save costs since much of the cost you spend for health insurance goes to pay for the overhead of private practice doctors. The beauty of the HMO plans is that they stress preventive medicine, so you can get your annual checkups free or with a minimal $5 or $10 amount. In addition prescriptions are usually either free or available for $2 per prescription, and emergency care is available to you anywhere you might be without extra cost. That is if you go to an emergency hospital, the hospital sends the bill to your HMO and you don't have to pay anything. Many surgeries and pregnancy costs, including Ceasarian operations, are also included.

3. The agent you go through to buy your health insurance can often make the difference between paying a high commission rate and paying none at all. Also agents who only represent one company will only be trying to sell policies for that one company. To get the best deal with an agent shop around for one who works with several health insurers, and where the companies pay the commission. This type of agent is known as an independent insurance agent. But if you know which insurer you want to go with, then just choose one who works for that company, and who is paid by the company, and see what kind of a deal you can get for signing up with his company. The agent earns his commission by signing up people, and will deal on what you are offered just like any car salesmen. Shop around for the best deal, and you may be surprised by what you find.

4. Check the small business pools for insurance bargains if none of these other areas fit your needs. Of course this means that you are involved in a small business, but those laws vary by city and state. Often you can join a local city of

---

commerce and qualify for business rates. The idea is to make yourself a part of a larger group so that you are not standing alone asking someone to insure you. The lone person has very little influence, but any group commands respect from insurers and health providers. The states of Connecticut and Massachusetts have even passed laws requiring that health plans for small businesses be made available to individuals as well.

HEARING LOSS

Need A Hearing Aid?
Where to Get Information to Find the Good Ones

You certainly can't listen to the companies who make them to find out what is the best hearing aid for the money. You need information from someone who is not going to make money out of selling you something. This information will tell you exactly who keeps track of hearing aid quality, and the information you will need to choose the best hearing aid for the money. Just write for the booklet "Hearing Aids, IB II-78a," from the Depot Officer, VA Forms and Publications Depot, 6307 Gravel Ave., Alexandria, VA 22314.

Worried About Your Hearing—Avoid Noise

You needn't lose your hearing just because you get older, or just because you work in a noisy place. In fact working in a noisy environment probably causes most of the hearing loss you might ever have. You can find your hearing damaged by exposure to either very loud noises over short periods of time, or even by lower noises over a long period. Getting used to loud noises, like machinery in a work place, doesn't stop the noise from hurting your hearing. If you are caught in a noisy setting, like near the plane engines at an airport, stick your fingers in your ears or cover them with your hands, and get away from there as fast as you can. Noises can also cause stress, insomnia, jitteriness, and headaches, so they are not to be ignored if they seem to be too loud to be comfortable.

If you have been in noisy places and you are worried about your hearing you can at least get some idea if you have had hearing loss. Ringing of the ears and hearing normal sounds which seem muffled are two of the regular signs of hearing loss. Although hearing aids can help correct some of the problem, there is no way to bring your hearing back to normal through medicine or surgery.

HEARTBURN

4 Keys to Avoiding Heartburn

With a good diet there is still the chance that you will suffer from heartburn occasionally. If you have a high fat diet you probably suffer from heartburn often, and it may take the joy out of your meals. Short of changing your entire diet, there are still things you can do to lessen your chances of getting heartburn no matter what your diet consists of. These keys will help to prevent stomach acid from coming up and causing the heartburn in the first place, and that is the only cause of heartburn.

1. After a meal take a walk for 15 minutes to a 1/2 hour, and it will give the food a chance to move out of your stomach. Also, since you are upright the stomach acid will stay where it belongs and you will not develop heartburn. If you have had an especially large meal, or your main meal of the day, you may want to walk for an hour, and it will also relax your mind and body and leave you in better shape for rest later. Do not go out and try any strenuous exercise right after eating, as that will simply make you feel bad and interrupt your digestion. Save the exercise for a couple of hours and it will be much more enjoyable.

2. If you are going to sit down or lie down just after a meal, make certain the upper part of your body stays above your stomach. You can do this with pillows under your back, or elevating the head of your bed, but keep your stomach down where it belongs and you will prevent the worst of your heartburn problem.

3. When you lie down for a nap after a meal, lie on your left side. It has been proven by doctors at the Thomas Jefferson University Hospital in Philadelphia that lying on the left side rather than the right side while sleeping significantly decreased attacks of heartburn. This works because the stomach is lower on the left side than the right side so that things stay down where they should and don't come up to the esophagus to cause you problems. This might not cure the entire problem, but at least it will decrease attacks on you.

4. Take a look at your meals and see if there is a particular type of food that always seems to bring on heartburn. If the problem can't be controlled any other way you may have to quit eating it, or cut back to small amounts. Common foods that cause heartburn are alcoholic beverages, spicy foods, acidic foods, and very fatty dishes. Many times just cutting back on these will cure the problem, and you won't have to entirely give up something that you love.

The Sleeping Position to End Heartburn

We get heartburn when the acids in our stomach come up into the esophagus. When we sleep, lying on the right side, stomach acid is able to wash into the esophagus and trigger an attack of heart burn. But, by lying on the left side, and elevating the head slightly, the stomach acid will stay where it belongs, and we can avoid the problem of attacks of heartburn in the night.

HEART ATTACKS

What to do If You are having a Heart Attack

Having a heart attack, particularly when you are alone, can be one of the most frightening things anyone can go through. And although more men than women have heart attacks, the numbers are huge for both sexes. Many people also have silent heart attacks that can only be detected through tests in a doctors office or hospital, but they still damage the heart. Of course there is little you can do personally about a silent heart attack unless someone is watching you at the time, but heart attacks of a higher level can be recognized by everyone, particularly by the person having them.

If you realize you are having a heart attack the first thing you, or someone else, should do is call 911 and tell them you are having a heart attack. This will usually get you medical help in just a few minutes. But in the meantime you want to do what you can to keep your heart beating and to keep yourself from passing out. The next step is to take as deep a breath as you can, to get oxygen into your lungs and blood, and then to cough violently and repeatedly several times. Then repeat the breathing and coughing until the paramedics arrive or you can get to a hospital. The coughing action squeezes the heart muscle, just like any muscle, and forces it to keep your blood circulating and keep you alive.

If you get to the point where your heart stops you will lose consciousness in about 10 seconds, and there is nothing you can do about it at that time. So as soon as you find that you are having a heart attack begin the breathing and coughing and you may just save your life.

HEART DISEASE

2 Natural Approaches to Fighting Heart Attack and Stroke

While you always have to go to a physician for treatment of heart disease, you rarely have to do so to take steps to avoid heart disease. Of course diet and exercise plans make up the bulk of things you can do yourself, but you still need to pay attention to the particulars. The wrong diet or exercise plan may be of no help, and might even hurt you. But when you get a good way to go, you can avoid diseases that all the doctors tell you are unavoidable. Of course they don't say that about heart disease. The problem is that they don't say very much about heart disease until you already have it. Well we are going to change that a little bit here, and tell you a couple of ways you can go about avoiding it in the first place.

The first approach is with a naturally occurring nutrient called L-carnitine, which is found widely in food. The wonderful attributes of this nutrient is that it strengthens the heart, relieves chest pain, and lowers blood fat levels. Since it isn't usually listed on food ingredient lists, you may want to buy a supplement from your health food store. The second approach is with the use of fish oil, which is also available is capsules, and contains Omega-3 fatty acid. Omega-3 fatty acid is an amazing nutrient that reduces the bad, LDL, cholesterol and raises the good, HDL, cholesterol. If you increase your consumption of fish, or fish oil, you can often avoid the use of cholesterol controlling medications. It is a good idea to do this even if you don't have a cholesterol problem in order to prevent it from beginning in the first place. These are safe and natural ways of dealing with the potential problems of high cholesterol, which causes heart attacks and strokes, and just keeping the heart healthy.

3 Ways to Beat Heart Failure

Heart failure is different from a heart attack because it is the heart itself that fails, where a heart attack happens because the arteries carrying the blood get blocked. You can get heart failure from any illness or infection that weakens the heart. This includes virus infections like measles or scarlet fever, or just getting older to the point where none of the muscles in your body work well, including your heart. If you can't treat heart failure it will kill you some day, but these 3 ways to treat heart failure are largely ignored but should be considered. After all, its your life we're talking about, not whether you should get a hair cut or not.

1. The first of these is a nutrient which is available over-the-counter. It is called coenzyme Q10, and while not used by American doctors, it is very popular with doctors in Japan who have prescribed it for 15 million heart patients. In a study of 126 patients, published in the American Journal of Cardiology in 1990, it was found to add several years of life in cases of severe cardiomyopathy. In cardiomyopathy the heart becomes too weak to pump blood around the body, and fluid collects in the lungs and throughout the body. Eventually the strain on the heart becomes so great that it just quits and you die. Coenzyme Q10 helps this by lifting the energy level of the heart back toward a normal range. An added bonus is that it can also improve the ability of angina sufferers to exercise, which can then help to decrease the angina.

2. The next is a nutrient which is a little more common, though not thought of as a heart stimulant. It is L-carnitine, and it also is available over-the-counter. This works very much like coenzyme Q10, and raises the energy level of the heart and of the cells of the body. Because its action is so much like coenzyme Q10, you should try each one, or a combination, to see what combination works best for you. If you have heart disease, or heart failure, you really need to do this under a doctor's supervision. But if you are just looking for something preventive, and you have no problems with your heart, there is no reason you could not try them as food supplements.

3. The third is L-Dopa, which is most commonly thought of as a drug for Parkinson's disease. However L-Dopa is just an amino acid that makes the body raise its level of dopamine. Dopamine is a natural body stimulant, and helps the heart to work more efficiently. This stimulation effect of L-Dopa, and dopamine, can effectively treat congestive heart failure, although no American doctors prescribe it for this use. Since L-Dopa is not available over-the-counter, you will have to find a doctor who is familiar with its effects in stimulating the heart, and obtain a prescription from them. Of course heart medicines are something you should never mess around with on your own, but finding the best doctor for your heart problem can be just as big of a problem. Also, since most people won't change doctors once they start a treatment, you need to find out the ways in which your own doctor treats serious conditions like heart failure before you get it. If you are not satisfied with the answers and approaches of your doctor, the time to shop around is before you are in any kind of any emergency condition, and won't have a choice of what is done to you.

8 Pains That Could be Warning Signs of a Heart Attack

If you ever have pains in your chest and wonder if you could be having a heart attack, then you need to learn this list so that anytime you have a real heart attack you will have the best chance of surviving. Almost all heart attacks are accompanied by pain, but many times these pains seem a lot like heartburn or an upset stomach. Also they may sometimes take several hours to develop. If you ever have a pain in your chest, or anyone you are with does, then go through this list, and it might just save your life.

1. The classic heart attack pain is pain under the breastbone, in the mid-chest area, or over the whole upper chest. This is what most people report at constricting pain over the chest, and a vice-like grip over the chest. If you ever have this kind of a pain have it checked out, and that means even if the pain goes away after a few hours. The natural relieving of the first pains over time is what fools many people into thinking they have just had an attack of heart burn instead of a heart attack, but delaying going to the hospital because of this kind of a process can cost you your life.

2. Pain in the jaw, neck, and mid-chest is also a very strong sign of a heart attack. Often these pains will not be as sever as the pains over the chest, but they are very good signals that something is going wrong with your heart.

3. Pain in the mid-chest accompanied by pains down the inside of the arms, though very often down only the left arm and shoulder. This is a symptom you often see quoted in many health books, and while it is common it also may not occur when you are having a heart attack. But pain in the chest and down an arm should sound an alarm bell for anyone suspected of having a heart attack.

4. Pain in the area of the upper stomach is certainly less common than in the chest, but any pain like this that persists for a few hours should alert you to the possibility that you may have a heart attack. Remember that heartburn in this area usually passes within a couple of hours. Certainly any such pain that lasts over-night is reason enough to go to the hospital.

5. Pain in the jaw, neck, and chest along with the chest area and inside of the arms should send you to the doctor immediately. This is a combination of some of the pains above, and simply shows a wider area of involvement of the heart attack, but not necessarily a more or less serious heart attack. Any heart attack is serious no matter what the symptoms are that send you to treatment.

6. Pain which is localized at the base and center of the neck, on the sides of the upper neck, and across the whole jaw area from ear to ear. This is a rather unusual area of pain, so far as mistaking it for pains from other causes, and if you are having a combination anything like this you need to see a doctor.

7. Pain limited to the arms. Particularly the left shoulder including the whole left arm, and the inside of the right arm from below the armpit. You should not mistake this pain for anything other than a heart attack unless you have

recently been involved in some heavy work or physical activity that might have put a lot of strain on your arms,

8. Pain between the shoulder blades is perhaps something that might be mistaken for an upper back strain. Again you must rely on your own experience to make a judgment in this case. If you have not have recent activity where you could strain your back, or have any history of this kind of pain, then the first time you feel it you must have it checked out medically.

50 Milligrams Daily of this Supplement Can Cut Your Risk of a Stroke, Heart Attack, or Related Death in Half

A Harvard Medical School study has found that taking 50 milligrams of beta-carotene every other day can cut the risk of heart attacks by 50%, in people who already have heart disease. Beta-carotene is also helpful in preventing strokes and other related causes of death which have the same causes as heart attacks. Beta-carotene can be found in health food stores, and in sweet potatoes, carrots, and cantaloupes. It is the substance that gives these vegetables their color, and you can take as much as you want safely because extra amounts just pass through the body.

4 Healthy-For-Your-Heart Eating Secrets

We have been talking a lot about nutrients which are good to your heart, or to prevent cancer, or to prevent or cure some other problem, but we have not gotten much into what you should eat to get a good combination of the nutrients you need for these problems, and heart disease is one of the biggest of the problems. To avoid heart disease, so the doctor's will tell you, you need to keep your weight down, exercise, stay away from saturated fat and cholesterol, and stop smoking. While that is all very fine, you still have to go on eating every day, and if you aren't given some alternatives to whatever you have been doing in the past, there is little chance that you are going to change in the future. Well at this point, and for this problem, we are going to change that. Immediately below are 4 foods that you should include in your daily diet to prevent heart disease, and why you should include them. The "why you should include them" is important because anyone can give advice, but you should never accept it without question if you don't know anything directly about how it is supposed to work. But read below and see what you think. If you are convinced then act on it. All of these secrets are well known to people who have already done the research, but if you haven't gone that far in your nutritional work, here is where you can get a good start.

The first secret is that garlic is the best protective food against heart disease that we have in our American diet. Heavy garlic eaters have better arteries and few respiratory diseases than those who avoid garlic. The countries around the Mediterranean where garlic is eaten most regularly, including Greece and Italy, have fewer heart attacks in their population than the United States. This is in spite of the fact that they smoke more heavily, and have higher levels of oils and fats in their diets. Because of the effect of garlic on heart disease, it is considered a blood purifier. The effectiveness of garlic in protecting the heart comes from its ability to prevent the LDL cholesterol in our diet from forming plaques on the arteries, or from forming clots in the blood that could cause a heart attack or stroke. If you are already fond on garlicky sauces, then you are already getting the benefits. But if your aren't, and don't want to include that much garlic in your daily diet, you can also get garlic capsules at the health food store which you can add to your morning daily supplement.

The second secret is that onions do much the same thing as garlic, but at the source. While garlic does its work in the blood, apparently onions do theirs in the digestive tract. Studies have found that a regular diet of onions will protect you from 2/3 of the cholesterol rise you get from eating foods high in butterfat. Not only that, but onions were tested both raw and boiled, and the effect was the same. Onions are especially important if you have a high cholesterol problem because they will remove most of your dietary cholesterol before it ever has a chance to enter your blood. If you are also using garlic, then the garlic will take care of the small portion of cholesterol that does get into the blood, and you will be doubly protected.

The third secret is fish, but not just any fish, only those fish who have high levels of nutrients called EPA and DHA. EPA is eicosapentaenoic acid, and DHA is docosahexaenoic acid, if you want to know their full names. The fish containing these two acids are trout, salmon, mackerel, and sardines, which are all common diet foods from some coastal peoples, and each of these populations are protected from heart disease. When fish oils were studied, and that included fish oil capsules, it was found that eaters of these fish had less clotting action than those who did not eat the fish. Not only that, but people like the Eskimo, who eat a lot of high fat foods along with their fish, still have very low levels of heart disease. The conclusion is that eating large amounts of these fish, or taking fish oil capsules, will protect you from heart disease by stopping clots from forming in your blood. If you are a hemophiliac however, I would talk to my doctor before I took anything that cut down the clotting time of my blood.

The fourth secret is beans, and that means beans of all kinds. People with high cholesterol saw their cholesterol levels drop when they were put on a diet high in beans. Beans don't exactly prevent you from getting high cholesterol, but they do help to lower it once you have gotten a cholesterol problem. Of course, why wait until you have the problem, and some of the damage, when you can prevent both. After all, if you have a diet rich in beans and never experience a high cholesterol problem, then you are way ahead of the game. The amount of beans to be eaten on a weekly basis is a little tricky. It has been suggested that one pound a week would be a good dietary goal. But if you can't handle that much, and that is not really very much, then at least get 1/2 pound a week. If beans tend to give you gas problems, there are anti-gas pills on the market that can help a great deal. You might also be able to find a method of preparation that decreases or eliminates the gas problem for you. But here is where I am going to have to violate my promise to you, we don't know exactly why beans have this effect on cholesterol, it's just that the effect has been found every time a study has been done.

I hope this little list of diet secrets has done you some good. It may sound a bit technical at times, but that is how nutritionists talk, and the information will always come in handy if you want to look up more information on any of the foods or nutrients we have just looked at.

4 Vitamins and Minerals That Protect You Against Heart Disease, and Can Even Reverse It

Underneath all of the diet planning you can do to protect yourself against heart disease is the assumption that you are getting nutrients that will have the desired actions. But sometimes, or even often, it is not possible to find a diet that will give you all of the necessary ingredients. For those instances when your need is especially great, or that you have anything other then a perfect diet, it is good to take supplements. And since we are especially interested in the nutrients that protect you from heart disease, that will be the major function of each of the 4 presented here.

1. Magnesium is the preventer of heart arrhythmia. With magnesium in the body at the proper level enzymes are released that keep the muscles of the heart contracting normally to keep blood circulating through the body. If you want some proof of this service just consider that people who are having heart attacks and going into arrhythmia are often given intravenous solutions of magnesium sulfate to get their hearts back on a normal rhythm. Furthermore, in parts of the country where water softening has removed most of the magnesium from the water, the heart attack rates increase. So to prevent the effects of heart disease the first mineral you should build your daily supplement with is magnesium.

2. For the next nutrient we are going to turn to thiamine, or vitamin B1. Studies of older people found that over half of those with heart disease symptoms had low thiamine levels. In heart operations, where the heart was stopped and

then restarted, twice as many patients with low thiamine levels had heart spasms when their hearts were restarted. Thiamine apparently contributes to the normal working of the heart, and in the prevention of circulatory diseases.

3. One of the best anti-clotting vitamins is vitamin B6, according to studies at the University of Illinois Medical Center in Chicago. The way that vitamin B6 works is by preventing the release of a chemical called ADP, that causes the blood platelets to stick together and form clots in the blood vessels. Once the clots have formed they can block small vessels and cause heart attacks and strokes. One of the good features about B6 is that its anti-clot effect may be active for two days or more after having a minimum dose. The problem in older people is that their diets are often so poor that then don't even get adequate B6 every two day, and one study found that 30% of those in a nursing home had low B6 levels.

4. For the last mineral we are turning to selenium. Selenium has such a particular effect on heart disease, that when it is absent it causes a very particular disease called Keshan disease. This disease is characterized by heart muscle damage, enlargement of the heart, racing pulse, weak heartbeat, low blood pressure, and edema. In fact 1/2 of those with all of the symptoms die. Selenium is perhaps the best heart disease preventive of those we have presented here since the range of heart problems is so broad if your levels are low. I would recommend selenium as a heart disease preventive, and as part of the therapy for anyone who has already developed heart disease (with the approval of your doctor of course).

No matter how strongly you feel about a nutrient or self cure, if you are under a doctor's care for an illness, check with them that what you want to take will not be dangerous to you. Many drugs prescribed by doctors are so toxic that to simply quit taking them will kill you. And the same goes to taking high doses of a vitamin or mineral that interferes with a prescription drug. Of course if you are convinced that a particular nutrient will help you, and your doctor won't do anything to help you, there is no reason that you can't go looking for a holistic or homeopathic doctor who will be more willing to incorporate your interest in natural healing with the drugs that you may still be required to take in the meantime. Hopefully such a doctor will be more willing to take you off of ineffective prescription drugs when and if a natural therapy is working.

A Blood Pressure Medication Without Side Effects

It seems inevitable that having a medication for high blood pressure means that you are going to have unpleasant side effects. Well there is one high blood pressure medication, and it isn't widely used, that doesn't have side effects, and is very effective. The medication is magnesium sulfate, and it is given by injection. One study found it to lower the risk of a second heart attack by 87%, but it is not familiar to most doctors. Ask around to find a doctor who knows about using magnesium sulfate to control blood pressure, and maybe you can save yourself some of the pain of the side effects of other blood pressure medications. Remember that low level of magnesium increase the risk of both heart disease and irregular heartbeat. Your minimum requirement of magnesium is at least 1,000 mg daily.

Heart Blockage? Protect Yourself After Angioplasty

A common treatment for blockage of the arteries to the heart is treatment by angioplasty, where a balloon is used to open up the blockages. After the procedure the main risk is that the arteries will again become blocked and another angioplasty of bypass will have to be done. It has been found that fish oil helps to prevent reblockage. This was investigated in Canada with great success. Fish oil is loaded with good HDL cholesterol which does not block the arteries, and even seems to help unblock those that have build-ups of the bad LDL cholesterol. Fish oil is available without prescription in health food stores. If you wish an even more direct source of fish oil you can eat fish on a regular basis. Asians, who have a much lower rate of heart disease than European Americans, use fish oils in their diets, and eat much more fish on a daily basis.

In the Canadian study half of the patients were put on fish oil for 6 months after angioplasty, and half were given olive oil capsules. At the end of the study it was found that the rate of blockage was cut in half for the group taking fish oil. These doctors also found that eating even one serving of fish a week decreased blockage by 4%, and felt that having a fish diet several times a week would probably be as effective as taking the fish oil capsules, but this has not yet been studied.

Even if you haven't had angioplasty, but especially if you have, a diet which includes fish more than once a week, and fish oil capsules. will provide insurance that you will not suffer from blockage or heart disease. This is not a complete guarantee, but it is certainly a big improvement over doing nothing, and can work very well even if you don't want to ever eat fish in any form. At least take the fish oil capsules.

Heart Cathertization? Is it the Right Test for You?

About 1 million heart cathertizations are done each year to diagnose blockages in the arteries of the heart. After passing a catheter up through one of the veins toward the heart, a dye is put in through it, and the dye indicates where the blockage is located, if there is a blockage. The only problem with this is that as many of 1/2 of these procedures may be unnecessary, according to a study printed in the Journal of the American Medical Association. Now while the heart cathertization is mostly safe, there are deaths from it, and in addition it costs between $2,000 and $3,000 to take. In order to screen out more people and get the same results it is possible to work with family histories, personal health histories, and take a treadmill test. If these were used more often a lot of money and trouble could be saved and those with possible heart disease would be just as well off.

Heart Problems? This Reduces Stroke by 79%, says a Harvard Doctor

A Harvard Medical School study of veterans has shown that low dose of warfarin can reduce the risk of stroke by 79% for heart disease patients. This is a remarkable finding because warfarin is used in heart disease to stop blood clots from forming in the heart and causing the heart to go into fibrillation where it just quivers without beating. Warfarin thins the blood, much as the milder aspirin does, but is more useful in cases where heart disease has already developed.

How the "Over 40" Woman Can Lower Her Risk of Heart Disease

Most women may not worry about heart disease since it is mostly men who seem to suffer from it and have heart attacks. But as women grow older their risk of heart disease increases. After menopause the chance that a woman will have a heart attack increases 300%, and is even higher than for men. Also heart disease in older women is more likely to be deadly than in men of the same age. If you are over 40 you need to do some things to lower your risk.

One of the best actions you can take is to learn to relax, and practicing relaxation exercises on a daily basis can be very effective. One of the best recommended forms is a yoga-like meditation, where you sit on the floor, cross-legged, straight back, close your eyes, and breath regularly and deeply for 5 to 10 minutes. Other relaxation exercises may be just as good, but this one requires very little room, and very little time to give you good results.

Other recommendations for lowering heart disease risk are to stop smoking, lose weight if you are overweight, and get regular exercise. Of course all of these are also effective for men, and if there is a man in your life then get him to do them with you. The togetherness might just help as much as anything else in keeping you healthy and active.

If You Take Saldane,
You Should Never Take These Two Drugs With It

Saldane is taken by many people to control allergies, and it is perfectly safe in normal circumstances. The problem you might encounter is that an elevated level of Saldane in the blood can affect the function of the heart, cause irregular heart beats, and might even cause heart attacks and death. When taken at the recommended levels all of these complications will be avoided, but if you are also taking either ketaconazole or erythromycin you are at risk. Ketaconazole is an antifungal drug, so that if you are taking it you may not think that it will have anything to do with your allergy medicine. Erythromycin is an antibiotic, and you might be taking it as insurance against complications from a respiratory disease while you are also taking the Saldane which is probably treating the real cause, an allergy. You will need to watch out for these deadly combinations since many times people are tempted to take old prescriptions they have around the house and have used in the past. Marion Merrell Dow, who makes Saldane, is changing its labeling to include a warning about these combinations, and notifying doctors as well at this time.

Is Angioplasty the Right Treatment for You

In angioplasty the surgeon takes a tiny balloon into a partially blocked artery and inflates it to squash back the blockage and let the blood flow through. Although a few people die from this type of procedure, it is pretty much same since they don't actually open up your chest to get at your heart. Oh, and it does work to relieve angina and increase the blood flow, but only temporarily.

The blockages are caused by cholesterol sticking to the walls of the arteries until it just closes them up. If too much of the arteries are closed they will do a bypass on you where they take an artery from another part of your body and make the blood go through that instead of through the artery that is all blocked up. This also works, although the clean arteries used in the bypass are usually clogged up themselves within a few years, and you have to do it all over again.

But is angioplasty the right treatment for you? Probably if your doctor recommends it, but if you aren't to that point yet then maybe there are some changes you can make that will keep you from getting there at all. The one that you want to go after most aggressively is to lower your blood cholesterol level. That alone will remove the substance that is going to clog your arteries in the first place. Other than that you need to give up smoking, if you smoke, and lose weight, if you are overweight. Both of these contribute to heart disease, and smoking puts so many poisons into your body that you can never be completely healthy if you smoke.

Is It Worthwhile Exercising to Prevent Heart Attacks?

Well, if you don't want to exercise under any circumstances, then I suppose it isn't worthwhile exercising to prevent a heart attack either. But for everyone else, take a look at the benefits and risks before you make up your mind.

If you ask a doctor what chance you have of getting a heart attack he will question you about your habits, and then add up the various risk factors you have and give you a number which he says is your risk of having a heart attack in the next 5 or 10 years. Risk factors for heart attacks that you hear about every day include smoking, overweight, a family history of heart attacks and diabetes. What you don't hear about so often is that not exercising and being inactive is also a risk factor. In fact the American Heart Association has just upgraded lack of exercise from a contributing factor in heart disease to a risk factor. Having a few of these risk factors makes it virtually certain that you will have a heart attack.

Just how important is exercise to preventing heart attacks? Well, if you don't exercise you are thought to be 3 or 4 times more likely to have a heart attack than if you exercise. This means that for every 1 million heart attacks in the United States in a year, about 750,000 to 800,000 will be of those who don't exercise, and 200,000 to 250,000 will of those who exercise. If you exercise you can get yourself out of those 500-600,000 extra heart attacks that the lazy are going to get in a year. That is not such a bad payoff for going out and sweating for 1/2 hour a day.

If you are now ready to say that you will exercise for the good of your heart, even if you have never exercised before, then what do you do next? That is a good question, and the AMA recommends that everyone get 30 minutes of exercise 4 to 5 times a week all year long. That works out to 2 to 2 1/2 hours of exercise a week, but make sure that you don't try to do it all in one day. You will be more likely to cause yourself to have a heart attack than you will be to prevent one.

Of course the quality of the exercise is also important. You need to do an active, aerobic, exercise that get your breathing up and causes you to break out in a sweat. If you do nothing more strenuous than bring yourself to deep breathing and breaking into a sweat each day you have done a good job. For this you can use walking, swimming, biking, tennis, and so forth.

But if you want an exercise that is less strenuous, and would still like the benefits, there is evidence that this can be done too. Gardening, dancing, and yard work will give you the same benefits if you give them some extra effort. Because they may not get your heart beating as rapidly, then you should do them for a longer time—perhaps 45 minutes to 1 hour each time over the week. They also need to be done just as often as the more strenuous versions.

For a last bit of encouragement, just remember that exercise will give you even more benefits than lowering your risk of heart attack. When you exercise your chance of getting diabetes goes down, as does your cholesterol and blood pressure. If you are over 40 and have been inactive, or have any history of heart disease, then get a doctor's evaluation before starting to exercise. Also stop smoking, but maybe the exercising will help you make up your mind about that too if you have the habit. Exercise is for the good of yourself, your family, and your friends.

New Study Reveals Nutrient
that Can Reduce Your Risk of a Heart Attack by 36%

A recent study of 87,000 women at the Women's Hospital in Boston has found that high intakes of vitamin E lowered the risk of heart attack by 36% from those who had too little vitamin E in their diets. This important study of women's health was looking at the health effects of vitamin E because of its ability to prevent free radicals from injuring the heart. Vitamin E can protect the heart and decrease your risk of serious illness from heart disease.

A large population study in Europe found that low blood levels of vitamin E were much more predictive of heart disease than measuring cholesterol levels of saturated fats in the diet. The conclusions were that a low level of vitamin E could predict heart disease 69% of the time, while high blood cholesterol was predictive only 29% of the time, and high blood pressure only 25% of the time. Recommended daily intake of vitamin E is 800 to 1,200 units.

Prevent Heart Disease

All the studies on heart disease have shown that it is usually associated with a lot of fat in the diet. In order to keep the heart healthy, and prevent heart disease, we need to restrict the amount of fat in our diets. Research has shown that the calories we eat must limit the fat consumed to 30%, or less. The easiest way of doing this, without measuring the fat content of everything we eat, is to make sure that we eat a lot of fruits and vegetable every day. It also helps that fruits and vegetables are usually a lot cheaper than fatty meats, and we feel better for eating them. You will also find that your digestion works much better eating more fruits and vegetables, and less meat and dairy products.

Risk of Heart Attack and Healthy Cholesterol

A study of Type A personality people indicates that your level of good cholesterol determines your risk of a heart attack. The Type A people were studied to see why they had a higher heart attack risk than more relaxed people. Type A people seem to be driven to accomplish goals which other people aren't, and they often die of stress related diseases like heart attacks. When the good cholesterol levels (HDL) of these people were measured it was found that theirs were 10% lower than other personality types. This meant that they had a 30% greater risk of a heart attack. This doesn't prove that the HDL level determines who will have a heart attack, but it does show that you need to be very careful about your HDL if you are a Type A person, and this is just another reason to watch out what level of HDL you have no matter who you are.

Smoker's Beware
Trying to Stop Might Give You A Heart Attack

While there is a definite increase in heart attacks due to smoking, and the increased risk is huge over a long time period, there is also the danger of giving yourself a heart attack if you are using a nicotine patch to quit, but have not completely given up smoking itself. At Sturdy Memorial Hospital in Attleboro, Mass., 5 patients were found whose heart attacks seem to have been caused by smoking while wearing nicotine patches. The FDA is looking into this now, but for your own safety don't use the nicotine patches if you are still smoking. There is no risk of heart attacks caused by use of the patch alone, when you are not also smoking, so if you have actually stopped smoking the patch can be a good aid.

The Vitamin That Helps You Prevent Killer Heart Disease

Since you are probably willing to do just about anything to prevent a heart attack that will kill you, then why not at least do something that is easy and might save you. All that you have to do is take supplements of vitamin C. You will need the supplements because you want an intake of vitamin C much higher than the minimum daily requirement, at least 500 to 1000 milligrams. In some cases you may want even more than that, but at least the 500-1000 mg is enough to give you basic protection from heart disease.

This recommendation for vitamin C comes from Dr. Linus Pauling, who has won the Nobel prize twice, and is more than likely right this time too. Vitamin

C is a powerful antioxidant which counteracts the free radicals which are involved in cardiovascular disease. By stopping the action of the free radicals you prevent your arteries from being blocked, or the walls of your arteries from being damaged.

In addition vitamin C has long been given credit for helping wounds to heal, probably also as a result of its antioxidant effects, and it will help to heal the walls of arteries already damaged thus preventing blockages. A third effect is that it elevates the level of HDL cholesterol in our body. Remember that HDL cholesterol is protective and does not cause heart disease.

All of the effects taken together add up to a powerful anti-heart disease medicine which can be had for pennies a day. If you prefer natural vitamin C sources, still be sure that you get enough vitamin C each day. Dr. Pauling did not test different forms of vitamin C against one another, so just make sure you at least get to the 500 milligram level with any of them to ensure protection.

What Effect Aspirin Really has on Heart Attacks

Aspirin has always been a wonderful medicine. It is cheap, can relieve headaches and body pain, and now is being recommended by many doctors as a preventive for heart attacks. But of course you would like to know if it really works to prevent heart attacks, and whether or not there is any risk involved in taking it?

The answer is that it does work, and at very low doses, which is good in preventing side effects. Besides relieving headaches and body pain, aspirin also keeps the blood from clotting at a normal rate. Perhaps it is this blood clotting effect that also helps the headaches and body ache, but no one knows if that is true or not. Anyway, because blood clots are one of the major causes of heart attacks and strokes, taking an aspirin a day can cut your risk by up to 2/3. The recommended dose for stroke and heart attack prevention is only 325 mg/day.

Because the dose is quite small there is little risk of any side effects. There are cautions however, if you have ulcers or other chronic stomach problems the aspirin might irritate them because the stomach is where the aspirin dissolves and begins its work. Aspirin has also been known to cause ulcers in people who took very high doses over a long period of time, but the doses were much higher than what is recommended here.

A large study by Harvard University found that women who used a low dose aspirin preventive therapy program has 25% fewer heart attacks than women not on the program. Doctors do not recommended though that aspirin be the only preventive program women use for heart disease. Women should also quit smoking, control cholesterol, keep their blood pressure down, and maintain an ideal weight.

As a final caution, don't feel that because one aspirin can help prevent heart disease, then ten aspirin should wipe it out. Overusing aspirin is more like-ly to result in bleeding in the stomach, and can even result in death by itself. But so long as you stick to low and controlled dosages, you should not have to worry. Always keep in mind with any medicine, that if you take enough of it you can always reach a toxic level, so don't be scared off by warnings of what will happen to you if you abuse it. So long as you stick to recommended levels you have very little to worry about from most medications. The way medicines are prescribed, the more serious your disease the more likely you are to be taking drugs which will have side effects. Just so long as the side effects of the drugs are less seri-ous than the expected effects of the illness you are suffering from, you will be given the drug even though there is a chance it may kill or cripple you.

HEMORRHOIDS

Non-Surgical Treatments You Need to Know About

First a word or two about what hemorrhoids are, they are the veins at the end of the anal canal that have protruded from the canal itself, either internally or externally. Hemorrhoids are very common in American society, and over half of those over 50 suffer from this problem at some time. Luckily far fewer than that are ever faced with the prospect of surgical correction.

American medicine has at times blamed hemorrhoids on the aging process, as if going from 49 to 50 increased your chances of having hemorrhoids from almost nothing to 50%+. But that is ridiculous, all of the diseases of aging have causes, and hemorrhoids is just the same. In our diet we have minimized the use of fruits and vegetables to such an extent that we really don't get very much fiber unless we go out of our way to look for it. Of course you can always take Metamucil, which has natural fiber, or bran as a supplement, but most of us don't unless we are suffering from constipation.

And there is evidence that it is this lack of fiber in our diets that is the root of the problem of getting hemorrhoids. When you have little fiber in your diet, but a lot of fat, the typical American diet, your food moves slowly through your diges-tive system and your stools tend to be dry and hard much of the time. In fact if you ask Americans how many have had constipation over the past year you are liable to conclude that constipation is another typical American disease.

But, back to fiber. Fiber softens stools, and makes food pass through the digestive tract more rapidly. Fiber also carries water, which is the softening agent, and because of which you will rarely have a problem with digestion or constipa-tion if you have fiber daily, and preferably with each meal. Without fiber your stools dry out and it becomes a daily strain to pass them, and constipation is always lurking around the corner.

The result, according to most doctors and nutritionists, is that you develop hemorrhoids after years of straining to pass your digested solids. The best preventive of hemorrhoids is fiber, preferably natural fiber from fruits and vegetables. And since you don't digest fiber anyway, it doesn't matter if its fresh, cooked, canned, or whipped into a drink. Have fruits and vegetables daily, and with every meal and you will probably never be bothered by hemorrhoids.

But suppose you already have hemorrhoids, what do you do. First off, if the hemorrhoids are inflamed your doctor won't want to operate because inflammation can be cured, although it might be painful for a while. The first thing for you to do though is to have bran with all of your meals. While this is a good idea anyway, it is a necessity when you are actually suffering from hemorrhoids.

But, going a step further, suppose your hemorrhoids are not only painful, they are also bleeding, doesn't that mean that you are going to have to have surgery? Not necessarily, and not necessarily surgery. Even if they are bleeding you should stick with the bran for a few days, as well as a lot of water. But if it comes down to surgery, because there is no other choice to get rid of the pain, try the most conservative before you actually go to getting cut. If the hemorrhoids are external, and protrude outside from the anus, you can probably have them frozen with liquid nitrogen. This will make the tissues die and fall off, essentially the same effect as cutting them out, but with much less pain. If they are internal you can have them tied off, and they will die and fall off, also getting the same effect but without cutting.

Make no mistake about it, if your hemorrhoids are going to be cut out it is going to be painful, and you are going to be laid up for a few days at least. Both of the other methods work just as well most of the time, and they are cheaper, easier, and safer for you to carry out as well. Always look for alternatives to the surgical knife before you consent to having something cut out of your body. And good luck.

HERNIA

A Problem Which Deserves Conservative Treatment

A hernia is actually defined as the protrusion of any organ through the wall of the area that is meant to contain it. As you can see, you can have a hernia anywhere, from the top of the head, to the bottom of the feet. But what we mostly think of as a hernia is the hiatal hernia, which is a break in the stomach wall that allows some of the intestines to protrude out of the front of the stomach, and that is what we will look at mostly here.

Hiatal hernias are probably the most common anyway since the muscles of the stomach, and the digestive system, are in a daily fight to take care of the food we eat. Of course once we have a hiatal hernia, or any hernia, it is too late to cure it with anything else except surgery. But at least we can live with it, 95% of the time, if we just take care of it as we should. This conservative treatment, which avoid surgery, uses such methods as losing weight, not bending or stooping, avoiding tight clothes to avoid pain, avoid alcohol and caffeine, not smoking, having light meals, taking after meal walks, elevating your head while sleeping, avoiding acidic foods like citrus juices, avoiding onions, and avoiding estrogen drugs. For the greatest number of you who face this problem, this list of actions will avoid the need for surgery. And you will probably have no other problem to contend with as a result of your hernia other than these types of behaviors if you are careful to follow them.

But suppose that you don't have a hiatal hernia as yet, and you would like to avoid having one altogether, what should you do? The number one action to take is to have a high fiber diet (lots of fruits and vegetables every day), and to add supplemental vitamin C, unless you are fairly certain that you are getting at least one gram daily. Once you have gotten a hernia, there is not much you can do with it except to live with it, but if you haven't gotten one yet, then go to a little trouble and try to avoid getting it altogether.

Hernias are not magical illnesses sent to you because you are bad, they are the result of poor eating habits that people in other countries with better eating habits avoid. Don't make yourself a martyr to a high fat diet, have fresh fruits and vegetables when you have any meal and you may never experience the problems and pain of dealing with a hernia. Why would you want to experience a hernia anyway when you can avoid it?

HIGH BLOOD PRESSURE

Lower Your Chance of Needing High Blood Pressure Medication by Simple Dietary Changes

High blood pressure is largely caused by what we eat and how we live our lives. Changing what you eat can prevent, and possibly even reverse high blood pressure by taking away some of the things that cause it. We get high blood pressure when we do something to speed up our heart rates or narrow the arteries that the blood must flow through. As we get narrower arteries then anything that causes the blood pressure to go up can bring on a heart attack or stroke. If the arteries get narrow enough, then even the normal beating of the heart will be enough to bring on an attack. Follow these dietary changes to help your heart, and lower your blood pressure.

If you do not already control the amount of salt in your diet, then cut back. The most common cause of high blood pressure is the salt we eat. Salt uses a lot of the bodies blood to stay in liquid form since it can't go through the body in crystals. As the blood gets loaded with salt it has to have more and more volume and increases the blood pressure. That is why anyone who has heart disease is put on a restricted salt diet. It has nothing to do with cholesterol or blocking up the arteries, but only with how high the blood pressure is itself.

Cut down on fats in the diet. This is on all fats, both saturated and unsaturated. Fats add many calories, which increases body weight, and causes high blood pressure. Make doubly certain though that you cut down on saturated fats, especially those that have the LDL kind of cholesterol, since they will clog the arteries. To cut down on fats not only should you cut back on your use of butter and margarine, but also on cheeses, red meats, baked goods, and bacon.

Control your use of alcohol. Although there have been some reports of a protective effect from drinking red wine, that is still no excuse for drinking more than 2 drinks a day. When you have more than 3 drinks a day (and that is 3 cans of beer, 3 glasses of wine, or 3 mixed drinks), you will get a rise in your blood pressure. Drinking more than 2 glasses of alcohol a day will also cause other physical problems, and do not have any greater protective effect on your heart in any case.

Increase your intake of potassium rich foods. Potassium helps to protect the arteries against the effects of high blood pressure. It is always good to use foods in season, they are fresher and cheaper than using canned or frozen foods, and they give you a change in diet every few months. Good foods for potassium are cantaloupe, squash, avocados, oranges, bananas, potatoes, tomatoes, and milk. If you have a little land where you live you can grow several of these yourself and have them fresh out of the garden.

Get more magnesium into your diet, it is also a protective mineral against the effects of high blood pressure. It is also found in several of the same foods that are high in potassium, and all that you have to do is pick the right ones for a good diet in both. Good magnesium foods are nuts, molasses, wheat germ, soy, milk, bananas, potatoes, and brown rice.

Use more fish instead of red meats. Fish is high in protein and low in fat, at least most fish is low in fat. The fat in fish is also the LDL (good cholesterol) kind, so that it not only cuts fat out of your diet but helps to protect you against any narrowing of the arteries you may already have. Fresh fish, and fish in season is best, but you should include haddock, mackerel, trout, salmon, and sardine. Not all of these are needed, but they should make up a good amount of your fish diet. Fresh fish is also less fishy when cooked, and cuts down on the odor problem that can smell up your kitchen.

Fiber, fiber, fiber! Of the things you can, and should, eat to protect yourself fiber is number one. Fiber keeps things moving in your digestive tract, and cuts down on how much of the fat you eat that gets into your body to add weight. A high fiber diet not only helps in high blood pressure, but cuts down on your chance of getting several kinds of cancer. High fiber foods are whole grain cereals and baked goods, fresh fruit and vegetables, and bran. If you do not eat fruits, vegetables, and grains with your meals you will not get enough fiber to protect you and keep you healthy. High fat and low fiber in your diet will also give you constipation and stomach upsets, but low fat and high fiber will prevent both of these most of the time.

2 Natural Ways to Lower Your Blood Pressure
Up to 53% in Only Eight Weeks

To lower your blood pressure that much in that short a period of time is going to take some effort on your part. For one thing you are going to have to change the way you eat, and for another you are going to have to change what you do with yourself during the day, and in the evening. Of course, if your blood pressure is normal you are not going to end up lowering it, but if it is very high, over 200, then there is really a chance that it will drop into a normal range in just a couple of months.

Now, assuming that you have this very high blood pressure, your doctor has already told you to stop smoking and to lose weight, and you have been put on medication. If these steps have not been effective as yet it is probably because you have not given them your full effort. That is where these natural ways come in, they will give you the push to get you over the edge.

The first way is to put bran in your diet, preferably oat bran, but bran in any case. A study of high blood pressure men, over 260 mg/dl, who were put on a diet with 18 tablespoons of oat bran as cereal or in muffins, had an 18% drop in blood pressure in 10 days, and a 26% drop in 14 days. The benefits continued to grow so long as the men kept taking their bran. While this is a lot of bran, when you are that high in your blood pressure you need therapy that gives you quick results. The bran had the effect of lowering the bad, LDL, cholesterol and raising the good, HDL, cholesterol. And if you are wondering what part of the bran is doing most of that work for you, look at your oatmeal the next time you cook it, it's the sticky stuff that helps. That stuff is called oat gum, and it works much better than just roughage alone in reducing blood pressure.

But I promised you 2 ways to reduce your blood pressure 53%, and so far we're not sure if the oat bran will go quite that far. So I want to have you do next is get up and go for a walk. In fact I want you to get up and go for a walk twice a day, every day. It doesn't have to be a real hard walk, but it needs to last 30 minutes. What these walks add up to exercise, and just because you are not huffing and puffing as you do it, it does not mean that your body doesn't like it. Exercise will lower your heart rate, and help to give you an appetite that will allow you to eat 18 tablespoons of bran a day. If you have been physically active anyway, then you probably don't have the high blood pressure problem to begin with, so I don't think you have been that active. I am suggesting walking because anyone, no matter how out of shape you are, can take a walk. It's even fashionable in many parts of the country for people to get out and walk around all the time. But if you have some problem where you can't do the walking, go for a swim, or ride a bike, or get a home exercise machine. To get the rest of the drop in your blood pressure you are going to have to get physically active.

2 Ways to Protect Against
the Effects of High Blood Pressure

High blood pressure does its damage by directly attacking the walls of the blood vessels until you have a stroke, which is caused by a break in the blood vessels. But even if you have high blood pressure there is a way of lowering the chance of death from 83% to just 2%, and in only 4 months. The total reduction in strokes is also reduced by 75%. All that you have to do ; is to take bioflavonoids and potassium to protect the walls of the arteries from the effects of high blood pressure. The bioflavonoid is responsible for reducing the risk of strokes, and the potassium for the decrease in the death rate. If you have high blood pressure

---

then it would be a very good idea to start using supplements of both bioflavonoid and potassium to protect yourself from these effects.

46% Cut in Risk of High Blood Pressure with Fruit

Now why would fruit lower your blood pressure by 46%? Well apparently it is the fiber in the fruit that does it, and we don't know if fiber from other sources is just as good or not. Apparently its a continuous affect from eating fruit fiber, because the 46% drop in risk was the difference in those who ate the most fiber and those who ate the least. Apparently the more fruit fiber in your diet the less likely you are to have hypertension. The Harvard study that found this out also found that the biggest overall risk of getting high blood pressure comes from being overweight, and the more overweight you are the more likely you are to develop high blood pressure.

What Household Spice to Use
to Lower Blood Pressure

Research in Europe has found that doses of garlic powder have a positive effect in lowering both cholesterol and blood pressure. Research is also being carried out in the United States, but it will be a long time before American doctors get to the point of recommending everyone eat garlic for these beneficial effects.

The beauty of it is that you don't have to wait for official research reports. With garlic available everywhere, in fresh, powdered, and capsule form you can take it for just pennies a day. For proof of the good effects of garlic remember that the Chinese have used it for 2000 years to do just the things our doctors are studying, and the Chinese have a much lower risk of heart disease than Americans eating a normal diet over here. If you take the effort to include a little garlic in your diet every day you may prevent a heart attack, stroke, or at least the need to take blood pressure medication for the rest of your life. Besides, garlic is a wonderful spice in many foods.

HIGH CHOLESTEROL

Amazing New Research
Shows Nutrient that Helps Lower Bad Cholesterol

One of the best ways to protect yourself from heart attacks and strokes is to lower your level of bad cholesterol, the LDL cholesterol, and raise your level of good cholesterol, the HDL cholesterol. There are many dietary plans that do this, but recent research has also found that a common nutrient will do it too. The nutrient is vitamin C, and it works by preventing our arteries from being blocked in the first place.

Research has found that LDL cholesterol has a small constituent which sticks to damaged walls of the arteries and blocks them up. Vitamin C also goes to these damaged artery walls, but there it helps them to heal up. Once they are healed they no longer attract the constituent, and stay open the way they are supposed to.

There is still the problem of how much vitamin C do we need to take to protect us from heart disease. The answer is probably 3,000 to 6,000 mgs a day, spread throughout the day. If you want to know why so much when the minimum daily requirement is just a few milligrams, the answer seems to be that our bodies need all of this vitamin C because they don't make it themselves. Almost all other mammals make vitamin C in their bodies, and those that don't have a naturally high diet in vitamin C. We have messed around with our human diet so much that it now contains little vitamin C, and we pay for it by having half of our deaths caused by heart disease.

The LDL constituent is called lipoprotein a, or Lp(a), and our bodies use it the way they do because we don't have the vitamin C in us that we need. You need a diet high in vitamin C, but you should also take supplements. If you have a high cholesterol problem, or atherosclerosis, make certain that your vitamin C level is high enough to do some good. If you are taking the right amounts you may be able to do away with your cholesterol lowering drugs, but only do so if your physician agrees.

Chinese Food Lovers' Cure for High Cholesterol

It is nice to know that if you love Chinese food you are probably lowering your cholesterol too. But just eating Chinese food is not the cure for cholesterol, it is the soy sauce, and things made with soy like tofu, that do the job. Studies found a 12% drop in cholesterol after only 4 weeks on a low fat, soy fortified, diet. And if you think that soy only comes in the form of a salty sauce and tofu, you need to think again. Soy flower is available in Oriental markets and can be used to make bread, muffins, and fruit bars. Soy ice cream can be bought in some supermarkets, and soy candy bars are available in many stores. To get the most effect from a soy diet you also need to cut out as much fat as you can from your diet at the same time.

Cholesterol Warning:
Popular Drug that Increases Death
From Non-Cardiac Problems

Everyone who takes drugs for cholesterol has been warned of the possible side effects, but it has now been shown that the drug Atromid-S actually produces a dramatic increase in deaths from non-cardiac problems. This effect of this drug is very strange. It decreases the rate of heart attacks, like it is supposed to, but it also increases death from other causes. If you are taking this drug now, talk to your doctor about an alternative. If you have been told that you need to take a drug to lower your cholesterol, don't take this one if there is anything else you can take. Talk this over with your doctor until you are satisfied.

Does Margarine Protect Against Cholesterol? Maybe Not

If you are using margarine in your home and staying away from butter because you are trying to cut your cholesterol, you might not be doing as much good as you thought. Even vegetable oil based margarine can raise your cholesterol after it has been treated with hydrogenation. And look at the margarine package the next time you go to the market—they all say they contain hydrogenated vegetable oil.

This hydrogenation process creates trans-fatty acids in the margarine, and it acts just like saturated fats from animals to raise your cholesterol level. You can cut the level of these trans-fatty acids somewhat if you use tub margarine rather than stick margarine, and liquid margarine is better yet. But any vegetables oils that have been treated to hydrogenation are still going to contain some trans-fatty acids.

If you really want to cut cholesterol there is no substitute for cutting fat out of your diet. While this might be painful, it is still the only sure way of lowering your dietary cholesterol. Red meats are also included in this order to cut fat. For the oils, or fats, that you still use, begin using canola oil. Canola oil is inexpensive, and is the lowest oil in saturated fats among all of the major vegetable oils available.

Natural Ways to Lower Your Cholesterol Without Drugs

The normal treatment for high cholesterol is to take drugs which lower it. It is now known that there are also natural ways to lower cholesterol levels, that work just as well as drugs, and have no side effects. To give you some idea of what may be done with natural treatments, let me give you two examples.

The first is inositol hexanicotinate, which is a combination of niacin and a B-complex type vitamin which protects the liver. In studies of this substance there were no side effects and the cholesterol levels were reduced by 20%. This is a much better way to take niacin, which in a pure form can damage the liver and has other bad side effects, because the vitamin part of it is protective. This is not something you are going to find in a health food store, so talk to your doctor about this if you need this type of medication. It has already been used in Europe for almost forty years, successfully.

The second is gugulipid, it is a natural extract from the plant Commiphora mukul, and has been used in India for over 2,000 years. It has been shown to lower cholesterol by up to 27%, and works by getting the liver to produce more LDL cholesterol. It can even be used in pregnancy, and no other cholesterol medication can make that claim. In a combination called Gugu Plus no. 860 P.S.E., combined with inositol hexanicotinate, it is available in health food stores, If your local health food store is not carrying it, you can ask them to order it from a company called Enzymatic Therapy.

No Cholesterol Foods, That Are Actually Bad for You

If you think that all foods that claim to have no cholesterol are good for you, you are badly mistaken. Cholesterol is not the only thing in foods that can clog your arteries. Fat is also a big problem, and saturated fat is the worst form you can get. Since fat is not cholesterol, a snack which has no cholesterol can still be loaded with saturated fat, and that is the problem with this kind of claim. Saturated fat is always bad for you, there is no good form of saturated fat, and any food with a lot of saturated fat will be bad for you.

What foods should you look out for? Most baked goods, real ice creams, potato chips, most crackers; the fats in these foods are often what you taste and what you have learned to love, but they are dangerous. If you feel you must have some of these foods, even the high fat ones, then limit when you eat them and how much you eat. A daily diet of saturated fats will add weight, clog your arteries, and can add risks of digestive problems.

The Real Reason People have High Cholesterol
It's Not What You Think

If you have heard of people who eat nothing but fatty foods, but who have no cholesterol problem, then you are on the right road to the real cause of high cholesterol. Contrary to what all of us have thought, its not the cholesterol in our diet that causes the problems, its the cholesterol that sticks around on our artery walls that does it. And cholesterol doesn't do this all by itself, it needs help from another substance called lipoprotein a, or Lp(a).

Lp(a) actually gives you the damage of high cholesterol by sticking to the walls of your arteries, and then collecting cholesterol until it blocks blood from flowing through the artery to the heart, or until chunks break off and block smaller arteries. We get most of our trouble from LDL cholesterol because that is the type of cholesterol that is most strongly attracted by Lp(a), and because Lp(a) is common in our bodies.

Some people are protected from the effects of cholesterol because their bodies either lack, or have very little, Lp(a). And in order to cure our cholesterol problem we need to either get rid of cholesterol (which isn't possible because even our bodies produce it), get rid of Lp(a) (which also doesn't seem to be possible), or find something that will prevent the bond of artery to Lp(a) to cholesterol from forming, and in that we do have hope.

It has been found by Dr. Linus Pauling and Dr. Rath that you can break the Lp(a) artery bond by taking vitamin C. If you take high doses of vitamin C it will prevent you from getting heart blockages, or any other bad effects of too much cholesterol in your bloodstream. A high dose of vitamin C, on a daily basis, is 2 to 3 grams. Remember that the normal doses in vitamin pills is in the area of 200 to 500 milligrams, and that you will need 4 to 6 of the 500 milligram pills for your daily dose.

What Your Doctor Probably Misses
from Your Cholesterol Report
You Need to Know Total Cholesterol Divided By HDL

You may very well want to know what all of this concern over HDL and LDL has to do with your chance of getting a stroke or heart attack. What it comes down to is that HDL is protective to your heart and blood vessels, and LDL is the kind of cholesterol that can cause these problems. LDL is deposited in the arteries and causes blockage, but HDL removes cholesterol from the body. Some researchers even believe that it can unclog arteries that have been blocked with LDL cholesterol.

The concern about LDL and HDL has been growing the last few years, but you can't just assume your doctor is measuring each of these separately when he gives you a cholesterol test. Always ask what each level is, and what it means—that is if he recommends a change in your diet or some medication. For your own information an HDL level of less than 35 is considered high risk no matter what the overall cholesterol level is. If the HDL is above 35 then you want to know what the ratio is of total cholesterol divided by HDL comes to—the lower the number the better so a high total cholesterol and a low ratio is much healthier than a low cholesterol and a high ratio. For example, a total cholesterol of 200 and an HDL of 50 gives you a ratio of 4.0 (200/50), but a total cholesterol of 200 and an HDL of 40 gives you a ratio of 5.0 (200/40), which is a higher ratio and indicates a greater risk to you.

HOUSEHOLD

Eliminate Toxins from Your Dishwater

Toxins in your dishwater come from the strong detergents that are used to clean dishes. Besides the heat of the water, dishwater detergents add strong chemicals like chlorine to cut grease and dried on food. If you have ever wondered why an automatic dishwasher can get off food that has been on a plate for a week, it is because of the chemicals it contains, and they certainly aren't just soap.

Because some of these chemical are so toxic, you need to make certain that all of them are rinsed off of your dishes every time you run them through the washer. The problem is that you may be so used to this kind of contamination that you don't notice the strange tastes you are getting. As a test hand wash and thoroughly rinse some plates and glasses. Then take some that have gone through your dishwasher, and place samples of water, juice, and other foods in side by side taste test fashion. If you taste any difference in the dishwasher washed dishes than you do in your hand washed ones, you can be fairly certain that you are getting contaminants from your dishwasher.

If this is the case there are a few steps you can take to eliminate these toxins from your dishes. If you can you might consider changing the dishwasher, since newer ones are usually better at getting rid of these contaminating residues. If that isn't practical then at least change your detergent types. It is possible that a health food store has a natural based form that has eliminated the harmful chemicals. You might even try something like borax that should be less contaminating. As a final solution you may even consider hand washing all of your dishes, and that is certainly possible if it is only one or two of you using them, or if you have the help of growing children who can be assigned the task.

But whatever you do make sure that you go through the taste test again before you just assume that everything has been taken care of. The idea is to be better safe than sorry.

IMMUNITY

A Vitamin to Maximize Your Immune System

For your immune system to be working at its best your blood must move as easily as possible through your veins. The defensive white blood cells travel in the blood, and the slower they are in getting to something that gets into your body, the more infections and illnesses you are going to have. A wonderful vitamin that helps your blood to flow more freely is vitamin C, but you must take much more than the recommended daily amount. To be an effective aid to the immune system you must take at least 1,000 milligrams, and up to 6,000 milligrams. You can't get an overdose of vitamin C, but if you want to take a dose of much more than 1,000 milligrams a day over a long period of time you should check with your doctor to be sure you don't have any conditions than might be affected for the worse by it. An additional benefit of high doses of vitamin C are increase in mental function as measured by IQ tests.

Kick Your Immune System Into High Gear

Your attitude toward life affects the function of your immune system. If you are in a good mood and feel able to cope with the world your ability to fight off disease, and get well from illness, is much better than if you are depressed and feel that the world is too much for you. In the prison camps during World War II thousands of soldiers died simply because they gave up on life and allowed themselves to die. Even today a Navajo Indian who feels he has been bewitched may simply resign himself and die. Your attitude to yourself and to life controls how well your immune system works. If you have trouble having a positive attitude about life, whatever the reason, than talk to yourself about it. Be alone, if you must, and talk out loud, yell, scream, and laugh. If this is a problem then write down everything that is a problem, get the grudges off your chest, and look at the good things in life—and every life has good things in it. By getting all of these bad, negative, things out of you, you can get your immune system working for the good of your body. It will no longer be necessary for it to overcome your bad feelings in addition to whatever illnesses it is faced with, in keeping you healthy.

IMPOTENCE

A Diet to Help, and Its Simple Too

Impotence is the inability of a man to complete sexual intercourse. It has many causes, and at least some of these are related to diet. If you have been having a problem with impotence it might be a good course to consider what foods your diet is made up of. Some simply make you feel sluggish, and affect your sexual performance as well as the rest of your physical functions. Fortunately not too many foods are believed to be a cause of impotence, but fat and refined carbohydrates are. These should both be cut back as part of our diet plan to cure impotence. Fat usually means red meat, but also includes fried foods. Refined carbohydrates are mainly sugar, and that means in baked goods as well as the sugar you put in your coffee and on your cereal.

Fortunately there are some foods that we can also use to increase our sexual performance. To begin with the nutrients, increase your iodine, magnesium, selenium and zinc. Iodine is available from seafood.

See, I told you this was a simple diet, and if it cures your problem is will be the best diet change you have ever made, or at least it should feel like it.

Natural Remedies to End Impotence and Premature Ejaculation Plus Increase Sexual Desire

When we talk about impotence and premature ejaculation, we have more than one problem in mind. If you have a problem with impotence, then you probably don't have a problem with premature ejaculation, but you may have one with a lack of sexual desire. Of course sex can be taken as a whole package, and that means to a problem in one area can very well show up in others. But let's deal with the odd problem first, premature ejaculation. This occurs generally because of poor timing between what you and your partner are doing. The object in any sexual encounter is for both of you to climax together. But it you go off during the petting and fondling stage this can leave both of you frustrated. But there are a few simple remedies to handle this, but you have to be willing to practice.

The first is that you have to have a consistent partner. If you go changing bed mates every day, then you may always be in such a state of excitement that you always have premature ejaculation. If so, you will probably end up closing off sex out of embarrassment and dissatisfaction, and you will still be frustrated. So let us say that you have a long time partner. This person is going to have some understanding and sympathy for you, or they wouldn't bother staying with you, and that is half the battle. If you are the only one who has the problem, so much the better. If you have sex frequently with one person the level of excitement normally goes down, and the problem may cure itself in that way. If not you may have to resort to a little trickery. You are going to have to keep yourself calm while you get your partner excited to the point that they are near climax, and then you step in and let them stimulate you. When you are ready, no matter how soon, just jump in and enjoy yourself. Of course it might not be that easy, and you can always resort to a drink of alcohol to depress your desire somewhat before you begin, but don't have more than one or two. Anyway, those are some basic techniques for premature ejaculation, and somewhere to begin.

But if your problem is lack of desire and impotence, you are going to have to do even more planning. Desire comes from the mind, if there is nothing physically wrong with you. Men and women are both generally stimulated by looking at naked bodies, or reading about people engaged in love-making. That is a start. Also talking with your partner about sex, or even creating fantasies works for many couples. In diet, cut out alcohol, cut down on coffee and tea, and never try to do it on a full stomach. All of these are turn offs to sexual desire, and they can also be big contributors to impotence. Impotence is the lack of sexual desire expressed in the inability to carry out the act of sex.

Impotence is most often caused by changes in body chemistry, but it may also result from depression, or surgery. When it is chemistry that causes it you can usually correct it by stimulating sexual desire, as noted above, and supplements of the B vitamins. You might also increase your other vitamin supplements, and get enough rest. If you are actively seeking to bring desire and potency back, you are going to have to have a healthy, active, and sexually stimulating life style. Take an active interest in sex and chances are it will take an active interest in you.

Simpler Treatment Which is Closer to Natural

The usual treatment for impotence is testosterone given as shots a few times a month. The only problem with this method of getting the testosterone, other than the shots themselves, is that you get a high dose when you get the shot, and it drops steadily until you get your next shot. While the shots work, it still means that your testosterone level has to be brought up well above your normal level at the time of the shot so that it doesn't fall below the level at which it will do you any good before the next shot.

Now there is a much simpler treatment which will bring your testosterone level to around a normal amount, and keep it there over a longer time, and there are no shots required. This method isn't available yet, but if you are in need of testosterone therapy you should inquire anyway through your doctor. What this new method uses are skin patches, the same as those nicotine patches which are used to stop smoking or nitroglycerin patches for heart disease. The testosterone patches are being developed by Theratech, Inc., in Salt Lake City, and they are being tested at the University of Utah in Salt Lake City. While the number of young men who need this treatment are very small under the age of 65, the need can occur at any age, and after the age of 65 as many as 20% of the males in the United States can benefit from testosterone therapy.

INCONTINENCE

Prescription Drugs May Cause Your Problem

While many cases of incontinence have no known cause, it is known that a large part of them are the result of taking prescription drugs. In general the larger number of drugs you are taking the greater your chances of developing a problem of bladder control. The problem is especially common among older women who tend to be taking medication for several ailments. With the custom in the United States of going to specialists for each problem, it is very likely that you will be prescribed drugs which are incompatible with one another. Because the kidneys have the job of breaking down chemicals you take into your body, they are

---

affected by every drug you take whether or not it is prescribed for a medical condition.

If this is the cause of your problem, and you are going to have to question your doctor to determine that, then you will probably be referred to a specialist in medications who will alter what you are taking to solve the problem. Generally this condition is cleared very rapidly in this way, but it can develop in anyone at any age, and the older and sicker person just happens to be the usual victim. Also remember that Americans tend to overmedicate themselves anyway, so if there is a way of avoiding drugs for a minor illness, you may also be avoiding an attack of incontinence as well.

INFERTILITY

The Latest Views on Curing Infertility

With everyone paying attention to women having rights to abortions, it seems almost odd that many women are desperate to have babies. And most of them are married or have long term male partners. Uptill recently, when a couple wanted a baby and there was no pregnancy, the woman would be tested for everything, and then maybe the man would be. If they wanted fertility drugs, they had to wait a full year after getting off birth control pills, and so on with a lot of other treatments that didn't make much sense and just made the process of getting help longer. But things have changed now, and by reading the next few paragraphs you can make the whole procedure faster and less trouble for yourself.

First off, doctors no longer believe that the woman is the most probable one to have a problem if a couple can't get pregnant. Now both members of the couple are brought in together and examined. This speeds up the process of diagnosis, and should no longer make the woman feel isolated and picked out as a problem.

Also when you go off of birth control you can be given fertility drugs after only 6 months instead of a year. The year rule didn't have any particular basis in medicine anyway, and doctors just finally decided that it caused more problems for couples than it solved.

Sperm counts do not any longer determine if a man can father a child. Sperm levels can be normal, but not have enough strength to penetrate an egg and cause pregnancy. So doctors will now have sperm tested for its ability to penetrate eggs if there is a normal sperm count and no pregnancy. Some of the automated machinery used for sperm counts has also added to weakening belief in it now. These machines sometimes count other stuff in the semen than just sperm, which give a count much higher than is real and covers up low sperm counts that really do exist.

Everyone has heard about different test tube methods of causing pregnancy. Using this approach eggs can be taken from the woman and fertilized in a laboratory, and then put back into the woman's womb. Although this is not quite a normal way of going about getting a woman pregnant, you end up with the parents you want, and mechanical difficulties with both the male and female equipment can be overcome.

Not all of the old solutions have been discarded though. Doctor's still advise couples to give up smoking and drinking before and during pregnancy. Recreational drugs should not be used in any form either. Each of these habits is known to affect the blood supply, result in low weight births, and in some cases in seriously ill babies. When a baby is born with a condition caused by recreational drug use there is no cure, and sometimes the baby doesn't even survive.

Some problems are so small that they can't be detected with regular medical examinations, but they can with those little fiber optic devices doctors use now. A cyst the size of a pin point can be seen in a tube and removed where originally it would never have been seen, and removal would have left an unusable tube anyway.

Diet may also be of help. Vitamin C protects against some of the effects of smoking. Studies have also found increased birth defects when mothers had less than 60 milligrams of vitamin C in their diets.

If you want more information contact the American Fertility Society at 2140 11th Ave. S., Suite 200, Birmingham, Alabama 35205-2800. Or phone at (205) 933-8494. And good luck.

INJURY SECRET

Use this Ice-Then-Heat Treatment for Best Results

Injuries are damage to the tissues, or cells, or your body. When you are injured, and the tissues are most damaged, they are open to infection, they bleed, and they are hot from the collection of blood at the point of the injury. When you are injured you need to control the injury according to what are the most dangerous, and frightening, symptoms you are going to have. The most immediate problem may be bleeding, and this can lead to a serious condition more rapidly than most anything else. To control bleeding apply direct pressure, but also apply ice. The ice will slow the blood flow, and the bleeding, and give your blood a chance to coagulate, When this has happened, and you are no longer bleeding (usually after 2 or 3 days if this has a serious injury), then you need to apply heat. The heat will increase the blood to the injured area and increase the rate of healing. If the injury has been serious enough to cause any serious bleeding, then don't try to apply the heat too soon, or it could cause more damage by increasing the area of swelling. Increasing the blood flow through heat also removes the waste products of the injury, but it can also aggravate it by increasing the pressure of the blood flow, so only use it when swelling has stopped and stop if the swelling is increasing while you are applying heat.

For the most part injured areas should be kept cold, though not extreme-ly so. The cold will allow the injured area to rest because the blood flow is slow-er, and will prevent secondary damage from excess swelling. For an emergency cold pack frozen vegetables, a half gallon of frozen ice cream, or a frozen fruit bar are just as effective as ice packs, and they can be eaten afterwards.

INSOMNIA

If you can't sleep at night then you have insomnia. But that is not all of the story, since insomnia can be short term or long term, and your treatment will depend upon which it is. But for all insomniacs, now that you have a sleep debt, and you owe your body some rest, what are you going to do about it? There are many answers, and the easy ones are often not the right ones. But if you don't know and try the easy ones you will never get to the hard ones that you need now and again. A good rule of thumb though for any sufferer of insomnia, don't try to use alcohol to help you sleep, it will only disrupt your sleep more, and can even contribute to breathing problems and more insomnia when you try to rest.

6 Tips to Stop Insomnia

This is a little checklist of ways you can go about stopping insomnia. It is meant that each of the tips is to be followed completely, so don't just do one or two and expect to be cured of your insomnia. Although an occasional sleepless night is certainly insomnia, you won't be able to get over it with these tips. But insomnia that lasts for a few days may be handled very efficiently by working all 6 into your schedule.

1. If you have a night without much sleep, or even a few, don't feel that it will make you unable to do your job, or carry out your responsibilities, the next day. Although some of your physical and mental abilities are affected by lack of sleep, most of the time a night of insomnia will not even be noticeable to the peo-

ple you work with. Even without insomnia many people are tired while at work, and the cause doesn't really matter. Also don't worry about it too much. The worrying may be worse than the problem. Just follow the next 5 tips and most of the time you will be fine.

2. Suppose you have a real worry that is causing the insomnia. You can't just make that go away by forgetting about it because it is a problem you are going to have to solve and live with. So what do you do? While you are waiting for a final outcome on the problem you are going to have to express it to get it outside of you where it can be shared. Talking it out with a friend or family member is best, but a psychologist or group treatment program works better for many people who don't want to go it alone. If you have trouble using either of these methods, there is another one which even psychologists often use, but you can do it alone. Sometime in the evening before going to bed, and for as long as the problem lasts, take some paper and write down all of your thoughts and feelings about the problem. You can keep this to yourself if you want, but keep each days writings for as long as the problem lasts. This will not only allow you to express those bottled up fears, but you will also be able to see where the problem is going after a few days. Also by getting it off of your mind you will be able to relax and sleep in peace. You will know that the problem is not being ignored because it will be there in the morning for you to deal with, just not in your consciousness keeping you awake.

3. Now that we have gotten your mind in shape for sleep, you need to get your body in shape too. At least one hour before going to bed have a snack (not a meal), take a walk or have a little exercise, and read a book. You needn't do all of these every night, but if you do at least two, you will have your body in a relaxed state.

4. During the day you are going to have to change your habits and your diet, at least as long as the insomnia persists. Give up caffeine drinks and smoking. Both of these accelerate your heart rate making it harder to relax. In addition smoking causes your blood vessels to get smaller so that your blood pressure will go up. Taken together you will have created a small case of anxiety for your body and make it harder to relax for sleep. All alcohol in the evening should also be eliminated. Alcohol slows the heart rate but it also causes your body systems to lose coordination and disturbs sleep.

5. If you are having trouble getting any sleep while in bed, then get up and do something to try to relax yourself. Lying in bed without sleeping will result in very shallow sleep, and leave you anxious, while doing some of the relaxing exercises in 3 may help your body to get itself ready to sleep. Of course don't get up and have coffee, smoke, or drink alcohol as any of those are likely to just make it harder to sleep later on.

6. Finally, keep a schedule. Try to go to bed at a normal time, and get up at a normal time. If you lay around all morning trying to make up sleep, you will just ensure yourself another night of insomnia. It is only by having a regular nightly pattern that you will be able to tell if you are getting better, and if any of the

corrections you are doing are working.

While this set of tips may not work in a single day, if you keep them up they will work for most people. Give yourself a couple of weeks of the 6 tips before you decide to go on to a doctor or to try another plan. None of these are anything that should be a big problem to anyone else, and all that you need to carry them out is some determination.

How Sleep Loss Affects Your Health

Any time you are suffering from insomnia you feel sleepy all of the time, as well as wonder about what the lack of sleep is doing to your health. Well, lack of sleep is not really harmful to you directly. That is, losing sleep does not mean you have cancer or will have a heart attack. The bad effects of sleep loss are what they do to your judgment and behavior.

You can more easily lose track of what you are doing, even if it is driving a car down the street. You can also miss seeing other cars or pedestrians, and could easily run into one or the other. If you sleep very little at night you can also fall asleep virtually anywhere—even sitting in front of your boss, or doing a job you are interested in.

If this is a problem of yours, and that means not getting at least 7 or 8 hours of sleep a night, then begin taking action toward a cure, and the sooner the better.

Jet Lag or Changing Shifts
Prevent Insomnia With a Pill

You can get your sleep schedule off so much when you travel, or work changing shifts, that no matter what you do you cannot rest at the right time so you can be alert when you want to be. There is now a pill that will help, and it has been tested in over 100 experiments in changing the sleep schedules of people, with a nearly 100% rate of success. The pill is called melatonin, and it can move your sleep schedule forward or backward whenever you wish. It also works very well for insomnia too because it allows you to set the time you will fall asleep, and it works. The pill is not yet available to the public, but a .5 mg. dose is enough to be effective. Melatonin is the hormone your brain produces naturally while you sleep overnight, so you will not be putting any foreign drug into your body when you use this.

Natural Cures for Your Sleep Problems

The best way to overcome insomnia is to do something for yourself that will let you fall asleep naturally. When you are sleepy you will be able to sleep, but if you have insomnia you never seem to get sleepy, so what do you do? Your first action has to be to make yourself physically tired. If you look in the books on how much people sleep, they always say that as you get older you tend to sleep less and less. But why should older people sleep less than younger ones. One answer may be that older people just are not physically active enough to get tired. If someone in their 70's or 80's is infirm, and just sits or lays around all of the time, it may take them 2 or 3 days to use up the energy that an active person half their age uses in 1 day. So the first action you must do is to exercise daily, but not necessarily too strenuously. Thirty minutes to one hour a day of any real physical exercise should be enough. This includes walking, biking, swimming, or gardening. Just give yourself this time and most of the time you will not have any insomnia.

Now that you have gotten your body sufficiently tired, you still need to get drowsy before you can go to sleep. Drowsiness is caused by a chemical in our bodies called serotonin, which increases because of the natural tryptophan that our body also produces. For several years tryptophan was prescribed for insomnia in the United States, but was banned in 1989 after a batch became contaminated. It is still banned and you cannot get it legally here. However, your body still needs the serotonin to feel drowsy, and it still has a supply of natural tryptophan circulating in your blood. To help raise the level of tryptophan, and serotonin, before you go to bed you need to eat a carbohydrate food such as bread, pasta, or a potato. The action of the carbohydrate will take everything out of your blood except of the tryptophan and you will begin to feel drowsy as the serotonin also increases.

There are also some nice herbal aids to sleep. The hops that are used to make beer act as relaxants. A beer before bedtime can help induce sleep, and if you don't like the idea of alcohol (which can disturb sleep), then use non-alcoholic beer. It is still made from hops, only the alcohol is taken out.

Valerian has been studied in 128 people and has been found to help sleep to be more restful, and to reduce sleepiness on waking, which is a problem for commuters. As far as effectiveness, it works as well as barbiturates in many cases, but without the side effects you get from the barbiturates.

Finally, try passion flower. Passion flower was used by the Aztecs before the Spanish invasion to help induce sleep, and as a pain reliever. The interesting effects of passion flower as a sleep aid are that it helps overcome the habit of waking in the middle of the night that many people have. This waking pattern is common in cases of depression, and depression is certainly common if you are having trouble getting a good nights sleep.

In addition health food stores have other over-the-counter natural remedies for sleep problems, and talking things over with these people may be very helpful to you. But first I would try the exercise, carbohydrates, and herbs, and most of the time you should not have any need for further medication for the problem.

Relax Tension to Overcome Sleeplessness

Many times when we have trouble going to sleep it is because we have gone to bed in a tense mood. When you are tense your body won't relax properly even if you empty your mind, and sometimes this can go on almost all night long.

Well, instead of just lying awake in bed for hours try doing some things to relax your body and allow yourself to fall asleep. Simple stretching exercises are very good, but it can also help if you take a shower first. The shower will increase the blood flow to your skin and help to warm up your muscles.

Some very good exercises to use to prepare your body for sleep are just slow stretching movements. Try standing with your feet a little wider apart than your shoulders, place one hand on your upper thigh and extend the other over your head. Then bend toward the side with your hand on your thigh—you can also bend that knee slightly to help stretch the opposite leg. Repeat this on the other side, and then on both sides four more times each. The combination of the shower and the stretching should be enough of an exercise to allow you to relax properly for a good night's sleep.

What to do About Chronic Insomnia

As a general rule of thumb, chronic insomnia is any problem in sleeping that lasts for more than two weeks. Of course it can also go on for years as well, but in this case it isn't really the insomnia that is the problem. While chronic insomnia may seem like a major problem, it is really the cause of it that should concern you. Chronic insomnia can be caused by a serious underlying disease, or serious mental illness such as extreme depression. For these types of problems sleeping pills and exercise plans are of little use.

The best, and sometimes the only, way to cure chronic insomnia is by finding the cause and treating that. While a cure of the underlying cause is best, it is often enough just to know what the cause is in order to cure the insomnia. The problem then becomes one of how do you find the underlying cause of your insomnia?

The most obvious answer, since there may be a serious disease involved, is to go to a specialist who will be able to diagnose you. While that is a good idea, the best specialists are located in diagnostic centers which can charge up to $1500 for an evaluation, and many insurance plans may not cover it. There are also self-help books available, and these may be of some help in putting you in the right direction.

These books usually give you ideas about reducing stress in your life. Stress reduction is the same whatever the problem it causes. The recommended program is to practice deep breathing exercises, meditate, think of quiet and pleasant places, and take quiet walks. While this is not a lot of detail on stress reduction, even if you do these successfully they may not work since the cause of your insomnia may be more a result of behavioral problems than of mental ones.

Behavioral problems mean that your body has just got out of the habit of sleeping when you want it to. The common cause of this is plane flights where your day and night periods change by several hours. Most of the time these correct themselves in a few days, but not always. If your body is tied more by sleeping and waking at certain hours than by the rise and set of the sun, your clock can have you up in the middle of the night and asleep in the daytime when you need to be awake.

There are a few behavioral modification methods to fix this kind of problem. For one thing you can use a sleeping pill to put yourself asleep at the right hour, and force yourself to wake up when you wish. This will help sometimes, but if it doesn't and you keep taking the pills you can become dependent on them. You can also do the same thing without pills, and this may work even better. All that you do is force yourself to stay up during your normal waking period, and then go to bed the next day at the sleep time you are trying to establish. You are usually so tired by then that your body will fall asleep, and the normal pattern will be established naturally.

If neither of these restore your sleep to the way you want it, then go one step further and begin keeping a sleep log. The sleep log will include your events of the day along with your period of sleep. A few weeks of doing this often reveals particularly bad times sleeping after specific events in your life. The events may be things you would not have expected such as meetings with your boss or golf games with your friends. But once you have found out the most probable causes you can avoid or change them so as to cure the insomnia.

These are just a few of the ways you can cure chronic insomnia. For an underlying disease you will need an examination by your doctor, along with treatment. But for every other cause there are things you can do directly as well as help you can seek from specialists. The only sure thing is that you cannot get over chronic problems, even insomnia, without taking some actions to cure the causes and treat the symptoms.

What to do About Temporary Insomnia

You can get temporary insomnia from jet lag, or a fight with your spouse, or from having a bad time at the office. Insomnia for a day or two is common when you have either had a hard or bad day, or when you are going to have one soon. The nice thing about this type of insomnia is that it is temporary, and it will go away on its own no matter what you do. But if you would like to give it a hand, and the insomnia has lasted more than a day or two, here are a couple of things you can do.

First, try an over-the-counter sleeping aid. Never do this for chronic insomnia, but for temporary bouts and use of no more than 3 days or so there should be no complications. The over-the-counter sleep aids are preferred to the prescription types because they are not addictive, and in lower doses. While you may think that higher doses are better, all that means is that you are giving your body a bigger dose of drugs. You should always go with the lowest dose that will do the job.

If over-the-counter doesn't work, then go to your doctor and try a prescriptive type. Because of their strength and ingredients these should only be used under a doctor's care. The doctor will watch out for addiction and help you to get off of the drug when its time. Often this is all that will work if you are dealing with a death in the family, or are suffering from a psychological problem such as depression.

For something in between you can try an aspirin, an antihistamine, taking a walk before bedtime, or reading yourself to sleep. These are what most people do to get to sleep anyway, and if it isn't one of your habits already, then it may help you to overcome a case of temporary insomnia. Try one and see.

IQ BOOSTERS

6 Types of Food Which can Increase Intelligence

Intelligence is the ability to reason and remember clearly and efficiently. If you are on drugs, even prescription drugs, or are taking any mood-altering substance your ability to reason and remember is changed, and you will score lower on intelligence tests. Because some drugs are known to lower intelligence, because they decrease our ability to think, it is logical that other drugs can help us think more clearly and rapidly. The drugs, or foods, that help us to think better are then capable of raising our intelligence levels. If you don't know something, or have never learned it, you won't know it just because you eat the right food. But if you once learned something, then eating the right food may help you to remember it, and be better able to use, and so to have a higher level of intelligence. It is those foods, and nutrients, that are going to give you a higher level of intelligence that we want to look at here. There are 6 types that are of interest, and each one is worth considering if you are concerned with how well you are doing when you need to use your intelligence to solve problems, and help you get ahead.

1. The first class of intelligence boosters we want to look at are those which help the neurotransmitters. Neurotransmitters are the pathways in the brain that carry your thoughts through your body. If your brain runs low in neurotransmitters, or you take in something that interferes with them, your thought processes will be slowed and you will be less intelligent when you are called upon to think. The most efficient neurotransmitter found so far is zinc. In animal studies, using monkeys, those with a low zinc level took 2 to 3 times the number of minutes to solve problems as those with a normal level of zinc, and their immune systems was depressed as well by up to 30%. While nutritionists do not think that American foods are low in zinc, it is known that many of the soils in our country are zinc deficient, and that our fertilizers do not add zinc to the soil. One simple solution is to just take zinc supplements, and 25 to 50 milligrams a day is enough for a good benefit. If you are still interested in getting your zinc from a natural source, 10 of the best food sources are also given (the numbers are milligrams of zinc in a 4 once serving, so you decide how much of each one you want to eat each day):

110 herring

14 wheat germ

10 sesame seeds

9.9 yeast

8.3 molasses

7.5 maple syrup

7.0 liver

6.7 soybeans

6.6 sunflower seeds

4.8 chicken

2. The next class of intelligence boosters has only one member, and works to help your memory. The first group was to help how fast your brain worked, and this is to help you remember what you have already learned at some

time before.   To find something that would boost memory, 40 middle aged peo-ple were given supplements of lecithin by the Neuromedical Centers of South Florida. The results were that 90% of the test subjects getting lecithin had a sig-nificant decrease in lapses of memory, and 60% of the test subjects on placebos had an increase in their lapses of memory. This is good evidence that lecithin is a necessary substance in having a good memory. It was even found that 40% of those getting lecithin were better emotionally, having a better feeling about them-selves and less anxiety, although this might have been due to the decrease in memory loss.   Choline is one of the main ingredients of lecithin and is thought to be the active fraction of memory sharpness. So if you have any problem in tak-ing lecithin supplements, then at least get the choline, and you should get all of the positive effects you are looking for.

3. When your brain is at work it burns energy, just like any part of your body. You use sugars to make your muscles work, but a protein called glutamic acid is used to make your brain work. When your mind is active it can run out of glutamic acid, and it will gradually slow down until it has to take a rest while the glutamic acid builds back up in the brain. This was the idea behind a test by doc-tors using children with I.Q.s around 65. After getting glutamic acid supplements for a year the I.Q.'s of these children rose by 11 to 17 points, and some of them moved their IQ. level into a normal range. With the positive effect of this test it was concluded that adults should take supplements of 1,100 to 4,0000 milligrams of glutamic acid, or 1-glutamine as another source, daily. These supplements are available in health food stores.

4. For general overall good health of the brain and its blood flow system vitamin C is recommended. Vitamin C has been found to be good for so many things in our bodies that discovering that it has a positive effect on IQ. seems to be expected. Raising IQ. may be only a side effect of all of the other good things vitamin C does. These include helping the immune system to be stronger, assist-ing wounds to heal faster, and helping the bones and blood vessels to be health-ier. The gain with vitamin C was measured at 5 points, which is about a 5% boost in IQ. for most people. When the IQ. effect was studied the group being tested was only given one glass of orange juice a day for 6 months, so it is possible that a higher dose or a longer period of time would result in a larger gain in IQ. You can take vitamin supplements if you wish, but natural sources are very common and can be used just as well. Ten of the best, and their milligrams are vitamin C, are given below.

3,000 rose hips

240 guavas

110 green peppers

55 strawberries

51 spinach

50 oranges

47 cabbage

38 grapefruit

35 lemons

32 green onions

    5. Vitamin B1 may be the champion IQ. booster, if you are willing to accept rat studies. The most extensive studies of vitamin B1 and IQ. have been done with rats, and the results are outstanding. Rats given high doses of vitamin B1 made record runs through their mazes, while rats put on low doses could barely make it through at all. Along with the rat studies, there have also been some studies of human, and these have also been very positive, with IQ. increases of 22 points in children given high doses of B1.

    Since B1 is found in many of the foods we eat every day you may think that you get enough in your diet. However, there are many ways that we destroy the natural B1 we eat so that it is not available to help us think clearly. Some of the things to avoid are refined cereals and bread, refined sugar, alcohol, smoking, coffee, raw fish, birth control pills, antacids after meals, emotional stress, and estrogen and sulfa drugs. If you do any of these, or a combination of them, you are probably deficient in vitamin B1, and need to change your eating habits or take supplements. If you want to take supplements you will need a 50 milligram dose per day of B-complex. Of course you should also cut back, or cut out, some of the activities that are depleting your B1 too. If you want to increase your B1 through your diet, here are 10 foods with the highest levels, and that do you the most good. The numbers are in milligrams in a 4 ounce serving. The recommendation is that you take a supplement and eat high B1 foods as well.

6.0 brewer's yeast

2.2 sunflower seeds

2.0 wheat germ

1.2 peanuts

1.1 soybeans

0.68 beans

0.60 oats

0.33 walnut

0.32 egg yolk

0.25 almonds

KIDNEY PAIN

2 Things You Must do to Save Your Kidneys, Or Even Reverse Kidney Disease

Kidney disease is not rare, and it always has a cause. Some of the most common causes associated with it are diabetes and high blood pressure. While this association has come to be accepted, accepting it does not explain it very well. So what if you have diabetes or high blood pressure, why should that cause your kidneys to fail?

The answers to your questions might lie in the diet you eat. If you have a good American diet you probably eat 8 ounces or more of high protein foods every day, giving you about 150 grams of protein in your daily diet. Is there anything wrong with that? There sure is, if you are concerned about your kidneys. Your kidneys have the job of breaking down all of that protein that your body doesn't need, about 2/3 of it, so it can be eliminated from the body.

Your body does this in the kidneys, and it puts a lot of strain on the kidneys to work that hard every day. Normally your kidneys can handle the workload without any problem, but if you develop high blood pressure or diabetes, the workload increases a lot. These diseases damage the kidneys, and the protein they have to process for your good American diet takes a lot more work to break down. The result is that the kidneys fail faster and more often then they would if you did not eat so much protein.

To save your kidneys you are going to have to cut down on protein. The World Health Organization only recommends 40 grams of protein a day, not 150 grams. If you tend to eat high protein meat and dairy foods with each meal, the easiest way to cut down might be to just have 1 or 2 meals a day which are all vegetables and fruits. If you do this you will feel a lot less sluggish through the day, as well as help your kidneys.

If you are already having kidney failure, there is still something you can do which might reverse it, and will certainly help it anyway. A report in the New England Journal of Medicine reported a study of patients with progressive kidney failure who were put on a low protein diet. In this study the patients were given only 20 to 30 grams of protein (less than the 40 grams recommended by the WHO), and were watched to see how they reacted. Of 24 patients in the study, 7 had their kidney failure stopped or reversed. The answer to reversing kidney failure, and its not a promise, is to go onto a low protein vegetarian diet. If you have any problems with your kidneys you should cut your proteins down. And even if you have no problems with your kidneys, it would be a good idea to have a meatless, low protein, meal every day.

KIDNEY STONES

Diet Changes to Help You Get Rid of Them

You might say that all kidney stones are the result of a bad diet, and you would be pretty much right. We cause our stones by our diet, and to a certain extent we can cure them the same way. At the very least we can help a bit by changing our diet. The diet will also help you to keep from getting more stones.

To help get rid of the stones we need to cut down on protein foods, sugar, and alcohol. But if you have calcium oxalate stones, and your doctor will have to tell you that, you also need to cut down on tea, coffee, chocolate, spinach, sweet potatoes, cucumbers, peanuts, grapefruit, beans and carrots. This is quite a list, so it would be a good idea to find out from your doctor just what type of stones you have before you begin revising your diet.

Now that you have cut back on all of those foods that are giving you the stones, and making them worse, what can you do besides that will help to prevent more stones from forming? For all stones you need to increase your fiber, magnesium, and water. And if you have the calcium oxalate stones, you also need to increase your B6.

There, that wasn't so bad. You need to cut down on a lot more of your food items then you have to increase, but you can live with that. Remember that repeated attacks of kidney stones can lead to the loss of your kidneys, and that would leave you on dialysis. Don't get scared, but get moving and correct the problem before it becomes something that is going to control a large part of your life.

Prevention With A Nearly Free Beverage

In Your Home Now, and Also Effective for Urinary Tract Infections and to Ease Joint Pain, Fight Constipation, and Avoid Wrinkles

The one beverage that we need every day, in large amounts, and which can do all of these good things for you is water. While you will be aware of the water in your body when you have edema, you should also remember that it is the water in our cells that makes our skin smooth when we don't have edema. Water also carries the waste materials through our digestive system, fighting constipation and flushing out organisms that can cause urinary tract infections. Kidney stones form when the water in our body is insufficient to keep the salts we eat in our food from forming crystals. So when we drink too little water, the salts form kidney stones that cause pain and may require surgery.

The best advice is to drink water throughout the day. If you are hungry, drink water or liquid with whatever you eat. Also drink water between meals instead of having a snack and you may not need any other diet to lose weight. You need to have about 8 glasses of water a day, one with each meal and one or more between meals and in the evening, and even more if you are active in the sun either working or exercising.

Something else to remember is that as we grow older our bodies store less water, and we don't drink it as much to satisfy our thirst. As you drink less water your skin will dry out, and the kidneys will have to deal with larger concentrations of salts and minerals (if you have older relatives or friends it is easy to find some who have very dry skin surfaces). The only way to solve this problem, since your natural craving for water will decrease, is to make it a point of your diet to drink 8 glasses of water every day. While this may be a bit of a problem, it will do you a lot more good than it can do harm, and avoiding an attack of kidney stones is worth drinking something your body needs a good supply of anyway.

KNEE PAIN

The Common Cause and What to do About It

Knee pain can come on you anytime, or it can be related to a particular exercise like climbing the stairs. In either case it is either related to some particular damage to the knee, such as bruising, or to some chronic problem such as arthritis. If you have bumped or fallen on your knees recently, then you probably have pain that doesn't easily go away. Athletes are particularly likely to get this kind of injury since the knee has been called the weakest part of the human body. The only thing about this kind of injury though is that it heals up. You may have to get fluid drained off of your knee and take anti-inflammatory pills, but the knee will heal up and be as good as new for normal use. If you are a football player, then you will probably have a similar injury some time in the future, and it may very well end any career that you have playing football. But for those of us who are not paid athletes, once your knee heals up, if you take care of it, you may never have another injury of this kind again.

But that now brings us to the other kind of knee injury, the other cause of knee pain, arthritis. You get arthritis when the bone around the joint that the bones of the knee fit into overgrows where it is supposed to be. The bone will actually form a little lip that keeps your knee from bending properly, and may press on nerves and blood vessels. Arthritis of the knee probably starts from some little injury around the knee, or reinjury, and that causes scar tissue to form on the bone. Only scar tissue on the bone, when it is around the joint, interferes with the bending of the joint.

If you have this there are only a few accepted cures. First, you can just live with it and take anti-inflammatory medicines when it hurts. Most people do that, and you can have a pretty much normal life that way. It is also a good approach if the knee doesn't hurt you all of the time.

But if the pain is more or less constant you may have to take a more aggressive method of dealing with it. You may need a daily supplement of pain killers and anti-inflammatories, or you may need surgery. While the pain killers and anti-inflammatories are available over the counter, the surgery will require the services of a surgeon. What the surgeon can do, and more of them do now, is use microsurgical techniques. He will make a little incision on your kneecap, insert some thin tubes, and proceed to trim off and remove the extra bone that has grown around your knee cap. In most cases this is a permanent cure, although there is always the chance that it may have to be done again in the future.

But suppose you have done all of that and nothing works, the pain is still there and you can't exercise, or even walk very well. The last medical cure is the most radical, it is the replacement of your knee with a mechanical knee. They actually have to remove your original knee joint and put in a metal one, which is attached to the bones of your leg. This is a permanent replacement, although there is always the chance that it might also have to be done again some time in the future. However, in most cases you will be cured.

The final advice that I will give you is use the least radical cure that you can. The more difficult the medical treatments, the more likely you are that your cure will be less than 100%.

LONGEVITY

5 Natural Ways to Purify Your Body
Get Rid of Toxins that Cause so Many Health Problems

While no one can predict just how long they will live, it stands to reason that less illnesses you have in your life the fewer chances you will have from dying of them. Everyone who dies, dies of something that may have been preventable. Of course some of the illnesses that kill us are a result of something that we did many years before. After all, you have to smoke for 30 or 40 years before smoking will kill you, and no one can tell you which cigarette it was that was the fatal one. We just carry on with our bad habits for as many years as we can, and then we die because of them. Well one of the ways to lessen the chances that this will happen to you is to use some preventive measures. The best preventive measure is to never be exposed to anything that might make us sick, but that is an option none of us can do. The next best way to go is to protect ourselves with the foods we eat and the vitamins and minerals we take to at least counteract as many of the threats that we can. The last way to go is the medical way. If we get to the point where we want a doctor to make us well again, then we have suffered damage that we may or may not be able to correct. In the hopes of preventing some visits to the doctor, here are 5 natural ways to purify your body and give you a long and healthy life.

1. Coenzyme Q-10, or CoQ-10, is a natural nutrient available as a food supplement, and in unsaturated oils such as corn oil and soybean oil. It is used to protect the heart and muscles of cardiac patients, and is effective for some kinds of muscle diseases. Although not widely used in the United States, 20 mil-

lion Japanese use it as a daily supplement, and UCLA is currently testing its effects on prolonging life. There are no known side effects. There are also no recommended amounts established, but taking an amount equal to a tablespoon of corn oil or soybean oil would probably be sufficient.

2.   Primrose oil has also created some interest lately as a prolonger of life. It it extracted from the primrose flower, and is known to lower blood cholesterol, which is an excellent preventive measure all in itself as far as heart disease. But it even has a wider application in relieving some of the symptoms of rheumatoid arthritis, and in laboratory studies it has been shown to kill cancer cells. Obviously primrose oil will take some years to be fully known, but its promise is great, and its hope is grand.

3.   Quinones, which are found in many different foods, are used in Japan to counteract memory loss in age-related diseases. These substances are in a very basic research state in the United States, although a Harvard researcher believes that they may have very strong anti-aging applications. Remember that nutrients that are found in many foods can best be supplied by eating a wide variety of food in your diet. The more narrow and limited you make your diet, the more likely you are to be missing essential vitamin and mineral combinations that will protect you from disease, and help you recover if you do get ill.

4.   AL-721 comes from egg yolk, and works to take cholesterol out of cells, and helps cells function better. Now this is very odd since egg yolk often thought of as the world's worst source of cholesterol, but maybe we have something special here. AL-721 has been studied in Israel where it has shown promise as an immune system booster. In a test, 70% of a group over 75 years of age had improved immune system function, and some of them were so invigorated that they felt 50 years younger. You may have to look around a bit to find this, but if you have a high cholesterol problem and low energy level it might be worth the trouble.

5.   Terazosin is a prescription drug used to treat high blood pressure. While known mainly as an alpha blocker, it is also being tested as a treatment for enlarged prostate glands. Happily it has been found to lower blood pressure and cholesterol levels along with improving prostate function. Because of these multiple benefits it has now been labeled as a good drug for the mid-life male. Of course we don't yet know what other uses it may have, so keep your eyes open for further announcements. By the way, if you are interested in it, it does have a side effect of mild dizziness and faintness, so show some caution when you use it.

Birthdays Can Shorten Your Life
But Who Are They Worse For?

Birthdays are either one of those traumatic events that kill people, or one of the days of happiness that people prolong their lives for, but in any case most people die around their birthdays. The psychologists think that birthdays are something that the dying prolong their lives to enjoy one last time, so maybe a birthday will actually lengthen your life, but who can say.

A study by the University of California found that more women died in the week after their birthdays than at any other time of the year, and more men in the week before. While this may be important, women still live several years longer in America than do men, so its only the week of the year that is important, not how many years either men or women live.

If you are seriously ill, and in danger of dying, it might be comforting to know that you have a good chance of living until the week before or after your birthday. But if you are not seriously ill, but in danger of something like a heart attack, perhaps you should consider your birthday a day of risk. For either men or women who are in reasonably good health, make your birthday a happy occasion and you will look forward to it and many more. If it is a time of depression and pain than you may feel like dying on your birthday, and maybe this study tells us that it can happen. Have a joyous birthday, live long and proper.

Foods to Eat to Beat Disease, Reverse It,
and How to Stop It From Attacking Your Body

Reversing disease with diet is always questionable since it depends on how much destruction a disease has done to your body. The higher the level of damage the less chance you will have for a complete recovery, no matter what steps you take. However, if you have the motivation to use a natural diet to control the diseases that threaten you, as well as the ones you may have, there is no reason why the same foods shouldn't have the same benefits. After all, doctors are now prescribing aspirin to prevent heart disease, and it have been used for years to treat pain of all sorts, so why not food as well.

To fight disease we need to get all of the natural sources of high nutritional foods that we can in our diets. We want our immune systems to work well to fight anemia, and anything else that attacks us. We need strong bones to fight osteoporosis and arthritis. Everyone wants to fight cancer and heart disease. and keeping our weight at a normal level along with our blood pressure, will protect us from many other diseases, and cure a few as well.

To go down the major list of food areas we will start with meat sources: fish for good HDL cholesterol; poultry for vitamin E and iron; in red meats, use only lean cuts of anything and have small portions; shellfish also for iron; dairy foods should always be low fat or fat free, and are also good for iron and all minerals and proteins; cruciferous vegetables like cauliflower and cabbage for vitamin C and fiber; yellow and orange vegetables for beta-carotene and iron; dark green leafy vegetables for vitamin C and iron; carbohydrate vegetables like potatoes and corn for B vitamins, minerals, proteins, and fiber; grains for proteins and minerals; beans for proteins and fiber; and citrus fruits for vitamin C.

While there are many other foods you can eat as well that are very good for you, so long as you eat a large variety of the best foods you can choose, you will be getting all of the disease fighting benefits that you can out of your diet.

9 Tips that Can Add
10, 15, even 20 Healthy Years to Your Life

The leading causes of death for Americans can be protected against with nine good health actions, we can take ourselves. None is impossible, but some are harder than others, so look them over and see which ones you can do yourself. It's a matter of life and death!

1. Stress—excessive stress increases the chance of suffering from heart attacks, accidents, and suicide. Find ways to minimize stress, relax, and take some time for yourself.

2. Exercise—a perfect way to lower stress, as well as help against diabetes and heart disease. Exercise doesn't have to hurt, just walk 30 minutes a day, or take up a variety of activities that can build up a sweat three or four time a week.

3. Weight—exercise helps to control weight by burning up calories and decreasing appetite. Over-weight people are more prone to have heart attacks, strokes, and suffer from diabetes and arthritis.

4. Diet—weight problems are caused by poor diets as well as by a lack of exercise. To have a healthy diet increase the amount of whole grains, fruits, vegetables, and fish you eat. Also decrease the amount of fat, cholesterol, and salt. Fish also contains substances which can lower your blood cholesterol.

5. Alcohol—a diet should not include a high level of alcohol. Alcohol has Calories and very little nutrition. High alcohol use, more than two drinks a day, can cause liver disease, accidents, and suicide.

6. Tobacco—the reason people use tobacco is usually for the lift it gives them, and they usually don't think about what it is doing to their body. Anyone who is a heavy user of tobacco in any form is at risk for cancer, heart disease, lung cancer, and respiratory disease. There are no health benefits to tobacco use in any form, only a probability of causing serious illness and death.

7. Environmental Hazards—tobacco can be an environmental hazard if you don't smoke, but someone near you does in the workplace. Other dangerous environmental hazards to watch out for are ultraviolet rays, chemical pollutants such as cleaners and solvents, and radiation in any form. These substances can cause cancer over time, or even poison you the first time you come into contact with them.

8. Seatbelts—while we don't have control over what we come into contact with at work, we all have the choice of wearing seatbelts when we ride in a car. By law all cars must have seatbelts, and everyone must wear them when the car is moving. Also all small children must have a safe car seat to ride in. Remember that all new cars will soon be required to have car seats as well, so make sure that your new car has one if you are in the market.

9. Sex—this is a lot like driving a car, but is much more personal. Everyone is afraid of AIDS, and there are other sexually transmitted diseases that can cause cervical cancer and sterility as well. Take precautions with anyone you are not sure of, and that should include anyone you have been in a relationship with for less than one year. It would also be comforting to be tested for AIDS at the start of any new relationship, and at the end of a year. Stay faithful to one person if you want to stay safe.

Recovery Secret
How to Imagine Yourself Healthy Again

The medical scientists at Case Western Reserve University have been studying a medical secret that anyone can do any time. It can help you to good health even if you are suffering from a serious disease, or have just had surgery. The idea is to imagine yourself healthy by thinking of the thing that is a problem, and seeing it as solved.

Cancer patients have used this to imagine their killer cells attacking cancer cells, and people with high blood pressure have used it lower their blood pressure without drugs. It is built on the idea that our attitudes cause a lot of our illness, or prevent us from being cured of it. When we are happy and in control of our lives we can get well much sooner than when we are depressed and unhappy.

To use this system successfully you must be as specific as you can in imagining what you want to happen. If you have a a broken bone you must think

---

of the bones as healing together, and if you have high blood pressure you must try to see your blood flowing freely through your body. This is something that works and that you can do on your own, but practice helps. There are also many groups around the country that do this type of treatment, and you can easily find one if you really feel the need.

Natural Life-Extension Secret
That Can Add 10 to 15 Years to Your Life

The secret to living longer is exercise, and you need to start today. It doesn't matter if you are 40 years old or 80 years old, if you want to add years to your life you have to get out of your chair and exercise.

Exercise is good for you because it gets all parts of your body in operation. Your heart rate increases, your bloods pumps faster, your breathing deepens, your muscles become warm, your joints loosen up, and your skin opens so that you sweat. These are all good things, and every time you do them you should know that your body is in reasonably good shape. And exercise not only lets you know that you are in good shape, because you are moving you can also tell if there is something wrong pretty much anywhere in your body. Look at exercise as your daily physical, and ask if your doctor would do as much for you. Doctors don't do daily physicals because their tools are too crude to find anything that happens in just one day, but you can. Also, sitting in one place all of the time can never tell you if there are any changes in you for the worse, but exercise can tell you that as well as whether there are changes for the better as well.

But, we will say, you are sold on exercising, but you have not gotten out for a while and you don't want to overdo it, what do you do? Well, the goal is to exercise 4 days a week, for 1 hour a day, but not all at once. Because you have been inactive you need to start out slowly. You also may need to see your doctor first and tell him what you are planning to do. If you are cured, you go ahead. To start, you go out for a 15 minute, leisurely walk the first day. Then repeat this every other day. After a week or two, walk a little faster and kick up the time to 30 minutes. Then every month increase your pace and your time until you are up to a brisk one hour walk, 4 days a week. To monitor yourself though, if you get so out of breath that you can't carry on a normal conversation while you are walking, stop or slow down.

Now that we have gotten in shape you can add other exercises to your plan, and do anything that is enjoyable, and which doesn't carry a risk of injury. Above all, avoid injury. If you get injured you will lose all of your benefits over a few months and have to start all over again.

Finally, this will actually add 10 to 15 active years to your life. The quality of life is just as important as the length, and the little pain that you have to endure for this exercise will pay off handsomely in keeping you independent and active for many more years. Exercise helps you to resist illness, as well as to keep your heart and lungs in good working order.

Regain Good Health, Vigor, and Have Abundant Energy

Are you wiling to use a 2,000 year old Chinese remedy for old age? It's one that a billion Chinese have sworn by for 10 times the length of time that the United States has been a country, and they believe that it gives all of the benefits that you are looking for.

If you haven't already guessed what I'm talking about, it's ginseng. However, ginseng is not only a Chinese remedy, it's also used all over Asia, and one of the major sources in the world is the United States.

But of course that is not what you are interested in. What you want to know is if it will really do the good things that are claimed for it. Well according to Chinese medicine ginseng helps to maintain good health in people of all ages, but is especially helpful to the aged, and it helps to maintain sexual vigor and potency, and finally it serves to give the body energy in abundance.

If you are willing to take the word of the Chinese population as to the value of ginseng, you will find that it is not very expensive. It is usually sold in Asian markets packaged as tea, with 100 servings costing around $7 or $8. There are also more expensive versions, but there is no reason to get into those initially. The taste is a little odd to Americans, but it is not at all bad with sweetener. Ginseng is also being marketed in a soda drink in deli type stores, but I do not know if you get the same dose as you would from the tea. For a dose I would recommend anywhere from one to three servings a day, depending upon the effect you are looking for. And if I were trying it I would certainly use it for two or three months with several doses a day before I would conclude that it wasn't doing me any good. Chinese medicines usually are designed to work very slowly over a long period of time, so you should not be looking for dramatic results in just a day or two. If you want to be able to measure changes that should take place keep a complete health diary for the entire test period. If there is no change after three months, then it is probable that the ginseng isn't going to do you any good. If it does help, then its a cheap source of healthful nutrients. And remember also that ginseng is sold as a nutrient, not as a medicine, so the stores that sell it will make no claims for any medical effects that the Chinese people commonly use it for.

Strengthen the Natural Disease-Preventing Organs in Your Body

While all of your organs are subject to disease, only certain ones are vitally involved with preventing disease. It stands to reason that if you can keep your defense line strong, it is less likely that disease will attack those organs or any other part of your body either.

The main organs that protect your body from disease are your skin, your digestive system, your kidneys, and your heart. Your skin is the first line of defense and protects you from all of those outside influences like bacteria and molds that are floating around in the air. Healthy skin simply kills off these attackers as it comes in contact with them, or resists them until they fall off. Strengthening your skin requires a good diet, keeping clean, and avoiding damage from the sun, or other cuts and scrapes. Whenever you get a brake in the skin you should be concerned about infection, and clean and protect the area accordingly until it heals.

Your digestive system is the next line of disease prevention because that is where all of the protective nutrients are removed from your diet. Many doctors consider the digestive tract part of the skin because it is continuous with the skin, and that gives you some idea on how to protect it. To stay healthy you don't want any breaks in the digestive tract (in the form of ulcers), and you want to keep food moving through it at a good rate through roughage to prevent local abrasions and infection. It is these local abrasions and infections that lead to chronic bowel diseases, and intestinal cancer. So eat your fruits and vegetables to keep your digestive system healthy.

The kidneys have been placed next because they serve to cleanse your blood of all unwanted waste products and return healthy nutrients to the body. The kidneys are just a filter system for the blood, but without their proper function you cannot live. The kidneys respond most negatively to medications and drugs, since they all have to pass through to be eliminated. Keep all unnatural medications and drugs out of your body if you want your kidneys to stay in good shape.

The heart was mentioned last, although it could just as well have been first. Your heart is responsible for circulating the blood, along with the functional parts of your immune system, through your body. When your heart loses its efficiency, your immune system stops operating effectively too. To keep your heart healthy, give it some exercise every day as well as the amount of rest it needs. Avoid smoking, which decreases oxygen in the blood and creates a constant state of congestive heart failure. Eventually smoking will lead to real heart failure, or cancer anyway. And keep the fats in your diet down, along with the cholesterol, to keep your arteries open and not starve your heart for oxygen.

The Type of Hospital to Avoid—Your Chances
of Dying are Increased 25%

No one wishes to die, and certainly no one wishes to die when they go to the hospital. It has now been reported by the AMA that if you are treated in a rural hospital, of less than 100 beds, instead of in a larger, big city, hospital, your chances of dying are increased by 25%. If you must go to the hospital, and it is not for an emergency, you are usually wise to think twice about going to a small, local, hospital rather than to a big city hospital for the same treatment.

LONELINESS

Is it More than Being Alone?

Loneliness is one of the worst tortures we can suffer, for it is the longing to be with and near someone, and the absence of anyone to be with or near. Of course it is more than being alone, all of us are alone most of the time without being lonely. It is only when you have no one who you can call on for a talk or a visit that it becomes terrible.

Not too surprisingly older people more often suffer from loneliness than those who are younger. As we grow older we can't help but lose family and friends to death, and many of those close to us retire and move off somewhere to be near family members who have also moved away. If we live long enough our life companions also die, and if we have never married and have a family this point of loneliness may arrive generations earlier.

But anyone can become lonely at any time. Loneliness is a feeling of isolation, and it is the reason that many of the lonely have long conversations with supermarket check-out clerks and bank tellers. These are captive audiences, and even though they may not really know or care about you, they have to sit and smile at you for a few minutes while you do business with them. But these are not good solutions, and will never solve your problem of loneliness. To do that you have to change your life.

Lonely people do not communicate. If you communicate with someone else in a personal manner, you care about them and they care about you. And therein lies the secret to getting rid of loneliness. Finding someone to care for, if there are no family or friends near, takes a personal investment by you. For one thing you have to get into a situation where there are people who want to communicate and share with you, even if they don't know you yet. And where will you find these types of persons. If you are religious, go to church. Churches are always glad to have new members come to them, and will do their best to make them welcome. Churches also have a constant stream of social situations, as well as volunteer work in which you can contribute your skills and get to know others.

If you are a senior, there are senior citizens centers in every community, and these people are always glad to have a new face join them. After all, as a group, older people are the loneliest in America. Go to the center, join in on the activities, and talk to other attendees.

If neither of these suggestions fit you, join a club. While it is not as easy to get to know someone in a club as in a church, these people at least have the potential to identify with you, and communicate with you.

Finally, volunteer for something you enjoy. This will give you immediate identification as a valuable person, and appreciation by the organization you volunteer for. The need for volunteers is everywhere: schools, libraries, the YMCA and YWCA, the Salvation Army, public gardens, museums, colleges, and community playhouses. Anyway, you should have the idea. Go anywhere you want and look for an opportunity to participate in life. Loneliness is usually something that just happens to people, it is not something that anyone plans because they want it. The cure is always to find someone with whom to share some part of your life.

But one further suggestion, suppose that you are restricted to your home, or even to a hospital, because of your health, what can you do? This is where you make use of the mails, or even the computer mails. There are always other shut-ins who want to have someone to talk to, write to one of them. If you don't know how to find them, call your local senior citizens center, and they will help you. Local churches will also help you, and they will also look in on you occasionally for helping out one of their members. There is always a way, so never stay isolated. Being totally isolated and lonely is bad for your health, and bad for your life. Get involved with others.

LOOKING GOOD

Crowning Your Way to a Better Smile

This is a problem that commonly comes up as you get older, but which you can have at any time. When you lose a tooth, or more than one, should you get a crown or a bridge, and what will it mean if you do get one?

First off, what they are. A crown is put over the base of a tooth that can't be filled, but which is too good to pull. A bridge is used to replace missing teeth in the mouth. If your dentist says that you need a crown or a bridge and you don't get one you could be in for trouble. The tooth you need the crown for is going to get worse, and you will lose it anyway. And if you don't get a bridge to fill in the space where you have lost teeth your cheeks are going to sag in and you will have trouble eating. The eating problem will put more pressure on one side of your mouth than on the other and you could get problems with the bones of your jaw next.

If you decide to get the crown or bridge here is what you can expect. For a crown the dentist will take you into his office and make some impressions so he can have the crown made up. Then, on your next appointment he will remove all of the bad tooth material and leave a strong base to attach the crown to. When the crown is attached it is simply glued onto the root, and you will be able to use it the same day. As far as appearance, crowns look very natural. They are usually made with metal bases, because that is stronger, and coated with a natural looking porcelain that will restore your appearance. As far as cost you will probably be looking at $500 to $1000, but many insurance companies will cover crowns.

For a bridge you are looking at a more complicated job. The bridge has to do the job of the teeth that have been lost and look good at the same time. It also has to be fastened to the teeth on either side of the missing one. Preparation to put in a bridge usually doesn't require much grinding, but the cost will be about the same as for a crown. The dentist will again measure and plan for the area to be filled with the bridge, and have it made. On your next visit you will get a porcelain bridge with metal supports on the sides. The metal supports will be glued to the teeth on either side of the missing one. You can also get a removable bridge if there is some problem with permanent gluing.

Whether you get a crown or a bridge it will improve your smile, but it will not be permanent. Crowns are stronger than bridges, but both will wear out after 5 to 20 years. Don't let that discourage you though, while you may know what you have in your mouth all anyone else will see is that you have a normal face and teeth. Take care of your smile and it will take care of you.

Feel You Look Older Than You Are?
Here's How to Look Younger

If you look in the mirror and think that the image looking back is older than you feel, it may just be that you have poor posture. One of the ways we judge how old a person is, is how they hold their bodies when they stand or walk. If you tend to slump your shoulders, allow your stomach to protrude, and sag your hips as you go about life you will look 10 or 15 years older than you may actually feel. On the other hand, if your posture is good, and you move about with an active and purposeful step when you walk, not only will you look better, but people will respond to you as they would someone 10 or 15 years younger than your actual years, and probably more like you feel about the world. If you don't care, it doesn't matter, but if you do, then there are four simple exercises that might help your posture, and the way you and others see you in the world.

1. Upper back straightener: in this one lie on your stomach, turn your hand down toward the floor and place them under your face. Then lift your elbows and count to five. Repeat this 10 times and you should get some strength in your back, which will help you hold your upper back in a more vertical line.

2. Semi sit-up: begin this by lying on your back on the floor and drawing your knees up until your feet are flat on the floor. Squeeze your stomach and buttocks tightly to give some tone to these areas. Fold your arms across your chest and slowly raise your your upper body off the floor (your head, neck, and shoulders), but keep the mid and lower back in contact with the floor. Hold this position for about 5 seconds, and repeat 10 times.

3. Knee lift: again lie on your back on the floor, and squeeze your stomach and buttocks. With your knees bent, draw your legs up until you can put your hands on your knees, and pull your knees slowly toward your chest. Hold this position for 10 seconds, relax, and then repeat 10 times.

4. Tilt the pelvis: lie on your back, squeeze your stomach and buttocks tightly, bend your knees and draw them toward you till your feet are flat on the floor. Pull your stomach in as tightly as possible and hold for 5 seconds, and repeat for 20 times.

If you faithfully take a half hour or so out each day and perform these exercises, you will have better posture, look better and younger, and feel stronger and better looking as well.

Facial Fitness Exercises to Erase Wrinkles

This is not something everyone should try, because some dermatologists question whether or not it works. Facial fitness exercises for wrinkles are based on the idea that sags in the skin are caused by the same things that make parts of the body and arms sag, weak and loose muscles. Whenever you go into an exercise program the muscles on your body tighten up and your body looks better even though you may not lose a lot of weight for a long time. There is also some evidence that loose muscles contribute to sagging of the skin on the face. Men who shave every day, and stretch their skin around to get all the little lines and corners of their face, seem to have fewer wrinkles than women of the same age. It is not known though if this is caused by differences in hormones in men and women or by the stretching that the men do.

But even with the doubts some dermatologists around the country are coming out with videos and programs promoting facial exercises as a cure for wrinkles. Others though are saying that these exercises will damage and loosen the skin—the opposite of what you want. Of course the exercise that men do to their faces would seem to be against the arguments of those dermatologists who are against it.

It is probably not harmful to the face to give it a daily massage and exercise the muscles. Stretching should not be too extreme, and a toner will help tighten the skin at the same time. If you give this a try and notice any damage then stop immediately. But for most of you it will probably do more good than harm.

LOSS OF APPETITE

What to Eat to Stimulate Your Appetite

Appetite is a funny thing. Sometimes your appetite can be so large that you eat all day, and you are never full, and at other times it can be so small that you don't eat much of anything for days, or even weeks. Now this great variation in your appetite is a normal thing, just so long as the swings from big appetites to small appetites even themselves out over a period of time, and that you have a normal appetite most of the time. But what happens if your appetite has gone away, and you don't know where to find it? You eat or you don't eat, or you eat certain things that you like but they don't even taste good. Your appetite may have gotten so confused by diets, dinners, and food binges that you don't know

---

when you are hungry anymore and when you aren't.

When those times come to you where you don't know where your appetite has gone, and you want it back, there are a few diet rules you can follow that might just help out. But before you start eating foods to increase your appetite there is one thing you are going to have to cut back on, and that is refined carbohydrates. What this really means is sugar, and it includes sugar in your donuts, cakes, and ice cream, as well as sugar in your coffee and on your cereal.

Now to help your appetite you need to get away from the idea that you need large meals 3 times a day. Go with small meals throughout the day, of both food and drink. Appetite is also helped by thiamine, which is found in bran cereals, along with zinc. Herbal teas can also help out in promoting appetite. The teas need to be made of fenugreek, juniper, clover, and yarrow. These are all available in the health food stores, but probably not in your local supermarket.

LOW ENERGY

Want More Energy? 20 Natural Foods that Boost Energy

The answer to a low energy problem might lie in your refrigerator. The foods you eat can make you feel tired, or they can make you feel good. Even without a perfect diet everyone eats foods that seem to give them energy, and also some that make them feel tired and sleepy. Here are 20 foods that can rid you of that tired feeling, and make you feel energetic and alive, and they are loaded with the right vitamins and minerals to do the job:

1. Atlantic mackerel—a 3 ounce serving for vitamin B-12
2. Baked Potato—one medium, with skin, for vitamin B-6
3. Bananas—one medium for vitamin B-6
4. Broccoli—a 3 ounce serving for beta-carotene and vitamin C
5. Brussels sprouts—a 3 ounce serving for beta-carotene and vitamin C
6. Cantaloupe—at least 3 ounces for beta-carotene and vitamin C
7. Carrots—a 3 ounce serving for beta-carotene
8. Cheddar cheese—one ounce for calcium

9. Chicken breast—a 3 ounce serving for vitamin B-6

10. Clams—a 3 ounce serving for vitamin B-12

11. Grapefruit—one-half for vitamin C

12. Kidney beans—one-half cup for vitamin B-6

13. Milk—one cup for vitamin D and calcium

14. Oatmeal—one cup for vitamin E

15. Peanuts-one ounce for vitamin E

16. Sockeye salmon—a 3 ounce serving for vitamin B-12

17. Spinach—a 3 ounce serving for beta-carotene

18 Sweet potatoes—3 ounce serving for beta-carotene and vitamin B-6

19. Wheat germ—one-quarter cup for vitamin E and vitamin B-6

20. Yogurt—one cup for calcium and vitamin B-12

LOW SELF-ESTEEM

12 Ways to Feel Better About Yourself

If you feel bad about yourself, feel that you don't have any friends, or are just depressed much of the time, it may be that you just have a problem of low self-esteem. While you may know that no one is perfect, it may seem to you that everyone has things better than you. Once you get this kind of an idea in your head you may have no idea how to get it out, and consequently spend days and months being depressed because of this common problem. The way to escape from this trap is to put into practice some or all of the 11 ideas presented here. If you do that you will not only have a high level of self-esteem, but your whole life, and outlook on life, will change as well. Read them over and put them into practice, and see how good you can be.

1. Start off by taking a positive attitude about yourself. Quit being overly critical of everything you do, and if you can't think of anything good to say about yourself, don't say anything at all. As a way of getting away from criticizing yourself too much, make a conscious effort to smile, relate to others, and just think good thoughts. You will be surprised how far this conscious attitude shift can go in raising your self-esteem.

2. Communicate to others about your feelings, dreams, and interests. There must be someone you know, or you can write to who would like to know

what you are trying to accomplish in life. If there is no one close to you then join a support group, you will often find them in the community services area at YMCA type locations where costs are minimal. If you know something you can teach others then volunteer your teaching, if you can't sell it, and you will find people who look up to you as a worthwhile person.

3. Take some time to see the good in others, and compliment them in some way. Do this verbally if you can, or you can show it in other ways through little thoughtful gifts that are acceptable in any situation. Don't be so forceful in your compliments that you sound insincere, really look for what you admire in others around you.

4. Smile to others around you, be friendly, and greet people around you, even if you don't know them personally. This may seem like a strange thing to do, but if you are walking toward a person on a lonely path around the city a smile, and a hello, will relieve the tension for both of you. If you are the one to act first you can congratulate yourself on turning an awkward situation into a comfortable one. This works especially well at all social gatherings where there are many people you don't know, and can often result in someone to talk to for an evening.

5. Don't be overly critical of those around you. Just as you don't want everyone who sees you to see only your bad points, do the same for people you see or meet in public. Anyone who consistently makes critical remarks about everyone else is soon dismissed as simply unhappy with life, and that is the opposite attitude from what you wish to convey. If you don't see anything complimentary at first, then don't comment at all and give the other person a chance to express themselves—you might be surprised at how attractive they are beneath whatever surface flaws you see initially.

6. Make an effort to look good. If you haven't had any new clothes in a while, then go buy an outfit. Also see that you are well groomed, since this makes a good impression whatever you are wearing. The idea is to make enough effort to improve your appearance so that you feel that you look good, or at least better than how most people have seen you. Even if they don't say so specifically, people will react positively to a nice and neat personal presentation.

7. Do something to please yourself. You can't feel good about yourself if you never do anything that you like. This may mean making some time for yourself each day or each week, but if you do you will find that you are accomplishing something that is more important to yourself than you can imagine. This can be a hobby, reading a book, cleaning your house, planting a garden, or anything else to which you give value whether or not anyone even knows that you do it.

8. Do something unselfishly for others. This may be volunteer work, or just good deeds. It can also be doing something special for your wife or children, or for a relative or friend, just because you know they will appreciate it. Try to make it come from the heart, and pretty soon it will.

9. Find a support group to get involved with. Clubs are very good, or the YMCA, or a professional organization. We are not lone animals, and to feel that

we are worthwhile people we need others around us who share our values. Everyone has interests, and sometimes you must look a little bit to find a group that has the particular interests you have. Especially good places to look are night school classes, trade magazines, community bulletin boards, and local newspapers.

10. Don't spend your energy comparing yourself to others. It doesn't make any difference what advantages other people around you have, you are unique, and others who share your uniqueness will want to be with you. Worrying about age, health, intelligence, and money in other people is a fruitless and endless process that can only depress you, and without benefit. Better yet, don't do any personal comparisons at all. Everyone has both good points and bad points, and there is no reason to spend time on either one.

11. Fulfill a dream you have had for many years. There is always something you have been wanting to do for a long time but have never gotten around to. Now is the time to do it! It can be dancing, writing, hiking, painting, or going to the theater. The point is that you should not wait out your whole life being frustrated about doing those things you really want to do. Also, do this again next year, and the year after, and in a few years you will find that everything that you are doing are things you really want to do for your own personal reasons.

12. Admire your talents, because they are yours and yours alone. There are always some things you are better at than others, and in which you take pride doing. These are true talents, whether or not anyone else has ever noticed them. Your talents are starting points to take you to where ever and what ever you want in life. Don't give them up, and don't ignore them. Practice them and use them, and enjoy them, and you will find that others will see you as the talented and remarkable person you have always been.

LOW SEX DRIVE

2 Vitamins Known to Help Athletes

Male athletes may not openly complain about problems of their sex drive, but strenuous exercise is known to depress testosterone levels and negatively affect the sex drive. If you are training hard athletically you can ensure that your testosterone level, and sex drive, stays at a normal level by taking vitamin C and vitamin E. Since these are good vitamins for most people, and important in staying healthy, they are doubly important for athlete, and anyone with hard workouts on a regular basis.

A Couple of Diet Changes that Can Change Your Life

Your sex drive can decrease from time to time without meaning that you will never be as passionate as you were before, all that it takes is a little stimulation, and maybe a new diet, and you should be as good as new. If you are on any kind of medication, or have been dieting to lose weight, or have any other stress in your life it is not at all unusual for your interest in sex to fall. As things return to normal for you and you feel better and more rested, your interest in sex should grow too.

But in the meantime maybe a dietary change can give a hand to helping your sex life a bit, if you give it a try. Now one thing good to know is that you don't really have to give up anything in your current diet to help your sex life. What you do need to do is add some things to your diet, and maybe cut out a few that you can live without.

So you should increase your intake of raw fruits and vegetable, vitamin A, vitamin E, magnesium, and zinc. Give it a try and it may give raw fruits and vegetables a whole new meaning.

MEDICATION

Foods to Avoid with Your Medicines

While many medicines give warnings about not mixing drugs or drinking alcohol when you take them, most don't mention foods that can cause complications or counteract their medical effects. One of the most common drugs we take for infections is tetracycline, but if you drink milk while taking it you will lose the antibiotic effects of the tetracycline. The calcium in the dairy products is the specific problem, so you should avoid all dairy products for an hour before and after taking the drug.

A commonly used anticoagulant is warfarin (sold as Coumadin or other trade names), but it is neutralized by foods rich in vitamin K. These foods include broccoli, cabbage and spinach. If you are taking this drug check your diet for high vitamin K foods and eat them in moderation.

If you are taking MAO inhibitors such as Marplan, Nardil, or Parnate you need to stay away from cheese and cheese products. This combination can cause high blood pressure, headaches, palpitations, nausea and vomiting.

As you can see the mixing of the wrong foods with your medications can result in serious complications. For any prescription drugs always ask your doctor if there are foods that should be avoided when you are taking them. This will make your doctor pay attention to this potentially serious source of medical problems,

10 Popular Drugs that May Harm You—and Why

All prescription drugs used in the United States are tested for years before they are freely prescribed for sick people. Testing is supposed to guarantee that they are safe and make you better when used properly. In spite of that popular drugs are always being found either do nothing, or, worse yet, can hurt you and cause diseases of their own. There are too many of these questionable drugs to look out for them all, and they come and go from year to year, but at least you can watch out for some of the most popular and possibly save yourself a lot of medical trouble. For each of these drugs try to find an alternative so that you can have effective treatment.

The first three drugs are diuretics which have been used for many years to treat high blood pressure. Over this time they have also been found to cause mineral deficiencies, cardiac arrhythmia, raised cholesterol levels, and increase the risk of heart attack—not lower it. The most shocking, deaths from heart attacks, have to do with the action of the drugs on heart rate. One natural alternative to these drugs is a low-fat, high-potassium diet, which lower blood pressure without additional drugs.

1. Hydrochlorothiazide

2. Chlorthalidone

3. Diuril

4. Zanax is a anti-anxiety drug which is now known to be addictive, and to cause mental instabilities. To relieve anxiety try any physical exercise, and keep it up until you forget the cause of your anxiety, even momentarily.

5. Halcion is a sleep aid which causes episodes of amnesia and mental disorientation. The best natural sleep aids are any activity which prevents you from thinking of your own personal problems of the day. This could be reading, making love, or watching television.

6. Atromed-S has been used to lower cholesterol since the 1970s, and has been effective at that, but it is also associated with death from other causes than stroke and heart attack, as well as gallbladder disease. Cholesterol can usually be lowered naturally through a regular program of exercise and a very low fat diet.

The next four drugs are widely used oral medications for lowering blood sugar levels in diabetics. They are also known to be associated with fatal heart attacks, which is one of the greatest fears of the diabetic. The diabetic, at the type

2 adult onset stage, may have no choice but to take medication specifically for the lowering of their blood sugar, but there are alternative available. For extra insurance, and to use a more natural method, you should also consider Chinese herbal medicine. This will require some additional trouble and expense, but if it is effective for you it may be well worth the trouble. Chinese medical practitioners can be found in most communities, and they are cheaper than western doctors.

7. Diabinese

8. Micronase

9. Glucatrol

10. DiaBeta

How to Get Free Medicines, Even Expensive Prescriptions

If you have trouble keeping up with the price of your medication try asking your doctor for samples of medications he is prescribing. While this will not normally work over a long period of time, it can often fill a spot of time when you are short of money, and can even let you try some medications for free that could cost you hundreds of dollars. All doctors get these medicines constantly from the manufacturers as sales promotions, and most doctors just end up putting a lot of them into a drawer until someone comes along and asks. Try it and see how it comes out, you might just save yourself a lot of money.

How to Read a Prescription Chart
Tells You What All the Scribbling Means

It is terribly frustrating to go to your doctor for a serious problem, be given a prescription, and then be unable to tell if the instructions your pharmacist gives you are really the same as those your doctor wrote down. Taking either too little or too much of something, and other similar mistakes in taking medication, can make you much sicker than you began, or fail to cure you even if you are given the right medication. This prescription guide will show you how to interpret the various instructions that your doctor places on your prescription, and can be used to check up on things any time you receive a new prescription for anything. Make a copy of this list to carry with you the next time you see your doctor.

a   before

aa   of each

ac   before meals

---

bid   twice a day

–

c   with

d   day

n, noct   at night

NR   no refill

OD   once daily

pc   after meals

po   orally, by mouth

prn   as needed

qh   every hour

q2h   every two hours

qid   four times a day

rep   repeat

Rx   take, prescription

–

s   without

tid   three times a day

ut dict   as directed

.

one

I

..

two

II

...

three

III

....

iv

four

....

MEMORY LOSS

Drugs to Avoid that Cause Short-Term Memory Loss

Memory can be affected by drugs and medications, and if you want to have a good memory you are going to have to avoid the drugs that affect you. A number one drug that attacks your memory is alcohol, particularly in high doses. Anytime that you drink past the point at which you have good control of your body, and that is more than about one drink in an hour, you are going to lose some control on your memory. If you drink heavily one day, your memory will even be impaired the following day. So the number one rule to a good memory is to control your alcohol use, and never drink before you are going to do something that requires a good memory.

The main culprits in medicinal drugs that attack memory are the anti-anxiety drugs and the sleep-inducing drugs. While not everyone takes these, everyone who does on a regular basis is going to have some memory problems. Some of these drugs to watch out for are Valium, Halcion, Librium, and Restoril. But any of these may affect you. Cold medications also have this affect. You need to look out for any drugs that make you sleepy, because this is a sure key that your memory is at risk.

If a doctor is giving you a drug which either makes you sleepy, or gives you an actual memory lapse, then talk to him about changing medications. If you are taking an over-the-counter drug that does this to you, you will need to act on your own. You can go to a doctor for a prescription drug to take care of your symptoms, but if you want to do it yourself you will just have to try some alternatives.

Remember that colds go away after a week anyway, so you could just suffer through. Also walks and warm milk may work just as well as sleep aids as a drug. Mild aerobic exercise is probably the best alternative to drugs for both insomnia and anxiety since the endorphins your body produces when exercising will leave you both relaxed for sleep, and calm and rational. If there is a problem with drugs and memory, then use other drugs, or use none at all and go to exercise.

How to Improve Your Memory in One Hour by Up To 50%

Most of the time your memory is a tricky thing. Your remember things that you really don't care if you remember, and you can't remember things that you really do want to remember. Memory is triggered by what happens around us, but we usually can't control what those triggers are, and so our memories seem to operate somehow independent of our will, and we never know what we are going to remember. We can only be sure that we will probably not be able to remember many of the things that we want to.

The way to solve this problem is to start out by paying special attention to those things that happen around us that are important. If you read something that you feel is important, then make an effort to remember it. How do you do that? While there are several ways you might go about remembering things you want to, one of the best is by visualizing. In visualizing we try to actually see what we want to remember. If you can create a picture of the information you are hearing, you will be able to look at the picture later, when you want to remember it, and recall details that you didn't even know you learned at the time. If you need a start in visualizing try beginning with an empty room with the name of the subject you want to remember. Then as you hear and see the new ideas place them into the room the same way that you would decorate any room. As you continue to place ideas in the area, look around the room once in a while to reinforce your memory. When you are done you will have a room fully decorated with the ideas of what you wanted to remember. And any time you want to remember a fact on that subject, all that you have to do is think of the room, and everything will be in it that you put there. To make this a successful way of remembering you will need to pay attention to what you are learning, and do a review of the room you have created every once in a while to make sure its still there. Eventually it will be there any time you want it, and no further effort will be required of you until it is of use.

Another effective method for memory, and one that can work very quickly, is to use what are called mnemonic aids. Mnemonic aids are little poems or rhymes that use the terms you are trying to remember. You will still have to decide what it is that you want to remember, but once you have made this choice, you can simply hang the words onto an easily remembered poem, and you will remember what it is that is important to you. If you have not tried this before you might be surprised to find out that your doctor or lawyer used just this method to remember some of the things he needed to get licensed. There is no shame in this method, and it can work very quickly. Once you have decided what it is that you want to remember, if no one gives you a rhyme to use, then make up your own, and then just remember the rhyme.

If you have a special problem, like remembering names, the processes of remembering them is the same. You will need to place the names of the persons in a room with their faces, or attach them to a poem that you can remember more easily. Names are one of the most easily forgotten things we learn, that we think we should remember. Because of this it requires extra work if we really want to remember them. To really remember a name of someone you don't see very often, you have to attach it to something that is more familiar to you. Think about the person and look for things that you see very often. If a woman's name is daisy, then think of the flower when you try to remember her name, and the next time that you see her you will think of a daisy and remember her name. If a man's name is Jerry, think of the "Tom and Jerry" cartoons when you want to remember him, and you will think of the name Jerry. So long as you can put that person in a setting that you see daily, you will remember their name when you need to. This may be a lot of work, but once you have done it once, you shouldn't have to do it again.

A couple of other ways for you to improve your memory quickly and painlessly are the old "tie a string around your finger" method, and put reminders around the house. The string method really doesn't require a string to remember, just do something out of the ordinary, and every time that you do it remind yourself of what you are trying to remember. This works best if you are not trying to remember too many things at once. The reminder method means making notes, of what you want to remember, and placing them around your house and car. Then every time you look at the TV or refrigerator, you will read what it is you want to remember. After a while you won't read each note out loud, but you will remember what they say. Also, once you have set up the notes, you only have to read them as you see them, you don't have to sit down and study the information any more in the way you study for a test. Putting it on tape and playing it over and over will work the same way, but don't make it too long, an hour or two of taping is enough to remember by this method at any one time.

Once-A-Day Natural Secret That Will Relax Your Nerves, Sharpen Your Mind, and Boost Your Spirits

Perhaps the one thing that you can do every day to help you the most is to take a multi-vitamin. A lot of the everyday things that bother us, like nervousness, dullness of the mind, and feeling down are just signs of low levels of some of our essential vitamins.

If you want to take some additional actions to help specific problems you might start with an extra dose of vitamin B12, which works specifically to help the memory. You will get it anyway in a multi-vitamin, but you may need a higher than minimum dose if memory is a particular concern to you.

The problem with too many of us, once we are out of school, working, and maybe with a family to support is that we forget to take time to keep ourselves healthy and active. While you may not feel like doing anything at the end of the day because you don't have any energy, the truth is that you probably don't have any energy because you don't take time to keep physically and mentally active.

Besides taking vitamins, which will help to correct poor eating habits, take time for some daily exercise (even a 30 minute walk each day will do). Exercise will clear the mind, boost your immune system, help you to lose weight, and burn off those feelings of frustration or anger that a day of working and commuting can bring on.

Staying interested in life mentally, which also helps the memory, attitude toward life, and the nerves is something you can do at home, in a library, or a museum. Your mind, just like your body, needs exercise to stay healthy. One handy way of using your mind, and which is available in the daily paper, is to do the crossword puzzle. Crossword puzzles can be very challenging, and may be just what you need. Other, excellent ways, are to read, or write, or even to play cards. If you read about things that interest you, and write regularly to friends and relatives you will soon find your interests growing and that you have more to say.

Start with vitamins, but don't ignore your body or your mind for a good memory and a healthy outlook on life.

MENOPAUSE

Estrogen for Menopause
Some Risks to Consider

Since estrogen replacement therapy is the most common type of treatment given to women undergoing menopause, it would be nice to know if there are any risks to taking it before you actually have to make that decision. But before you consider the risks you should know that estrogen does help prevent osteoporosis, and if that is your major concern then you will have to balance the risks with the benefits.

But now to the risks. Risks vary according to what type of person you are physically. If you are a heavy woman, then not getting estrogen increases your risk of breast cancer. But if you are a thin woman then getting estrogen therapy can double your risk of breast cancer. This makes it a very complicated decision as to whether or not you should have estrogen therapy.

Before you make up your mind about a final decision you should also consider whether you have any of the more well defined risk factors for breast cancer. These are probably far more important than estrogen therapy as causes of breast cancer. the major risk factors are age, family history of breast cancer, early maturation, and late first full-term delivery. If you fall into one or more of these categories, then whether or not you use estrogen therapy may not be very important. The same goes if you have none of the risk factors, in which case estrogen therapy could either protect you from breast cancer or be your biggest risk factor itself.

It Might Just Be the Best Time of Your Life

So many women fear the menopause will be an unhappy time for them that they don't bother to look about themselves and see that their friends and relatives who are at this point in their lives are really quite happy. The stories of menopause being a terrible time in a woman's life are false, and now a study by Mill's College in California has systematically gone out to debunk these fears. Women in their early fifties have been found to be more contented and satisfied than at any other time in their lives. These women were no longer angry at the men in their lives, but expressed tolerance and closer to their life ideals then before they had gone through menopause.

The problem with the fear of menopause is that it is always those women who were looking forward to it who were quoted, not women who had already gone through it. You need to learn to trust this change of life, and you may find it a time to look forward to rather than a time in which adjustment will mean unhappiness or problems with defining yourself. Accept what is inevitable, and don't listen to your fears, instead look at the facts and discover that you have nothing to fear and much to look forward to.

Menopause Relief Natural Secrets that Work

Hot flashes are one of the major problems for women going through menopause, and when they are troublesome the usual treatment is estrogen therapy. But if you are trying to avoid estrogen therapy for some reason, and there are risks to using it, then you will want to know what else there is for you to do?

You can just endure the hot flashes, and many women do, or you can go at it the way the University of Texas did in a study and look for a simple feedback method that will work. Out of all of the feedback methods they tested, the one that was most effective was just simple deep breathing. Most everyone is familiar with using shallow breathing as feedback to relieve pain during childbirth, but deep breathing is usually used to calm people down. When you use deep breathing to control hot flashes you are forcing oxygen into your blood and offsetting the loss of estrogen your body is experiencing. Consequently there is no risk whatsoever in using this method to relieve the hot flashes, and it has no restrictions according to age or physical condition either.

Even if you are taking estrogen, if hot flashes are the only reason you are taking it you may be able to cut out the estrogen therapy with this simple exercise.

To use deep breathing first inhale as deeply as you can, hold the breath for a moment or two, and exhale slowly. Continue deep breathing for as long as the hot flash continues, and repeat the exercise each time you get an attack.

MIGRAINE HEADACHE

14 Million Missed Diagnoses in the United States

How can there possibly be 14 million headaches misdiagnosed in the United States? It is both outrageous and silly to think that that many people could have their migraine headaches missed. Migraines are one of the easiest headaches to diagnose, after all they all have the classic symptoms of the sufferer seeing spots of light and facial numbness, or at least that's what we are always told.

The answer to this little mystery is that we have apparently been lied to for these many years. You can have a migraine headache and not have the spots of light or the facial numbness. In fact 2/3 of migraine headaches do not have these symptoms.

Like all medical problems, migraine headaches can range from very severe, where we have all of the symptoms, to very mild, where they are still migraines, but there are none of the symptoms we think they should have.

Another problem is in the difference between men and women. Most of us think that women get migraines and men do not. While this isn't true, it still means that many men won't report the symptoms that would allow their migraines to be diagnosed, and the symptoms of some women may be ignored because they are thought to exaggerate the symptoms they have.

For a little self-diagnosis consider this: if you have a headache that emanates from one side of the head, you feel naseous, and have vomiting and sensitivity to light and noise, then you probably have just had a migraine. Even if you have several headaches, but never experience all of these symptoms, even if you have just 2 or 3 at a time, it is a good bet that it is migraine.

If you have migraines, do your best to get them diagnosed. Treatment includes both relief of the headache, and even prevention of future migraines, is available through prescription drugs. There are no over-the-counter drugs on the market that are going to cure this problem, so it is something you are going to have to depend on your doctor for treatment.

MUSCLE CRAMPS

The Home Remedy Your Doctor Probably Doesn't Know About

We don't really know what causes muscles to cramp. Some of the causes suggested are a build-up of acid in the muscles, or a lack of oxygen because of use, or strain on the muscles, or even a lack of some vitamins and minerals in the body that have gotten used up or depleted. But whatever the cause, the general medical remedy is rest, soaking, and muscle relaxants. While these certainly work very well, there are also home remedies that a doctor will not usually discuss with you, and may not even be aware of.

It is been found that a supplement of 300 IU. of vitamin E can prevent up to 99% of the muscle cramps people normally suffer from. This was discovered by taking 125 patients who had a history of muscle cramps, giving them 300 IU. of vitamin E daily, and watching to see their rate of muscle cramps. Only 1% as many muscle cramps were seen as had been there before the vitamin E was taken.

There is one theory about why vitamin E will prevent your muscle cramps, and that is that it helps to keep the blood flowing smoothly and steadily. The idea is that muscle cramps are caused by the blood slowing down and pooling in parts of the body (claudication), and that vitamin E prevents this pooling. Now if this is right it means that the vitamin E, by preventing pooling of the blood, helps keep the muscles better oxygenated and better nourished, since both oxygen and muscle nourishment are carried in the blood.

This is something you will have to do at home, and you certainly can't prove that it helps prevent muscle cramps. Unless, that is, you do it the way they did in their original test. If you have a history of regular muscle cramps, and you begin taking 300 IU. of vitamin E every day, and then you don't get any muscle cramps, you can consider it proven that it helps. This is the sort of non-scientific proof you use every time you take aspirin to prevent heart attacks, and about the same as what researcher's used to prove that aspirin prevents heart attacks. If it works for you it's worth using, but only you can determine if it works, since you are the one who has to take it.

MUSCLE PAIN

Natural Ways to Get Rid of
"Morning Aches" in Your Body

Morning aches can come from many things, they can be caused by arthritis, hard work, general tiredness, or be just the little bit of stiffness that most everyone has who gets up to an alarm in the morning. Of course they usually aren't very serious since they will fade all on their own during the day, but it would be nice if you had some ways of getting rid of them before you have to go out for your days activities. Well all I can do is offer some suggestions since the ones that will work for you depend upon the cause and seriousness of your own morning aches.

For everyone I strongly recommend a warm morning shower when you first get up. You may still be half asleep at that time, but the warm water will help you wake up, as well as increase the blood flow to your muscles and skin. Even parts of your body that are still will start to loosen, and the shower need be no more than 15 minutes.

Now once you have showered, if you can spend another 10 minutes, you need to do some slow stretching exercises. Stand straight and bend your upper body from side to side and rotate your trunk to loosen yourself at the waist. Then sit on the floor with one leg bent in and bend your upper body forward and try to touch your toes. Change legs and do the same exercise, and then do each one at least one more time. All of the stretching exercises should be done slowly, and don't do any early morning aerobics for at least an hour after you get up.

By now you should be feeling pretty good, and if you are you can just go about your business. However, if your stiffness is caused by arthritis you may want to take an early morning aspirin to rid yourself of further discomfort. If you do not have to go off to work, but have some additional time, then after breakfast go for an early morning walk of 30 to 60 minutes. That will thoroughly warm and relax your body, and the speed doesn't matter.

At this point there should be no more morning aches and pains and you should be ready for your day. Of course the same sequence of acts can be repeated at the end of the day if you come home stiff and sore too.

3 Simple Stretches
that Relieve Muscle Stiffness in Seconds

If you are one of the many people who spend their days sitting at work, or unable to move around enough to stay limber, there is help with three simple exercises. Before doing these exercises you should warm up a little by walking for a little while, until you feel warm, and then do the stretches at a comfortable pace, and hold each one for no more than 30 seconds. They will leave your back and legs feeling loose and comfortable.

Stretch 1: stretching the major muscles of the body is a good place to start. First lie down flat on your back on the floor, on a soft surface. Start by exhaling deeply, and with your arms at your sides; then slowly bring your arms up over your head, flatten your back to the floor and breath normally. Then role onto your stomach and stretch out your legs; bring your arms down under your shoulders, and keep everything flat on the floor. Hold this position for five seconds.

Stretch 2: this is a leg stretch in which you start from a standing position and lunge forward with one foot. Put the foot out far enough so that your back knee can come down and tough the floor. Keep your back straight and raise both hands over your head, and exhale deeply once, and then breath normally. After a few seconds do this exercise leading with the other foot.

Stretch 3: this is a lower back stretch in which you lie on your back on a soft surface (like a mat or carpet). Then bend your knees up toward your chest and hold them there just below the knees with your hands. Keep your head on the floor and breathe normally while you hold this position.

NAUSEA
An Herbal Secret Which Prevents Nausea

Nausea can come from many causes. You can feel badly from a stomach flu, or get car sickness, or seasickness, but what it all comes down to is that you feel like throwing up. Since once you have gotten to this condition of nausea there is little to do but suffer through it, a better solution is to take something in advance to prevent it.

About 10 years ago doctors began looking at ginger as a preventive for nausea, and found that 70% of a test group taking ginger had decreased attacks of nausea. Ginger even works with pregnant women, and is better than anti-nausea medications because there is no danger of overdose, and it has no effects upon the baby.

Ginger is now being studied for possible use before surgery, and during therapy for cancer. In both of these cases nausea can be life-threatening, and taking other medications often does not work. The effective amount of ginger required is only as much as you would get in a piece of ginger cake, and it is available cheaply in both health food stores and supermarkets. If you are in any state of illness, or seasickness, begin taking ginger and you may save yourself a lot of distress and discomfort.

NECK AND SHOULDER PAIN

A Guide to the 5 Minute Cure You Can do Anywhere

Of course we can't really cure neck and shoulder pain, since you can always bring on another attack, but we can at least cure it for the time being. Now some neck and shoulder pain can't be cured in this manner, especially when it comes from an injury like arthritis in the shoulders or a slipped disk in the neck, but it can be helped. So pretty much any case of pain in the area can feel better if you take 5 minutes to do something about it.

Pain in the neck and shoulders relates from tightness of the muscles that presses on the nerves and cuts off blood circulation. So, if you do an exercise that relaxes the muscles, and encourages blood circulation the pain will go away and your neck and shoulders will feel better.

The Exercises: If you are driving, or otherwise restricted from free movement, the exercise consists of turning your head from side to side, and hunching your shoulders up as far toward your ears as you can. Do each of these movements 5 times, and hold the hunched position for 10 to 15 seconds at a time. This will relieve a lot of the tension in your neck and shoulders and give you some instant relief. The only problem is that you will have to repeat this exercise every 30 minutes to an hour until you can stop and get a better range of motion. Now when you can stop whatever you are doing, and have no room to move, you can get a little longer relief by adding more movement. Stretch your whole upper body out, reaching with your arms toward the sky, and then swinging your arms at the shoulders. If you have another 5 minutes, take a walk. The combination of these exercises will loosen everything up, and get the blood flowing much better. If you can do the whole range of exercises you will probably be in good shape for a couple of hours at a time. And, of course, repeat as necessary.

This is no wonder drug for a painful neck and shoulders, but it is a means of dealing with a problem many of us have every day, and don't believe we can solve until we get home from work and can put our feet up on the sofa. A little effort at work, or in the car, might make your workday and your commute a lot more pleasant.

NERVOUSNESS

This Free, Once-A-Day, Natural Secret Will Relax Your Nerves, Sharpen Your Mind, and Boost Your Spirits

There is a boom in America and its helping everyone stay healthy in a simple natural way. The boom is bicycling to work. Bicyclists can easily travel 10 to 15 miles in an hour of commuting, which is pretty close to the travel time in a car, and get all of the benefits of exercise at the same time. Bicycling is especially good for those who don't have time for other exercise, or who want to lose weight and calm their minds at the same time. Commuting to work will not cost very much, and it will leave your nerves and your mind feeling more relaxed and more alert than you can imagine. This exercise also stimulates your brain to release chemicals that will leave you feeling good about the world, and good about yourself at the same time.

NIGHTMARES

Nightmares Scaring You as an Adult Not Uncommon

If you had nightmares as a child, and pretty much everyone has, then you know how much of a problem they can be. If you are still having nightmare as an adult, then they are probably frightening you more than they did years before. Why should you, as an adult, still have to suffer from nightmare? Those are supposed to be something that kids have, and that they get over as they get older.

Unfortunately the causes of nightmares do not know what getting older is supposed to do for us as well as we do. While we think that getting older means

---

we should have no more nightmares, if we are still under the same types of pressures we had as a child, then we will continue to get nightmares. In fact adult nightmare can be much worse than anything we suffered as an adult. Whether it was the subconscious knowing that our parents were in the next room, or what, adults have nightmares that leave them panicked and screaming in bed.

Nightmares seem to run in the family, so if other people in your family have them don't be too surprised if you do too. And nightmares in children are often tied to such events as going through puberty or the death of a parent. Even if a parent has not, but some other person known to the family, a child may develop severe nightmares. Children fear most the threat that they may be left alone in the world, because they do not really know how to deal with anything personally until they get into their late teens.

Adult nightmares are tied to much of the same causes. Stressful events as an adult such as death or job loss can trigger nightmares. Unfortunately for an adult there is not the opportunity of just growing out of the problem and getting over it. If your subconscious has been scared by a severe problem in your life, you may develop nightmares which frighten you out of bed.

If this is your problem, and it is something that won't go away such as the death of someone close to you, then the best way of taking care of it might be through taking care of yourself. Before going to bed do things that you know are going to relax you. Take a bath, or a walk, or get a massage. Doing deep breathing and meditation are good, but you can also write yourself out. This is a technique which purges your soul by having you put into words all of your feelings, good or bad, about everything that is bothering you. This "journal" technique is used by weight loss clinics and psychologists to allow their patients to express themselves. When you use it to get rid of your nightmares you are using an established technique of psychology, and it can remain entirely personal if your problem goes away. If you can't get rid of it no matter what you do yourself, then you have something to start with for professional help. In most cases your needs will never go that far, and you will be sleeping peacefully after a few months. If you express your problems out loud on paper, they will not be left behind in your mind to torture you as you sleep.

NOSEBLEEDS

The Best Way to Treat a Nosebleed

Most nosebleeds are caused by the breaking of the little blood vessels at the front of the nose, and there are some very simple ways of caring for them that work, and some very popular ways that don't work. Since your nosebleed is at the front of your nose, putting ice on your nose or the back of your neck won't do any good. Neither will pinching the bridge of your nose, that will just make your nose sore. The best way to control your nosebleed is gently clear your nose by blowing, this will get out any clots that have formed, and then gently pinching the end of your nose. This will slow the flow of blood and give the damaged blood vessel a chance to stop bleeding. Most nose bleeds will stop on their own within a few minutes in any case.

Preventing nosebleeds is another problem. Most nosebleeds are caused either by direct irritation, like blowing your nose over and over again when you have a cold or hayfever, or in hot weather when your blood pressure builds up a little from your body trying to get rid of extra body heat. If you are prone to either of these two causes you can probably prevent most nosebleeds just by being careful at certain times. If you have a cold or hayfever take some cold medicine that will dry your sinuses. This may make your nose feel a bit dry, but it will pre- vent the nosebleeds. A dab of lotion around the tip of the nose might also keep it from drying out so the tip of your nose won't become irritated and start bleeding. If heat is your problem then the only thing you might be able to do is keep your body temperature as cool as possible in hot weather using cold drinks and by being inactive in the middle of the day.

NUTRITION

6 Healthy Choice Answers You Should Know

      The first step in making a healthy diet is to be able to tell which is the best nutritional choice when we are faced with two foods that are very much alike. Health food stores often tell us one thing, and the U.S. government and the food companies often tell us another. Now while we would like to believe the health food people are always right, the truth is that sometimes they aren't. People in the health food business can be just as interested in money as the people in the regular food industry. So we are really left up to our own knowledge to decipher which of the choices is the healthiest, in many cases. The answers given here are not meant to give you all of the information that you will ever need in choosing your diet, but they will at least get you started and give you something to work on. Whenever you come to any questions on your diet, such as the ones asked and answered here, always look deeper than the claims of either side and make the choice yourself instead of letting food salesmen do it for you.

      1. Which is the best vitamin choice for you, natural or synthetic? Answer: the best vitamin choice is the one that has the dosage you want for the lowest cost. While natural vitamins may have other trace elements with them that synthetic vitamins do not, the actual vitamins themselves are exactly the same from either source. Health food stores will try to tell you differently, but the whole point of synthetic vitamins is to duplicate the chemical structure of the natural vitamin, and synthetic vitamins are thoroughly tested on animals before they are allowed on the market as supplements. Also many natural vitamins use the same binders, dyes, and emulsifiers as do the synthetics so you get the same exposure to these non-nutritional additives whichever choice you make. If you really want natural vitamins then get them from a natural choice, such as the fruit or vegetable where they have high concentrations and can be worked into your diet.

      2. What is the single best choice for calcium, ricotta cheese, milk, broccoli, or cottage cheese? Answer: ricotta cheese is by far the best natural choice for calcium of these 4 foods. Ricotta have 335 milligrams of calcium in a 4 once serving, and that is four times the amount found in a 4 once serving of cottage cheese, and more than in either a cup of broccoli or an 8 ounce glass of milk. If you are looking for a natural source of calcium to prevent osteoporosis, cottage cheese is the worst choice of the four.

      3. For a thirst quenching, and healthful, melon what is the best choice between cantaloupe and watermelon? Answer: cantaloupe is the winner all around. It has 2 times the fiber, 4 times the vitamin C, and 10 times the vitamin

A of watermelon. An added bonus is that a serving of cantaloupe is usually cheaper than a serving of watermelon during the summer months.

4. Which is the healthier choice for frozen desserts, frozen yogurt, ice cream, "lite" cream, or ice milk? Answer; while there is a lot of overlap, ice cream usually wins. This somewhat surprising result though only holds well for the chocolates. Chocolate ice cream may have more butterfat, but may also have 1/2 the cholesterol, 40% less sodium, and fewer calories overall. Of course if you like fruit deserts you are probably best off with frozen yogurt. If you can restrain yourself to a single scoop, then it really does not matter very much which choice you make since the nutritional effects will not be very large. You also have to make choices based on the amount you expect to have in a serving, and the total calories, and other nutrients, in that serving.

5. What water should you and your family use, tap water or bottled water? Answer: while you may live in a city where the tap water is undrinkable, in most cases tap water is as good or better than bottled water. Tap water is not only prepared by your water department, but in the preparation and delivery it is constantly watched and tested. If anything is found that is wrong it is corrected immediately. Bottled water, on the other hand, comes from many sources and you cannot ever be sure what the degree of quality control is. Some bottled waters have been found contaminated with bacteria, kerosene, and mold, and the level of contaminates allowed by bottle water companies are often higher than public drinking water standards. If you want a further thought to discourage you from buying bottled water just consider the cost. Bottled water can cost 1200 times the amount of tap water. If you really want the bottled water experience without the cost, find a public artesian well in your area and pay it visits when you want water. These are not all that uncommon, and the water you get is generally comparable to bottled water.

6. Is it safest to have your meat well done, to kill bacteria, or should it be cooked medium? Answer: there is evidence scattered around that overcooking meat, to the point of charring or even get it well done, actually adds harmful substances to it. Well cooked meat has been found to have larger amounts of cancer causing agents than meat cooked only to a medium well done level. The study was done by the National Cancer Institute, and just points out what you may have already heard about cancer causing agents in smoked and barbecued meats. Meat can still be barbecued, but not in the smoke and not over direct flame. Remove the meat while it is still pink inside, except for chicken and pork of course. But for beef make sure that it is not overcooked and burned. Overcooking also goes with pan fried and oven cooked meats as well. Even though you don't have the flame and smoke, just the fact that it has been cooked to such a high degree means that there are cancer causing agents in it.

9 Nutritional Myths that Can Hurt Your Diet

Nutritional myths are not just things other people believe about their diets that aren't true, it is also things you are told that are wrong as well. While you would not believe that a dragon will come down and eat you, you might believe that some foods actually make you lose weight by eating them, and that is very debatable. Nutrition is still a very experimental science, in spite of its history in American medicine and the immense interest the American people have in it. What to eat, how much, and when to eat it are such individual questions that no 2 people eat the same diet. Diets that are very near one another may kill some people and cure others, but that is because each of our needs are different, and particular to each of us. But because you are so unique and special as to your own diet needs, giving you the wrong information can result in your eating exactly those foods you actually want to avoid. And how do you know? Only if you are given the best information available, and even that is not sufficient unless you continue to listen and read as new information comes out and old pieces of advice are cast away.

1. **Myth**—late night meals are more fattening than meals at other times of the day. **Fact**—if you are overeating, it doesn't matter when you eat because you will gain weight. Of course this makes common sense, calories not burned will be stored on your body. But there are a couple of special cases you need to keep in mind. If you skip early meals to cut down on calories, you are more likely to develop a low blood sugar condition that will inspire you to eat heavily at night, which will lead to a weight gain instead of a loss. Also if you are already obese there is evidence that a meal eaten late in the day is more likely to be stored as fat than food eaten earlier in the day.

2. **Myth**—food in the supermarket that are labeled "lite" or "light" are lower in calories than foods not so labeled. **Fact**—this particular term is not regulated by the FDA, or any government agency. It is also not standardized in its usage by the food industry. Light can refer to color, or weight per serving, or taste, as well as to the number of calories or amount of cholesterol in the food. Unless you can actually find what the term is applied to, it is best to ignore it. For a hint on finding out the application take a look at the nutritional labeling that most foods now carry, and if that doesn't quite do it then look at other products of the same type which don't have the label. With a little bit of work you can usually find out what it is all about, and then decide whether or not it is of interest to you.

3. **Myth**—chicken is lower in fat than red meats (beef and pork). **Fact**—while this is true in many cases, there are also many exceptions, and you cannot accept this as even true in most cases. First, if you don't take the skin off the chicken, and it is cooked in oil, the chicken will usually have more fat than a piece of red meat. But even with the skin off, much chicken has more fat. A skinless chicken thigh has 11 grams of fat, verses a piece of pot roast of the same size which has only 9 grams of fat. A pork tenderloin of the same size has only 5

grams of fat. To minimize fat from red meat, "select" grade has the lowest amount of fat per serving, and "choice" grade is next. Now if you are concerned about cholesterol, there is no gain either way. The servings of chicken and beef both have about 25 milligrams per ounce. If you want to cut back on fat and cholesterol you need to cut your serving of meat from any source, and go more to vegetable and fruit dishes for your meals. Most vegetables and fruits are without either fat or cholesterol, and will help you lose weight and cut your dietary cholesterol at the same time.

4. **Myth**—2 percent milk is healthy for you because it is low in fat. **Fact**—actually 2% milk is not really so good for you, as milk goes. It still has 130 calories in an 8 ounce glass, along with 5 grams of cholesterol. You are much better off with 1% milk, but the best to use is nonfat milk or low-fat buttermilk. If flavor is a big concern, but you still want to cut your fat and cholesterol as much as possible you can mix 1/2 gallon of 1% milk with 1/2 gallon of nonfat milk, and get a 1/2% milk that has only 1/4 the fat of the 2% milk you were using before. You will also find that the little bit of fat still in the milk goes a long way to giving you the taste you have gotten used to.

5. **Myth**—bran muffins are the healthy way to go for a light and nutritious breakfast or snack. **Fact**—unless you are baking your own bran muffins, you have no guarantees that what you are eating is low in calories, or fat, or even that it has very much bran. In-store, and bakery, bran muffins can have up to 400 calories, along with 13 grams of fat. They are often cooked with hydrogenated oil (saturated fats), sugar, and eggs, and have very little of the bran you are eating them for. Remember that bakeries and markets are looking at shelf life and appetite satisfaction when they sell food, not at what you may be buying it for in the first place. You are more easily satisfied by eating something with a generous dose of fat and sugar in it than you are by something of the same size and cost that does not fill your stomach. If you want to do the best by the bran muffin, make your own, of if you must buy them, get one that has a lot of bran, little fat, and no more than 90 calories per ounce. That seems like a lot, and it is, but its about the best you are going to do with a bran muffin. Most low cal way to get your bran is having a bowl of bran cereal with nonfat milk.

6. **Myth**—fresh vegetables are better for you than are frozen vegetables. **Fact**—flash frozen vegetable, frozen just after harvest, often have more vitamins than do the fresh vegetables in the supermarket. The reason is that the freezing process pretty well preserves all of the vitamins, although you may still lose something in texture. On the other hand, fresh vegetables which have spent days being shipped in and marketed can easily lose 50% of their vitamin C, as well as other vitamins that can oxidize. If you want to be really sure of getting the best vegetables, nutritionally, then start a garden of your own and search out the local farmer's markets in your area. If you harvest your own, and buy local vegetables in season you will get the best nutritional quality possible at any price in your area.

7. **Myth**—frozen yogurt can be eaten as a source of beneficial intestinal bacteria. **Fact**—this belief is a confusion of frozen yogurt with regular yogurt. The

regular yogurts in the market are indeed good sources of beneficial bacteria, but the frozen yogurts have been pasteurized (as required by law), and most of the bacteria has been killed. Now if you are going to eat frozen yogurt as a substitute for ice cream, you will get some benefits in addition to some beneficial bacteria. Frozen yogurt has almost no fat, and far fewer calories than ice creams, and so are worth having from that viewpoint in any case. As far as bacteria go, and remember that all of these numbers are much lower than in regular yogurt, Haagen-Dazs is best with 130 million per gram. The ranking on the others is; Colombo with 15 million per gram, Frusen Gladje with 5.3 million per gram, Heidi's with 140 thousand per gram, and Yoplait with a measly 41 thousand per gram. Of course frozen yogurt does give you calcium, so it has nutritional value beyond just getting you away from the higher calorie ice creams.

8.   **Myth**—vitamins can be taken instead of eating a balanced diet. **Fact**—while vitamins can supply many of the nutrients we need, they do not provide the combined balance we require to stay healthy, nor do they contain the complex carbohydrates or fiber that are also necessary. A well balanced diet contains abundant amounts of the antioxidant vitamins E, C, and beta carotene, which lower the risk of cancer and heart disease. But even so it is not certain if it is these vitamins themselves that are protective or if it is something else in the foods that carry them that does the job. The only sure way to have a healthy diet is to have a balanced diet of the appropriate foods (high in fiber, fruits, and vegetables, and low in sugar, fat, and refined flower products). Naturally supplements should be used whenever you feel you need one, or where you can't incorporate enough of the proper foods into your diet for any reason. But they are still supplements and cannot replace all that you need from food.

9. **Myth**—fresh water fish are a safer food to eat than are salt water fish. **Fact**—while fresh water fish may seem to be in a cleaner environment, because you can see the clear waters, actually most fresh water areas are much more polluted than are the oceans where salt water fish are caught. In fact the farther away from the polluted shores of coastal industry the fish are caught the more healthy they are for you. For the cleanest fish choose cod, haddock, flounder, pollack, tuna, ocean perch, and salmon. None of these are fresh water fish, and all should be reasonably clean. One other consideration is that the trout you find in your supermarket are grown in fish farms, not caught at your local lake, and they should have no pollution. Since fish are not watched as closely by the federal government for cleanliness, you should look at them yourself to make sure of freshness and cleanliness. A fresh fish should have clear eyes, and no strong, fishy odor. The odor part goes for other seafood as well. If something smells bad, don't eat it, take it back to the store for a replacement or a refund.

Avoid Chewable Vitamin C for Your Teeth

While vitamin C is good for you in almost any quantities you want to take it (unlike vitamin E that can give you an overdose), it is not necessarily good for your teeth. Chewing vitamin C upsets the acid balance in your mouth and can erode your tooth enamel. The most susceptible are the teeth in the back of the mouth, and even the vitamin C in some fruit juices can have the same effect.

Calcium for the Bones! Take It the Right Way

Most of the calcium supplements come in the form of calcium carbonate, which can be just fine if taken in the right way. For calcium carbonate to help you it has to be dissolved in the stomach before it can get into your blood stream and go to the bones. The only way it will dissolve is in stomach acid, but if you are in the habit of taking calcium on an empty stomach you may not have enough stomach acid to allow your body to make use of it.

Stomach acid decreases naturally as we get older, although the level can be low in anyone at any given time when the stomach is empty. To get the maximum benefit out of your calcium supplements take them with your meals. Its even a good idea to take them with milk or yogurt, which also give you calcium, and you will be getting the maximum absorption possible.

One other thing to think about is the time of day. If you take your calcium in the morning or in the middle of the day you may still be lacking calcium when you need it the most. As we sleep the body continues to use calcium, and if the level in our blood is too low, calcium will be taken from the bones. So to avoid any contribution of night-time calcium loss to osteoporosis, take your calcium supplements at night just before you go to bed. If you want some protection from calcium loss at night but don't feel that you want to take calcium tablets, then at least have a glass of milk just before your bedtime. A glass of milk at night is worth more than just something to get you in the mood to go to sleep, it can also protect you from calcium depletion as you sleep.

Guide to Building a Low Cal Salad to Fit Your Diet

Eating salads is an excellent way to cut calories and lose weight. Unfortunately you can also build salads that will bust your diet just as if you ate nothing but deserts, which is doubly discouraging if you would rather be eating a desert anyway. The way to making your salads so that they fit your diet is to learn.

For the Best Juice, Get the Best Juicer
What to Look For

Whether you just get an occasional craving for fresh juice or you want it to have a good and nutritional diet, you need to keep a few things in mind when you go about choosing which machine to use. If you are just interested in juicing oranges than a juicer is your simplest, cheapest, and best choice. But if you are interested in getting the juice out of vegetables as well as fruits you are going to have to resort to a juice extractor to get the full benefits you are looking for.

In general juicers work with juicy and pulpy types of fruit than you can even squeeze some of the juice out of. Extractors work by crushing the vegetables, and then extracting the juice by a centrifugal action, which requires a much stronger machine. Because of that the extractors are more expensive than the juicers. In either case your juicer/extractor should cost you less than $100, unless you are going for a top of the line model.

A few things to keep in mind when you go about making your own juice for the first time. Juicers and extractors do not produce the nice and clear liquids you are used to seeing in the supermarket. The supermarket juices have been allowed to set so that all of the pulpy material can settle, and the clear juice is then taken off of the top just as they do when they are making wine. If you want a nice and clear juice at home, just set it aside for an hour or two after you make it, and drink the clear liquid on top. If you want the pulp, or don't care, then drink it as you make it. The taste of pulp does not hurt the taste of fruit and vegetable juices anyway.

It is also good to use fresh and firm fruits and vegetables for your juicing. Overripe, and dry, material won't go through the juicers and extractors very well. Also dried out material doesn't contain as much juice as when it is fresh. After all, juice is almost all water, even when it has a lot of pulp.

For the best results use fresh fruits and vegetables, and after you make the juice drink it as soon as you can. If for some reason you can't drink it right away , then it is best to refrigerate it. If you leave it at room temperature overnight it is best to throw it away and start over. Fresh juices will spoil just as fast as fresh milk. There is no reason to save a dime and drink something that is probably bad for you, and won't even taste good.

How to Store Vitamins to Keep Them Strong

When you buy bulk vitamins it always seems like a good idea to store your supplements in the refrigerator. After all, the refrigerator is dark, cold, and everything else you want to keep fresh gets put in there. If that is what you do you are making a big mistake, and could very well be damaging just what you want to protect.

When vitamins are exposed to moisture they will absorb it and lose potency. Because refrigerators are not dry places, but are very wet and very cold, everything you put into a refrigerator is going to be exposed to moisture. When this happens to your vitamins they absorb the moisture, and are weakened.

For a much better choice put the vitamins into a cool, dark, dry cupboard, but make sure it is away from the stove and not exposed to direct sunlight. Heat will do the same damage to vitamins that dampness does. With this precaution your vitamins should last many months at full potency.

Liver! Should You Eat it?
Why and Why Not

As a child you were always told to eat your liver because it was good for you. Now that you are an adult do you still eat liver? Probably not, because most adults don't like liver, and most won't eat it. But should you eat it? Is it good for you in spite of having a taste you don't like? Here are some of the answers.

Liver is both good and bad for you, so you will have to decide whether or not you will eat it, and how often. It is good for you because it is a good source of iron, vitamin A, vitamin B2, and other nutrients. If this is all liver had in it than you should certainly eat it occasionally whether or not you like the taste.

However, the bad things in liver are cholesterol and fat. Just 3 1/2 ounces of beef liver have 482 milligrams of cholesterol when it is pan-fried. It also gets 1/3 of its total calories from fat, which is a large amount of the fat you should have in your diet each day.

So how do the two balance off? If you like liver you should not have it more than a couple of times a week. If you don't like liver, and have no particular medical needs for its nutrients, then skip it and use multi-vitamins. If you don't like it but have a need for iron and B-vitamins then you should have it every week or two unless you also have a cholesterol problem that it would make worse. Think it over because the final choice is yours. By the way, you can also get liver extract pills that can give you some of the benefits but cut down on the fat and cholesterol. This gives you a little more flexibility in making the best choice for you.

Magnesium, the Overlooked Miracle Nutrient

Magnesium does seem to be the nutrient that nobody gets very excited about, at least up to now. But it doesn't cure colds like vitamin C, or give you the boost of B12, and you don't hear of anybody dying from a deficiency, so what is it about magnesium that makes it important? This will surprise you, but magnesium is involved in our bodies' fight against heart disease, kidney stones, depression, stress, and PMS, and is an energy booster besides. Now if we are willing to slow down a little bit and take a better look at magnesium, we can see why it does all of these good things, and can we really believe them?

The good things that magnesium does for us must be part of the way it works in body, and of where we find it. Most of the magnesium in our body is in the cells, along with potassium. In the cells and body fluids it helps our body enzymes to work properly making it possible for us to use proteins, burn carbohydrates, grow bone and muscle, and have a good nervous system. It also helps you to maintain your proper pH balance in your body, and helps to build strong tooth enamel by working with calcium. Because magnesium is involved in so many of the operations your body has to do to be healthy, you can see that not having enough is going to show up in many ways, but why in the ones it is claimed to control?

Heart attacks are clearly one of the big ones since they kill more Americans than any other disease we have. A lack of sufficient magnesium is known to lead to faster hardening of the arteries and more blood clots. Magnesium is also part of the control system for the heart rate, and low magnesium levels lead to more irregular heart rates. Without enough magnesium in your diet you are also more likely to have second heart attacks that will kill you even if you have survived the first one.

Part of the same things that help you prevent and survive heart attacks, magnesium also helps in better performance in athletics. It is used in the system of energy burning in the cells, and also helps to carry oxygen to the muscles. You can see that these are also important in helping you to recover from heart attacks.

Kidney stones prevention and cure need magnesium to keep the calcium levels in the blood low, and if the stones are small enough it can also help them to dissolve. But now that you are convinced of the value of magnesium, how much do you need and where should you get it. Well a daily diet of between 200 and 450 milligrams would take care of everyone, and you can certainly get it by tablet from health food stores. The store-bought magnesium is quite inexpensive, but you may want to get most of your magnesium from your diet. If you do want your magnesium from your diet, here is a table of 20 excellent sources, and a couple of ideas of how to go about getting all of your magnesium this way.

20 of the Best Sources of Magnesium

Tofu	3.5 oz.	119 mg magnesium
Dried Figs	10	111 mg "
Avocado	1 medium	104 mg "
Sunflower Seeds	1 oz.	100 mg "
Lima Beans	1 cup	97 mg "
Raisin Bran	1 cup	97 mg "
Wheat Germ	1 oz.	91 mg "
Acorn Squash	1 cup	87 mg "
Almonds	1 oz.	86 mg "
Kidney Beans	1 cup	85 mg "
Brown Rice	1 cup	84 mg "
Spinach	1/2 cup	79 mg "
Cashews	1 oz.	74 mg "
Baked Potato	1 medium	55 mg "
Peanuts	1 oz.	49 mg "
Walnuts	1 oz.	48 mg "
Bananas	1 medium	33 mg "
Dates	10	29 mg "
Peanut Butter	1 Tbs.	28 mg "
Corn	1/2 cup	26 mg "

This table just shows some of the immense range of foods that can be eaten to get your magnesium. Any diet high in vegetables, or that uses nuts as an essential part, should have no trouble in supplying enough magnesium for any preventive purpose. The problem diets in America are those which use very few vegetables, and this table should serve as a message as to what is needed to ensure good health. Since magnesium is of such importance, don't try to rely on supplements to get all of your needs. Any daily diet that lacks all of the vegetable that are high in magnesium is also going to be deficient in other nutrients as well. A varied diet with several servings of vegetables and nuts daily is the healthiest and best for you.

Tap Water Taste Good?
It May Not be Good For You

Just because your tap water tastes especially good, it is no guarantee that the water is good for you. Water tastes good for many reasons, and one of them is that it may contain lead. Lead is found in many older city water systems in the pipes and soldering that carry the water to your home. Lead was also used in the past for cups to drink wine out of because it made the wine taste better, and it might also make your water taste better too.

Lead is very dangerous to have in your diet. It goes to your bones, and can attack your brain and central nervous system. Children who get enough lead in their diets grow up mentally retarded, and adults develop nervous diseases and deterioration of the mental abilities.

Even if you do not think that you have a lead problem you can't be certain, and it is wise to take some precautions to protect yourself. In daily use hot water can dissolve lead from your pipes and give you a bigger dose in your drink, so heat any hot water you want to use on your stove. Lead can also build up in the pipes over a period of non-use, and before you use any tap water you should flush the system for a few seconds to get that concentrated lead out of them.

If you can inspect the pipes around your house do so, or hire someone to take a look at them and see if lead solder was used on them. You will probably find lead solder if you have copper pipes. Copper pipes are probably best replaced with PVC (plastic) if it can be managed. If not then, besides flushing, you should also invest in a filter system that removes lead from the water, and only use water for drinking that has gone through this filter.

For information about water from the city, check with your cities water district and ask them what the content of lead is in the city water. They should not only give you this information freely, but may also give you some additional information about the dangers of lead and what to do to avoid them.

Big News
Take Time Release Vitamins for Poor Nutrition

Because time release vitamins sound like they will keep vitamins coming into your body over a long period of time it is easy to believe that they will do you the most good. However, studies have shown that they are really the worst way to take your vitamins, when compared with the other three popular ways of taking vitamins.

The best way to take vitamins is with vitamin solutions. This will get you the best absorption, so that you will actually get the benefit of what you take. The next best is with chewable tablets, and the third best is with regular tablets. Each one of these three gives you a better vitamin absorption than time release vitamins.

If Your Food Tastes Bland, You Need Zinc

That's right, a zinc deficiency in your diet can make your food taste bland. Think of all of the older people who complain about how poorly their food tastes, and you always thought that it was just part of the problem of aging. Actually older people change their eating habits, and many simply end up not getting enough zinc in their diets. But taste is not the only, or the most serious problem, in having a zinc deficiency. Zinc is also necessary to have a healthy immune system. So if you want to enjoy your food, and avoid infections, then get your 15 to 30 milligrams of zinc a day either from your foods or through supplements.

Message in Your Vitamins With Exercise

Exercise is always recommended for weight loss, and general conditioning, but it should also be recommended for anyone taking vitamins too. A study of active exercisers and sedentary couch potatoes taking vitamins found that the exercisers got the most benefit from their supplements. The test was done with joggers and non-joggers who were taking vitamin C and vitamin E over a 2 month period. At the end of the 2 months it was found that the immune system of the joggers was in much better shape than the immune system of the inactive group. While the jogging itself might be responsible for part of the improvement, the vitamins were also felt to play a very positive part in increasing immune system efficiency.

Should Iron Supplements be In Your Diet?

Iron supplements are usually included in nutritional programs because iron carries the oxygen in the blood. Therefore the more iron you have the more oxygen your blood will have, and the healthier you will be. Unfortunately this logic is wrong. You don't need very much iron on a daily basis, since it is not lost from the body very rapidly, and recycles in the blood. If you are a woman who is menstruating, or anyone who has given blood lost blood for some reason, you probably have a small need for iron. But for most people you probably get enough iron in the red meat and protein foods you eat to take care of your needs.

Now the real reason you shouldn't take iron supplements, at least for men, is that they have been shown to increase the risk of getting a heart attack. While it is not exactly known why iron does this to you, it doesn't really matter since a heart attack is such a serious medical problem, as well as that it can kill you. This was first found out about in 1981, and recent studies have confirmed it. Although women haven't been studied to see if iron supplements do this to them also, it would be a good idea for women to avoid iron supplements as well. The only exception to this is when your doctor prescribes iron as a supplement, and they often do so in cases of anemia. Otherwise everyone should keep the extra iron out of their diets.

The "30 Plus 40 Plus 50" Rule for Good Health

This rule is very simple, and can be a big help to those people who would like a rule which is easy to remember, and can make a big impact on their health. The "30 plus 40 plus 50" rule says to eat:

30 grams of fiber every day, minimum,

40 grams of fat each day, maximum, and

50 grams of protein each day, maximum.

The Vitamin That Can Make You Sick -
If You Overuse

If you have been using megavitamin type treatments, or just feel that if a little bit of a vitamin will do you good then a lot of it will be better, you will have a problem with your vitamin supplements. Some vitamins, like vitamin C, can usually be taken in large doses because they are water soluble, and the extra amounts just pass through the body. But if you are also taking the other kind too, the fat soluble vitamins, then they will have to be broken down by your kidneys whether or not you need them. And you can get overdoses, which are just as bad as not getting enough of the vitamins you need.

Vitamin B6 is one of these fat soluble vitamins that you have to be careful of. Many people take B-complex supplements because they counteract many of the affects of aging, and make us feel better and live more comfortably. However, if you take too much vitamin B6 you may be getting more than you want in a vitamin. High doses of vitamin B6 can cause muscle weakness, pains in the fingers and toes, muscle pains, and general numbness and hypersensitivity. You may think you are suffering from many different things while all you really have is too much vitamin B6.

Watch the recommended amounts of vitamin B6, and other fat soluble vitamins. The recommendations are made with safety factors in mind so that increasing them by even 5 or 10 times will probably be no problem. But if you are using 50 or 100 times, or more, of the recommended daily amounts of B6, or any other fat soluble vitamins, you could be causing your own worst problems. If you are into taking large doses of vitamins, and include any of the fat soluble vitamins then consider cutting down on them. If you have any unexplained aches, pains, or illnesses, then cut out all megadoses of fat soluble vitamins and you may just find the quickest and cheapest cure you are going to have.

Trouble Getting Your Iron? Maybe You Are Blocking It.

It's true, you can have enough iron in your diet, but not be getting enough in your body because you are blocking its proper digestion with some of the other foods you are eating. The iron blockers are English tea, antacids, and dietary fiber supplements. Now assuming that you aren't going to stop using all of the food items, what you do need to do is make sure that your iron rich foods, and supplements are taken at different meal times, or times of the day. There is one additional step you can take and that is to make sure that you have vitamin C rich foods along with your iron rich foods. Vitamin C promotes the absorption or iron, and will counteract some of the problems caused by the blockers.

What to Avoid to Keep Your Body's Vitamin Levels High

Our bodies need high vitamin levels to resist disease and keep us healthy. When we are sick we even take extra vitamins to help with the cure, but if we are doing certain things while taking those vitamins we can end up worse off then we were before. For instance, your vitamin C level is affected if you smoke.

Smoking depletes up to 40% of the vitamin C in your body, and can leave you open to colds and other infections. Since vitamin C also helps in healing from simple injuries and operations, smoking will slow up the healing, and make it more likely that you will get an infection in the injured area.

Smoking isn't the only problem activity that depletes the bodies vitamins. Drinking alcohol depletes vitamins B1, B2, B12, and C. Steroids attack your body's calcium, and antibiotics and oral contraceptives affect the B vitamins. And being a vegetarian isn't all good either since it can lead to lower vitamin B12 levels. Since most people do one or more of the activities a multi-vitamin tablet each day seems to be a rather good idea. If you are still worried you can either stop the activity that depletes the vitamins, or take specific supplements for what you are doing. In any case taking precautions against vitamin and mineral depletion is a good protective action you can take.

What is "A Recommended Daily Allowance?"

Every time you buy something at the market which has a list of its nutritional ingredients, it also lists the RDA (Recommended Daily Allowance) of each of the nutritional ingredients. Many will say 5% or 10%, some will say 150%, and many of them will just have a star or a dash. The importance of these ingredients is obviously related to this RDA number, and where it comes from.

RDA is meant to be the amount of each nutrient needed to prevent disease for a vitamin or mineral deficiency, but only for the average person. Too much of something can cause disease in some cases, just the same as too little, but even two or ten times an RDA will not make you sick. Because your body stores many nutrients, and each person's needs are somewhat different, the RDA is only an approximation of what your particular needs are. Our government sets the RDA numbers high enough to prevent disease in practically everybody. But while low vitamin doses will not always make you sick, most of the time we don't know how high the doses have to be to also affect your health negatively.

However, nursing mothers need much more calcium than the RDA, as well as growing children, and if you are very inactive due to your job or age, then your needs are probably somewhat less. To be sure that the amount of required nutrition you are getting is what you need, you have to take a personal interest in your own nutritional requirements—don't depend entirely upon the government, or upon doctors who do not know you personally. Generally it is a good idea to have an intake of several times the RDA to make certain that your body gets enough of the nutrients it needs.

Another criticism of the RDA is that it is normed to healthy people. This may be stated as, if you are healthy, an RDA of each of the nutrients will prevent you from developing a deficiency disease. This sort of overlooks the vast number of people in America who are not healthy. For instance there are 10 million alcoholics, 35 million allergics, 27 million hypertensives, and 56 million with diseases of the heart and blood circulation. This adds up to an awful lot of people who aren't healthy, and for whom the nutrient requirements are probably not filled by an RDA. This huge population probably makes up 1/2 of the people living in the United States, and all that they will get from their RDA is an inability to deal with their physical needs, or to heal properly from their illnesses.

Besides pregnant women and growing childrens need for certain nutritional elements can increase or decrease according to whether you have a chronic disease or are getting over an illness or operation, or even if you are a competitive athlete. Don't depend upon the RDA to protect the nutritional requirements of your body, at least not without also looking into any special needs or problems that you may have personally.

Also remember that there is no RDA for calories, since that depends entirely upon your activity level and age. Although no RDA is listed for water, everyone should have 6 to 8 glasses of water per day. Water is necessary to keep your digestive system in good order, and your blood flowing efficiently through your veins and arteries.

Whenever you are taking supplements always keep an eye out to avoid overdosing. Just because vitamins are something your body needs doesn't mean that you can't get such a high dose that you make yourself sick. A megadose, the level at which you can get overdosed, starts at 10 times the RDA. So 10 times or more of the RDA is going to have a negative effect upon you in many cases. Therapeutic doses, that you might take for a specific problem are usually less then 10 times the RDA. If you want to take dose levels of any vitamins at more than 10 times the RDA consult a doctor or nutritionist before you begin. Overdosing yourself with any nutrient can be just as dangerous as overdosing yourself with a prescription drug.

Vitamin C seems to be a particular problem in regard to the RDA. The RDA for vitamin C is only 60 mg, but the dose recommended by many lines of research, in particular Linus Pauling's, recommends that you get at least 1,000 mg, and some even recommend 6,000 mg. Now while this is not exact, high doses of vitamin C apparently result in an improved immune system function, better blood flow (which decreases its potential to build blood clots and clog arteries), increased mobility of the white blood cells, and increases in mental function as reflected in IQ tests.

It might also be wise to think of the food companies in regard to RDA levels. If the RDA's are low enough, most foods can claim to supply them in many areas, even if they have very little nutrition to offer. Don't believe for a minute that higher RDA's will not cost the food companies money, and that they would actively resist any increases in RDA levels by our government. Of course if you decide to go onto a supplement program, check each nutrient you are adding, and if they warn of possible overdose, then keep your intake at 10 times RDA or lower and you should be within a margin of safety.

What to Put in Your Tea
So Your Body Absorbs More Calcium and Iron

Like a cup of tea in the morning or afternoon? Most tea doesn't have anything resembling nutrition in it, at least so far as American teas are concerned. English tea has a little tannin, like they tan leather with, and some caffeine. Herbal teas do away with the caffeine, and Chinese medicine is practically based on herbal tea of many kinds. But this little additive can be used in any tea, and it helps you absorb both calcium and iron, which is not a bad idea. The additive is just simply lemon. So for a little nutritional boost to your tea break add a slice of lemon or a dash of lemon juice.

Why Pink Grapefruit is 20 Times Better
for You Than White Grapefruit

On the surface there is no difference between white grapefruit and pink grapefruit. After all, both come from the same type of plant, and they are very closely related. But as it turns out there is a very large difference in the two, pink grapefruit has much more vitamin A than white grapefruit. Of course this may not mean much to you if you have a diet rich in vegetables and fruits, but if you are on a diet, it can be very important. It can also be very important if you have some serious diseases, and you are looking for a therapeutic diet.

Vitamin A is usually thought of as the eye vitamin. And deficiencies of vitamin A are known to result in deterioration of eyesight. That is one of the reasons that vitamin A is always added to milk nowadays (during the Depression many kids lost eyesight because they were deficient in vitamin A, and all kids drink milk). But that is not the only reason for wanting a good dose of vitamin A in your diet, especially if you are a teen-ager or an older adult.

For teenagers, vitamin A is a fighter of acne and the effects of acne. While you see many American kids with bad acne problems, you rarely see Asian teenagers with the same problems, and that is because they have a diet which is much richer in the vegetables that have vitamin A, and have much less fats and sugars in their diets.

For older adults, especially those who have had, or may have cancer, vitamin A is an anti-cancer vitamin. Vitamin A will decrease the effects of radiation therapy, and can help in preventing cancer to begin with. These are just some of the reasons to choose red grapefruit when you go the market. A simple decision, but one that can help you live a longer and healthier life.

OILY HAIR AND SKIN

A Hint that You have too much Oil in Your Diet, and What to do About It

The normally healthy person will have a certain amount of oil in their hair and on their skin. After all, the oil in the hair keeps it from drying out and getting brittle, and the oil in the skin protects you from infectious bacteria that lands on you from out of the air. You don't want to have completely dry hair and skin or your hair would be constantly breaking off, and your skin would always have sores on it.

But that is true only for the normal oiliness of your hair and skin. If your diet contains more oil than necessary, and that is very easy to do with our American diet, you may have oily skin and hair almost all of the time. Just think of the last time you had an especially fatty meal, say of pork spareribs. Even if you bathed just before the meal, a couple of hours afterward you are likely to find your skin oily and smelling like the spareribs, and within a few hours your hair will start to feel oily as well. This will happen anytime that you have a meal in which most of the calories come from fat.

But, even supposing that your meals are moderate, but still fatty, will you continue to have oily skin and hair? And the answer is yes. Your body doesn't store oil, except as fat, but it does use all of the avenues it can to get rid of excess oil that you have eaten. Of course oily skin and hair doesn't mean that you are actually sick. While that may come later, it only means that your body is over-loaded with oils.

On the other hand, any time that you fail to bathe for more than 2 or 3 days you will develop a bad case of oily skin and hair, as well as a certain amount of body odor. But, even if you do, the solution is the same.

The most obvious solution is to wash it away, which works very well unless you continue to have a lot of oil and fat in your body, and the oiliness will return. To get this problem entirely under control you are going to have to go on a diet, and start exercising. The diet you have to go on is not one to make you loose weight, it is one that ensures that you have a perfect nutrition. The diet must be low in fat, and high in fruits and vegetables. That alone will get rid of most of the skin and hair problem.

But the other action you are going to have to take is to start exercising regularly. At least every other day is necessary, and daily is preferable. Now this is not just exercising, and it doesn't matter whether or not you get your heart rate, or breathing, way up. In this exercise you want to get your body sweating freely, and you want to keep it up for 15 to 30 minutes. This will clean the oils off of your skin, as well as open your pours and clean them as well. Of course your hair won't sweat, but your scalp will, and that is the source of the oil in your hair.

As soon as you have finished exercising, go and shower. You will have no more problem that day, and only a very minor problem the next day. By the day after tomorrow you will start to notice the oiliness again, and you repeat the exercise and shower routine.

There is no more effective way to deal with oily skin and hair than changing your diet, exercising, and showering regularly. Incidentally, you will also feel 10 times better about yourself when you don't have these problems, and your skin is healthy and clean.

OSTEOPOROSIS

A Drink a Day to Keep the Doctor Away

Drinking alcohol does so many bad things to you, how can a drink a day possibly keep you healthy? A study at the University of Pennsylvania has found that it can anyway. The study focused on postmenopausal women, and found that 3 drinks a week decreased their risk of both heart disease and osteoporosis. These good effects were a result of the alcohol raising the level of estrogen in the women, and estrogen protects women from osteoporosis and heart disease. Remember that these diseases stay very low in women until after menopause, when their level of estrogen decrease. Rather than taking estrogen supplements, having a drink every other day helps to restore the estrogen levels to those before menopause, and protect against heart disease and osteoporosis. The study did caution women not to take more than 6 drinks a week or the alcohol itself could begin to cause problems.

New Ways to Strengthen Brittle Bones

Bones become brittle when they lose calcium. When this happens, and older women are the main victims, the bones become brittle and break more easily. That is really the major problem with osteoporosis, when women get broken bones more easily they end up being less able to take care of themselves and more of a problem for other people who try to help them.

Because there is no exact way to cure osteoporosis the usual treatment has been to take calcium supplements. If this is what you have done you know that the calcium supplements decreased your chance of spinal fractures by 2/3 over the first year. But the problem remained, and you still had a very great chance of getting one of these fractures later on.

Well a new drug has been found that can strengthen those brittle bones even more than calcium. It is called calcitriol, and it is a form of vitamin D. Remember those stories about children in New York many years ago who got rickets because they didn't get enough vitamin D, they are still true except that now they can apply to you.

Calcitriol works just as well as calcium in decreasing spinal fractures the first year, and it seems to be even better in the second and third years. It is still being tested for osteoporosis, but it is available by prescription in the United States. In tests in New Zealand calcitriol has been found to cut fractures over the whole body by 1/2. The reason it is still being studied is to find out if there are any side effects in long term use. None have been found so far, though, although some women do get some nausea, but only about the same number as who get it when they take calcium.

Other then using these drugs to treat osteoporosis after you get it, you might consider trying some things before you get it. If you are a woman over 50, it would be a good idea to take supplements of both vitamin D and calcium, as well as watch your diet to give yourself natural forms. Don't overdose on the vitamin D, so just aim at something around the minimum daily requirement.

7 Foods that Strengthen Brittle Bones

Some foods which can insure a high calcium level in the body are yogurt, milk, tofu, sunflower seeds, broccoli, soybeans, and cheese. These are all foods commonly available in the market, usually reasonably priced, and high in calcium. It can be seen that there are several foods derived from milk on the list, and in general dairy foods have a high calcium content. However, because calorie content may also influence choice, it is of interest to anyone planning a high calcium diet: Yogurt, 1 cup, 294 mg CA, 123 Cal.; tofu, 4 ounces, 148 mg CA, 44 Cal.; sunflower seeds, 1/2 cup, 87 mg CA, 406 Cal.; broccoli, 1/2 cup, 74 mg CA., 23 Cal.; soybeans, 1/2 cup, 68 mg CA., 20 Cal., and cheese, 1/2 cup, 66 mg CA., and 117 Cal.

While decreasing brittleness with a high level calcium intake it is also necessary to take vitamin D supplements. It is recommended that at least 1,200 milligrams of Calcium, along with 375 units of vitamin D, be taken daily. Eating one serving each of the foods listed above will supply 795 milligrams of calcium, and 729 calories of energy, or about 1/2 to 1/3 of the total calories most people will require in their diets.

One of the major causes of bone loss is that your body is unable to use the calcium you eat. As you grow older your stomach produces less stomach acid, and the foods which contain calcium are not digested as well. To help you get the calcium you eat into your system you need to pay attention to what you eat. Milk is the simplest and most direct form of calcium. Skim milk is the best form because the fat in whole milk cuts down on the amount of calcium your body will absorb. If you are taking calcium supplements, then take the most absorbent form you can get—such as calcium citrate. Calcium carbonate in another common supplement form, but is less easily digested when your stomach is empty, and should be taken with meals. Calcium should be taken with carbohydrates like milk, cereals, and breads, and not with high fiber foods like fruits and vegetables which decrease calcium absorption. Whatever you do in your own diet, try to eat as many foods high in calcium as you can every day, because that is the natural way to protect yourself from osteoporosis.

Osteoporosis and Contraceptives
What is the Connection?

Even though osteoporosis does not usually begin to develop until after age 50, and women usually stop taking oral contraceptives by their 40's, there is still a close association between the two. if you began taking oral contraceptives by your 20's, and continued taking them for at least 10 years, studies by the Creighton School of Medicine in Omaha have found that you have increased your bone marrow mass by 11.3%. This means that you have gained some protection from developing osteoporosis.

The cause and effected relationship between bone mass, which fights osteoporosis, and oral contraceptives taken 20 or 30 years before seems to be in the management of your hormone levels through which the contraceptives prevent pregnancy. Normally through the month your hormone levels go up and down by very large amounts, but with oral contraceptives they are changed and the changes are minimized. That is why the increased bone mass takes place in your 20's, and persists throughout your life. It also means that at some point in a normal menstrual cycle your body either stops depositing calcium, or even reabsorbs some calcium that it has already laid down. The result of having a normal menstrual cycle, which you will have if you don't take contraceptives, is an increased risk of developing osteoporosis in later life. This sounds like a good argument for all women, but especially those not taking contraceptives, to take supplementary calcium, and that is also one of the preventive measures you commonly see recommended in medical literature to prevent osteoporosis.

Osteoporosis and the Older Female

Why do older women always seem to complain about aches and pains? Most women above the age of sixty who are do not have a diet high in calcium suffer from osteoporosis. Osteoporosis may start out as a slight twinge in the back, but may later show up as a broken hip. Osteoporosis is practically the greatest problem of older women in the United States.

Osteoporosis develops when the bones lose calcium. As calcium disappears, the bones lose strength, become brittle, and can even break. The joints and muscles are also affected, and many pains in the joints and other parts of the body are also caused by osteoporosis. To correct osteoporosis women need to eat foods with a lot of calcium.

Caffeine Effects and Osteoporosis

Caffeine does not increase the risk of osteoporosis, except under certain circumstances. But in other circumstances it does increase your risk of osteoporosis, and you need to know the difference if you want to avoid developing this crippling illness.

Osteoporosis develops in older women, after menopause, as their bones lose calcium. But why do their bones lose calcium? It is because their bodies simply dissolve the calcium out of the bones and use it for something else. This dissolving, or leaching, action takes place after menopause because your body chemistry changes at that time, and estrogen stops being produced, which apparently protects you from developing osteoporosis at a younger age. Now caffeine comes into it in this way. The caffeine increases the rate at which calcium is leached from the bones, and therefore increase the risk of breaks from osteoporosis. A study by Harvard Medical School found that women who drank 4 or more cups of regular coffee a day had a 300% increase in hip fractures from osteoporosis over those women who did not drink the coffee. This was a study of 85,000 nurses, and is pretty good evidence that the caffeine in coffee is a high risk source of caffeine.

But now that you have decided to give up caffeine to prevent osteoporosis, you need to think again. It is not all caffeine that does this. Not that the caffeine is any different when it comes from another source, but it acts differently on your body when it comes from tea rather than from coffee. You see tea also contains fluoride, which helps to strengthen the bones, and as far as can be determined the fluoride in the tea counteracts the caffeine, and there is no increased risk of osteoporosis in drinking tea with caffeine in it.

So if you are a woman of any age who is concerned about the risks of osteoporosis, and what you can do to prevent it, here are some ideas. First, give up drinking regular coffee, particularly if you drink 4 or more cups a day. Instead go to decaffeinated coffee or tea. If you refuse to give up your regular coffee, then at least limit your intake to no more than 2 cups a day, and even at that remember that you are increasing your risk of osteoporosis by some percent.

Stop Bone Loss With 1500 milligrams
of This Mineral Daily

Bone loss in a loss of calcium from the bones. The most common cause in women is menopause, in which they stop producing estrogen, and calcium begins to leach from the bones. But bone loss can also occur during child bearing, as the many women who have dental problems afterward will testify to, and general inactivity. Just as exercise results in larger bones for muscle attachments, a lack of exercise will result in a wasting away of the muscles, and a loss of calcium from the bones at the same time.

The most direct way to counter this loss is to take calcium supplements, or at least assure that you are getting 1500 grams of calcium daily. A study of women over the age of 70 found that even most of them could be helped with calcium supplements, and a high calcium diet.

If your diet is good, and you are otherwise healthy, you probably have no need for extra calcium supplements. But if you are undergoing any stress or restriction that keeps you from normal activity, or from having a full and balanced diet, calcium supplements to make up the difference are necessary to your long term health.

OVERACTIVE CHILDREN

Diet of Foods to Avoid Calms 63%

Anyone who has an overactive child knows how hard the active level to control with medication, since there is always the danger of over medication or under medication. For this reason it is much easier to simply avoid foods that set children off into an episode of hyperactivity. The foods named here have been found to help 63% of overactive children when they were removed from the diet.

You can try changing your children's diet by taking these foods out since there is no danger involved, and another food can be substituted for each one removed to ensure good nutrition.

Always to be Avoided	Sometimes to be Avoided
chocolate	eggs
cow's milk	citrus
foods colored	wheat
synthetically	beet sugar
nuts	cheese

OVERWEIGHT

Build Muscle and Lose Weight With this Nutrient

When you build your muscles you automatically increase the number of cells which burn the calories you eat, as well as those you have stored as body fat. Studies have shown that the addition of chromium to the diet increases the rate at which muscle develops, as well as the rate at which fat is burned. This results in a leaner, firmer, and more efficient body. It even helps in the replacement of body fat with muscle, and has been studied in athletes as a non-steroidal means of increasing performance. The most biologically active form of this nutrient is found in chromium picolinate, and all that you need as a supplement is 200-400 mg per day.

Don't "Yo-Yo", even If you Hate Your Weight

Yo-yo dieting is not only hard on you psychologically, it is also hard on your body. If this has been your pattern in life it is better to come to an understanding with yourself and either allow your weight to rise, or get it down where you want it and keep it there any way that you can.

A Yale University study found that yo-yo dieting may increase the death rate from all causes, and as much as double the death rate from heart disease. And don't think that large numbers of pounds have to be involved to make it yo-

yo dieting. If you gain and lose 5 pounds ten times, the effect on death rates is the same as if you have gained and lost 50 pounds.

Before you decide to undertake your next diet look deeply into yourself and see if you have the motivation to commit to a life long control that will get you off the yo-yo. If you do decide to go ahead, then stay clear of crash dieting programs and go for one that has a built in maintenance plan that you can live with so that you won't fall off into binges and watch your weight go back up again. There is practically no success rate with crash dieters, so if that is all that you are willing to do, then give up the effort and learn to live with yourself as you are.

Guide to Building a Low Cal Salad to Fit Your Diet

You want to lose weight so you eat salads regularly. But in eating salads you find that you still must count calories all of the time or you can't even lose weight with them, what is wrong? It's obvious that most of the things that go into salads have very few calories, so you should lose weight easily if a large part of your diet is made up of salads. But that is wrong-many times what we put into our salads are just as fattening as the non-salad foods we are avoiding. What you need is a simple guide so that once you make up a salad you will know that it is only a few hundred calories, and not the 1,000 or more that a salad loaded with high calorie items can have.

Dressings: to be used in limited amounts, and only as a topping, avoiding salads which are premixed. Salad dressings are the single greatest culprit in turning a low cal salad into a high cal meal. Most salads taste better with a dressing, and most dressings are based on oils, which are fats, and are what you are trying to avoid. With dressings, figure about 150 calories for 2 tablespoons, and for low-cal types about 75 calories for 2 tablespoons. Stick to the low-cal types, or have only 1 tablespoon of the regular dressing. Always measure your dressing out by the spoonful, never just pour it on or you will probably have anywhere from 6 to 8 tablespoons, and up to 600 calories just in dressing.

Regular salad dressings 150 calories per 2 tablespoons

Low-cal salad dressings   75 calories per 2 tablespoons

High Calorie Ingredients: these are ones that you should limit by putting on a minimum amount, or just using for topping over the low calorie base. The high calorie ingredients are:

avocado   95 calories per 1/4

bacon and bacon bits   70-90 calories per 2 tablespoons

garbanzo beans	90 calories per 1/4 cup
cheddar cheese	114 calories per1/4 cup
croutons	132 calories per 2 tablespoons
eggs in any form	100 calories per 1/4 cup
macaroni salad	120 calories per 1/4cup
pasta salad	120 calories per 1/4 cup
potato salad	100 calories per 1/4 cup
sunflower seeds	101 calories per 2 tablespoons

Low Calorie Ingredients: these ingredients have from 1/2 to 1/10th of the calories of the high calorie ingredients. Consequently you can use from two to ten times as much of each of them on your salad before you will reach the calorie level of the high calorie items. The base of every salad should be made up of the ingredients in this category, and if you do that you can be quite certain that you will be losing weight with your salad based diet. It also help that these foods are cheaper per serving than either the high calorie ingredients or the salad dressings.

marinated artichoke	**35 calories each**
kidney beans	58 calories per 1/4 cup
bean sprouts	9 calories per 1/4 cup
beets	23 calories per 1/4 cup
bellpepper	10 calories per 1/4 cup
broccoli	27 calories per 3 florets
carrots	25 calories per4 sticks
cauliflower	25 calories per florets
celery	8 calories per stalk
coleslaw	25 calories per 1/4 cup
cottage cheese	55 calories per 1/4 cup
cucumber	4 calories per4 slices
green peas	29 calories per 1/4cup
lettuce	16 calories per 2 cups
raw mushrooms	10 calories per 1/4 cup
raw onions	10 calories per 1/4 onion
sweet pickles	30 calories per 6 slices

radishes	5 calories per4 radishes
scallions	20 calories per 6
spinach	20 calories per 2 cups

Here is Why Your Teen- ager is Dieting

Everyone does not diet for the same reasons, and this goes especially well for teen-agers. Most teen-age girls who diet are not overweight, but most teen-age boys are. In each case they diet for different reasons. Teen-age girls diet mainly to improve their physical appearance, but they may also have emotional or personal problems. This is why you get more girls than boys in those compulsive diets for which they have to be hospitalized. For teen-age boys the reasons are usually to develop a heavier, and more muscular, body. Teen-age boys usually want the large muscles of their fathers and the famous athletes they see on television. The added problem for the teen-age boys who were dieting is that they were usually overweight to begin with, so any gain they did make in weight did not give them a better body image. Both boys and girls of this age group are concerned with physical appearance, but what they do as far as diet has more to do with how they see themselves than with how others see them. If you can get your teen-ager to accept a table of appropriate weights for their height and build, rather than rely upon vague opinions by their friends or strangers, then fewer of them will be dieting and more will be dieting for the right reasons.

New Weight Tables : Revised Upward 5%

You must be saying to yourself that if this isn't a trick then you aren't as overweight as you thought, and you don't have as much to lose either. Well this is true, and the weight tables have been revised by insurance industry themselves. The changes were made from a study center in Switzerland, so they certainly weren't looking to help Americans feel better about their weight. Also the insurance industry wouldn't do something like this if it meant paying out more claims for people dying of heart attacks because they were overweight. The reasons Americans get this boost in their acceptable weights is that even though we weigh more than people in other countries, we also exercise more and take care of ourselves better, so that we come out just as good in survival as our less heavy neighbors. You still may not be satisfied with the way you look at the heavier weight, but at least you can be happy that the extra weight isn't increasing your chance of getting a heart attack.

Revised Weight Table -----MEN - Age 25 and over

Height (+ 1 inch for shoes) Feet Inches	Small Frame	Medium Frame	Large Frame
5 2	117-126	124-135	132-148
5 3	120-129	127-139	135-151
5 4	124-132	130-143	138-155
5 5	127-135	133-145	141-159
5 6	130-139	136-150	144-163
5 7	134-143	141-154	149-169
5 8	136-148	144-159	154-174
5 9	143-152	149-163	158-178
5 10	147-157	153-168	162-182
5 11	151-164	157-173	166-187
6 0	155-165	161-178	172-193
6 1	159-170	165-183	176-198
6 2	163-175	170-189	181-203
6 3	168-179	175-194	186-208
6 4	172-183	180-199	191-214

Weight (in pounds)

WOMEN - Age 25 and over

Weight (in pounds)

Height (+ 2 inches for heels) Feet Inches	Small Frame	Medium Frame	Large Frame
4 10	96-103	100-112	109-124
4 11	98-106	102-115	111-128

5	0	100-109	106-118	114-131
5	1	103-112	109-121	117-134
5	2	107-115	112-124	120-137
5	3	110-118	115-128	123-140
5	4	113-121	118-132	127-144
5	5	116-124	121-139	131-149
5	6	119-129	126-141	135-153
5	7	124-133	130-145	139-157
5	8	128-137	134-150	143-161
5	9	132-141	138-154	148-165
5	10	136-147	152-158	152-171
5	11	140-151	147-162	155-176
6	0	144-155	151-166	160-181

The Amazing Natural Supplement that Will Speed-Up Your Body's Fat Metabolism Function for Faster Weight Loss

The rate and efficiency with which your body burns fat has a lot to do with your ability to lose, or maintain, your weight. It is even possible to have a state of undernutrition causing less fat to be burned than could be done with normal nutrition and this nutrient. The nutrient that helps to determine how fast your body burns fat is L-carnitine, and it is essential to have in your diet for your body to use its fat reserves. The L-carnitine carries fat molecules across cell walls to where it is burned for energy. It has been shown to decrease blood fat levels, thereby clearing arteries while eliminating fat, and to increase the rate at which fat is used in those with normal diets. To ensure an adequate supply of this nutrient in your diet you should take a nutritional supplement of 500-1,000 mg per day.

To Lose Weight Permanently:
Cheat on Your Diet

No one can stick to a diet forever! How long did you stay on your last diet before you broke down and gorged yourself? And after that how long did it take you to get back on the diet, and how long did you stay on it before you gave it up as a lost cause? To go through all of this process your diet probably lasted from a few days to a few months, and whatever weight was lost was probably regained within a few months, or less.

The problem with diets is that they are too boring and too strict. You are asked to give up everything you like forever so that you can enjoy a slim body, but you can't enjoy the slim body if you can never again eat anything you want, and so the diet fails.

There is another way to go that will give you both the body you want, and still allow you to eat the foods you love, but in moderation. In this diet plan you go on a basic 1500 calorie diet 6 days a week, and allow yourself a cheating day on the 7th. On the cheating day you can eat whatever you want, and this is where you should eat all those things you love the most.

There is one other requirement to the cheating diet way of reaching your perfect weight, you must also exercise, for it is in exercise that you burn off those cheating calories, as well as where you keep your body looking well as you lose weight. The requirement is to exercise 3 to 4 times a week, and sufficiently to burn off an extra 3500 calories a week (that is the amount of calories needed to lose one pound). This will require about one hour of exercise a day average, but days can be combined just so long as you don't try to do it all in one or two days a week.

For the diet itself, although you can use any plan that is well balanced and low calorie, it must be low in fat, and you should drink 6 to 8 glasses of water a day. Water will help your body work and help to fill you up. It is a good idea to make fresh fruits and vegetables a big part of the diet, and to eat small meals throughout the day, don't just skip meals to cut calories. If you must snack, snack on celery or carrots, or have an apple. To make it really work, plan your cheating day so you get what you want, and after you reach your ideal weight you can have two cheating days, but not back to back.

Want to Lose Weight- Turn Off the TV

If you have both a television and a weight problem it's possible that television watching caused the weight problem. Recent studies, on teen-agers so far, have found that watching a single 1/2 episode of a television show lowers your metabolism by 14%. As you also know it is hard to watch television for an evening without having something to eat now and then, and the most popular things to eat while watching television are chips and sweets, both high calorie foods. The study on teen-agers concluded that a daily diet of television could result in a gain of several pounds each year, with the lowered metabolism and the higher food intake. It has also been found that if you are already overweight, your metabolism will drop 16% while watching television verses 12% if your weight is normal. Aside from staying off of snack foods in the evening, it would be a good idea to make sure you have an hour of activity outside for every hour of television watching you do, then you might be able to at least come out even.

PAIN

A Household Chore that Relieves Shoulder, Arm and Hand Pain

What do you mean, scrub my floors for relief? If I could scrub my floors I wouldn't have any pains, and since I am in pain there is no way that I can get down and do something like that. The whole point in having arm and leg pains is that you can't do much of anything that require you to use your arms and legs. Everything hurts all the time. So what do you really want me to do?

This is certainly a first reaction to many of you who have arm and leg pains so severe that they keep you up at night, and hurting all of the rest of the time. You already can't do any thing because of these pains, so how can you help to get them to feel better?

Actually this is an entirely serious plan for rehabilitation which has been used by Yale University for 15 years, and it works. The idea behind it is that is you don't use a part or your body, like an arm, because it hurts, the arm will get weaker and weaker until you lose all use of it. The only way to make it stronger is to use it, and you must use it even if it hurts. Any muscle that hasn't been used for a while is going to be sore when you first put it back into use, but that will pass with time.

Scrubbing floors is not really of much use to your legs, but it can help tremendously if the pain is in your arms or shoulders. By getting down on your knees you give the sore areas the best possible exercise, and strengthen them the fastest. While you need to check out any new exercise program with your doctor, if you have a medical condition, you can still go out and spend 3 minutes a day scrubbing floors.

But why scrub floors? This is something women have been trying to get away from for years, and men have never been much good at. Basically the value in scrubbing floors is that it puts pressure on your arm. It makes the arm muscle do some work, and that makes the muscle stronger. By making it stronger each day, you will eventually make it well if you keep it up long enough. Also this works just as well for muscles that are just sore or those which are sore from surgery.

But what if the soreness is in your legs? Then you have to use the same idea, but come up with something that will work for your leg instead of your arm and shoulder. The first thing that comes to mind is to walk. Walking does all of the things for your legs that scrubbing floors does for your arms and shoulders.

On the other hand, what if scrubbing floors is not something you can do because of your social consciousness? Then you will have to come up with something else. Maybe some light hitting of tennis balls against a backboard, or maybe swinging 2 pound free weights around in your hands for 10 minutes a day will do just as much good and fit into your schedule too. The idea is that you don't let an injured part of your body go more than 2 weeks at a time without exercise, and if it isn't injured then everything gets exercise at least 3 times a week. If you want to live free from muscle pain then you are going to have to make the effort to get out and use your muscles. Muscles that aren't used wither, and become useless. If you use the muscles, then strength will come and pain will go.

A Breathing Technique
that Stops Pain Dead in It's Tracks

There is a pain control technique that has been taught to pregnant women for years, and most of the time we don't think of it as something that just anybody can use who has a problem with pain. It consists of rapid, shallow breathing, or panting, and it forces oxygen into the blood. Perhaps it stimulates the brain to release a few endorphins along the way, but it has enabled many women to undergo birth contractions without medication, and it does it by relieving much of the pain that goes along with the process of having a baby.

Now this will help with virtually any form of pain, but it will be most effective in relieving headache pains, and in getting you over acute pains. If you have chronic, long term, pain from an injury you need a more permanent method that doesn't take quite so much energy.

There are a couple of ideas about how a simple breathing exercise can banish pain, and they might help you in finding other methods that work as well, but which fit your own pain problem more exactly. The first is that taking pure oxygen also is used to stop pain because it raises the oxygen level in the blood, and may slow the rate of blood flow through the body. While this might be true, pain travels along your nerves and doesn't have anything directly to do with your blood flow. The other is that yawning can also be used to stop headaches, and yawning also gets oxygen into the blood, and it also stretches the muscles a little bit and loosens up the neck.

So stretching the muscles might help with yawning, but it doesn't with oxygen, and it certainly doesn't with panting either. Frankly, I like the first theory a little better, any method you can use that will bring your blood oxygen level up

---

a little bit is going to stimulate your brain to release some of those endorphins that make runners and athletes feel good, and they are going to relieve your pain for as long as they last.

Actually, I have given you 3 ways to relieve pain, and all of them should work for you no matter what the source of your pain. If your pain is of a more chronic type, try getting an oxygen tank and raising your blood oxygen level over a longer time period that way for the same effect. But if you can be active, take a good walk and it may have the same effect for a whole day at a time.

Nature's Miracle Pain Reliever
Rub on Your Pain for Fast Effective Relief

There is a pain reliever on the market that you should know about. It's called capsaicin, and it comes from red chili peppers. It's also only manufactured by one company, Zostrix, but it is sold over-the-counter. Because it comes from hot peppers it burns when it is first put on the skin, and that is the way it is applied, a cream that is rubbed onto the skin. After a while the burning goes away, along with the pain. Getting used to the first feeling of burning may take a while, but it can be used for any skin, joint, or muscle pain. It is also sold in two strengths, regular and HP, the first time you use it try the HP. Also put on a very thin layer over the painful area.

Capsaicin is thought to work by blocking the pain transmitters around the painful area. It does this by first stimulating them, giving you the initial burning feeling, and then stopping them from passing the pain transmissions to the brain. To get effective use you will have to make repeated applications of the painful area so long as it is a problem, and then cut them down as the pain passes. Capsaicin should work rapidly on simple surface pain, but will take longer for cases of chronic or deep pain. If you have one of these conditions results may take days or weeks, and you should only be using it under a doctor's supervision. When you are applying capsaicin don't touch your eyes, nose, or lips because it will sting. Also don't use it just after a bath or shower because your skin will be hotter then and heat makes the burning worse.

It has been tested on chronic itching problems such as neuropathy and dermatitis, and although it takes time it has proven to be effective. It also works for neuralgia and arthritis as a surface treatment. It is even being tested for chronic headaches and herpes, but you are not advised to do this yourself because effectiveness is not proven, and it has to be put into the nose for the headaches. The irritation of doing that is going to be too great unless you have a very good reason. Capsaicin is not likely to replace aspirin for mild headaches since it comes with an initial price of burning that you have to get used to. Try using the low-dose form for some joint pain or skin irritation, and if it is effective you are in good shape. If you get some relief but are not quite satisfied try the stronger, HP, form. And if you get irritation but no relief, then try something else. By all reports it works very well once you get past the initial burning feeling on the skin.

Pain Control After Surgery
can Protect You From Cancer

Studies at UCLA have found that post-operative pain can actually contribute to your getting cancer. In a way that is not understood pain after surgery apparently suppresses the immune system. The study was conducted on rats, and it was found that those rats who received no pain relievers grew cancer cells at twice the rate of rats who were given morphine to control their pain. For us this means that your doctor should work very hard to control your pain after surgery in order to protect you from getting cancer at some later date. Since cancer can take up to several years to develop, you may never know the exact cause of your cancer. But if you have had a life of physical pain you are probably more susceptible to developing cancer at some time in your life than someone with the same physical problems who has had an effective pain relief program.

PHOBIAS

5 Secrets to Ridding Yourself of Fear

Of course you do not want to rid yourself of all fear, because fear keeps us cautious in dangerous situations and can save our lives. But fear which is greater than the danger we face can keep us from carrying out our normal days routine. If you have a fear of the dark, or of high places, or of flying then you may have a fear you can live with or you may have a phobia. Phobia is the name given to fears that are so great, and out of proportion to dangers, that they keep us from having a normal life. Those people who are afraid to go out of doors, or who are so afraid of germs that they spend all day washing their hands and cleaning their homes have very serious phobias which have to be treated by psychologists. It is healthy to keep in mind that fears and phobias run in families. If you have a close family member who is suffering from one of these, then don't be surprised if you or some other member of the family develops a fear or phobia too.

But if your fear is somewhat less severe, and your life pretty much normal, then you may be able to cure yourself by following some of the secrets here.

---

1. The first method of overcoming fears and phobias is baby steps. If you are going to a psychologist or a treatment group you may be given the same treatment, but if you have someone close to you who will work with you then you might as well try it yourself. This method takes time, so don't be discouraged if you need several months, or even a couple of years before you are cured. You also can't use this method if you are totally paralyzed by your fear. If you can't go outside of your house, or climb two stairs because of a fear of heights, then don't try self-therapy. But if your fear is not complete, then you have a chance of dealing with it in private. This idea is to take your fear, say a fear of the ocean, and to gradually develop trust and confidence in yourself. If you can't go into deep water, but you can wade in the wave splash at your ankles, then (having someone with you for support) go a step or two deeper into the water each week or each month. The idea is that you will eventually get used to the thing you fear, and will no longer feel that it is deadly to you for whatever reason. Most of the time, when we have fears and phobias, we don't really know what it is that we are really afraid of, and those things that we fear are not very dangerous with even a little bit of care. Using this method will overcome most fears and phobias, and don't be discouraged if you still fear something a little bit, so long as you are able to handle it and carry on a normal life.

2. The direct physical approach makes use of the fact that our fears and phobias are just things that our bodies do. If our bodies don't react, then we have no fear. While this doesn't ignore the mind, it does help a lot in carrying out the first type of self-cure. To prepare for this cure you might try learning some deep breathing exercises, and taking a regular walk of 30 minutes to learn what your body feels like relaxed. Once you have done a little preparation, you will need to start practicing whenever you feel your fear. The whole point of using this way of dealing with your fears is to learn to relax your body when you need to so you can face the fear, and overcome it with time. If your fear is of heights, then go up a little higher than you can without fear, and practice breathing and relaxation for a few minutes until you feel comfortable. Repeat this as often as possible until you can go up higher, and until you lose the fear completely. This can take a long time, but since just taking these little steps can overcome fears anyway, the relaxation exercises will speed up the process and help you to act without being fearful. When you have finally gotten to the point of a nearly complete cure, but still have a little fear, physical control can help you whenever you are in need. With practice no one will even know that you have a fear of anything, or that you are treating yourself in front of them.

3. The facing your fear approach, while not really gradual, can take time to really work for you. The idea of this method is first to name your fear as accurately as you can, and then to take it head on, but with a support group. The idea of this way of dealing with fear is to have more support than you have fear, and a need to do a job may have the same effect on you as a bunch of friends or psychologists. If you don't have a job that forces you to face your fear or lose your job, then you are going to get some supportive people around you, you can't do this alone. Once you have gotten your people around you then start attacking the

fear directly. If it is a fear of flying, then take flights with them, and if it is a fear of heights, than go up high with them. You can talk about your fears, and you can stop before you panic, but face the fear and use your friends to help you overcome it. This won't work with extreme fears, or where you don't have anyone to help you, but for many minor fears you can get almost instant relief. If you decide to use this method of getting rid of fears, than take your time, at least several weeks, and don't worry about the time involved. Fear can last for many years, and a few weeks or months of work to overcome a fear is a cheap price to pay for a normal life.

4. The indirect confrontation method is not something you usually hear about, but it is in common use. The idea behind it is to get you so familiar with your fear, with others around you to give you support, that the fear disappears. To do this you need all other ways of facing your fear except doing it directly. If you fear heights, then watch movies about high places, talk about high places, and go into higher places where you are not fearful. If used alone this method will take a long time to cure you, but if you use it to prepare for the one or more of the first three methods, it can speed up the whole process. If you have trouble finding ways to face your fears indirectly, you may have to do a lot of talking and maybe some group therapy. This is what a lot of group therapy is about in any case, so don't feel that you are doing anything unusual if you decide to use the indirect approach. This approach can never solve your fear alone, since you must face it directly in order to really overcome it, but by experiencing the fearful object frequently in a safe place you can grow so familiar with it that when you do come face-to-face with the fear, you will know how to act and that it can't really hurt you.

5. Overcoming fear through your thoughts is a little different than actually facing the source of the fear. Although you may think that your fear is a reaction of your body, it really begins in what you think about it, and how you think about it is something you have learned. What you want to do now is to un-learn your fear, and then you will be ready to begin facing it and curing yourself. Begin by putting yourself in a situation that brings you just the smallest amount of fear. Then look at what you are fearful of, and especially at why you have no need to fear. If your fear is of the ocean, then go to the ocean and take a step into the water. If you start to feel fearful stop, and start looking around you. Your foot is in only a few inches of water, other people are in the water enjoying themselves, and the water is calm and shallow for many feet beyond where you are standing. If the fear continues look at the whole thing over and over, and repeat it later if you need to, but don't give up. Over time you will begin to accept the safety in what you are fearing, and to understand that your fear is something in you and not in anything in the outside world.

Combine this with some of the other fear treatment methods, and you will soon find that you can deal with many things that you couldn't even bring yourself to think about before.

PMS PROBLEMS

What Men Can Do to Help Women Cope with PMS

While many women don't seem to be bothered by PMS, when women are bothered by it, it can ruin a relationship. If someone close to you is suffering from PMS symptoms they are probably moody and irritable at the least. Here are 5 ways of handling PMS that can defuse the condition, and make it possible for both of you to live in the same house over this period.

1. If you give the woman some space you may find that there is no problem for the two of you. PMS makes many women very unsociable. Because they would prefer to be left alone, they may attack those who try to make them feel better. If you are around a women who does not want to be around you just before her period, then let her use her time to read or rest as she sees fit. There is no law that says a person has to be entertained or involved with others (no matter how close), 100% of the time.

2. Though most women will want time to themselves during this time of month, there are times when they will also want some affection. This doesn't mean sex, and your normal diet of sex might have a bit of a setback for a few days. If you know that your woman has PMS symptoms, and she still comes near you, then it is a good bet that she would like some attention. A hug, or better yet a back or foot massage might make her feel a lot better at this time.

3. Because PMS can make regular duties seem overwhelming, try to take over some extra responsibilities around the house for a few days each month. If you detect symptoms of PMS, then get the kids out of the way and take care of the meals, even if it means eating out and doing your own cooking for a little while. Don't make a big deal out of this, but do make an effort to see how much the PMS is bothering her, and do as much as you can to help. This will not only help her to feel better, but it will be a direct expression of your own affection and will be appreciated later on. Finally, do not put heavy social pressures on her when there are PMS problems. A big party or other social event is the worst thing you can do to her if she doesn't even feel like being sociable with her own family.

4. Take over some of the diet planning at this time so that you have good balanced meals. This does not mean 3 meals a day either. Meals are better if taken in snack form about 6 times a day, and alcohol and caffeine should be avoided. The alcohol and caffeine, and even sugar, can be problems because they change our moods, and mood altering is a big part of the problem with PMS. Try to get emotions on a stable level so far as diet goes. If, in spite of what you do, she breaks into tears at something unimportant, don't worry about it. Go back

to comforting and just try to give her room to express herself.

5. If, in spite of all you do, she still seems to be out of control, and blames you for everything, then be forgiving. If her PMS is so extreme that she can't control it you are going to have to be all that much more understanding. By this time you should know something about her mood swings with PMS, and you know that she does not mean to hurt her family just because she is having a period. You must be all the more calm and helpful when she is at her worst. And if you can give her the run of the house, and just pretty much get out of the way, then your temper will keep in check too. The watchword for this problem is "forgive." Forgive her everything, for she shall be normal in the morning. Well maybe in a day or two, but she will be normal soon, and you will have the person you love back, and in her right mind too.

PMS Relief Natural Secrets that Work

If you are one of the women for whom PMS pain is a problem there may be a simple solution at your supermarket. Try drinking at least four glasses of milk a day the week before, and the week of your menstrual period. This is a natural way of getting an extra dose of calcium, and it is the calcium that decreases the menstrual pain. Research has found that 1,300 milligrams of calcium a day (the four glasses of milk) result in less premenstrual irritability, anxiety, crying, depression, water retention, and pain during the menstrual period. Of course you can get the extra calcium through a pill or powder instead of in milk if you wish, but try it during your next menstrual cycle and see if it works for you as it does for so many others right now. Once you have gotten your PMS symptoms under control, women over the age of 25 are recommended to have 800 mgs of calcium per day to prevent their return. That way you won't have to go through a high dose program every month, but simply avoid the whole process as you need it.

The Nutrient that Lessons PMS
Irritability, Anxiety, Crying, Pain, and Water Retention

Many women have PMS problems so bad that they must take medication. Now a common nutrient has been shown to relieve 54% of the women taking it, in a London University College Hospital study.

The nutrient you need is starch, and eating starchy snacks every three hours through the day will keep a woman's blood sugar levels high, and relieve the common symptoms of PMS. Good foods to use for this are rice, potatoes, bread, and cereal. Don't increase your total calories though. There is no need to

do that. Just eat a small serving of one of these foods every three hours, beginning an hour after you get up and stopping an hour before you go to bed, and see
if your symptoms are relieved.

PREGNANCY

4 Exercises to Make Your Pregnancy Easier

These are exercises you should begin doing at least 3 months before you
intend to get pregnant, and even earlier if possible. The idea behind them is to
get your body in good shape for all of the changes it is going to go through during the pregnancy, as well as to help you have an easier delivery and a quicker
recovery. While you can do these exercises perfectly well yourself, if you do feel
that you want professional guidance this same basic plan is taught at the YMCA
and YWCA.

1. Modified sit-up: as in any sit-up, this one is meant to strengthen your
stomach muscles. You do this sit-up from a standing position rather than lying on
your back. First place your feet about 3 inches from a wall, and your back flat
against the wall. Then bend your knees slightly and slid your forearms down the
wall. At the same time contract your abdomen. Then stand up and relax, but
repeat the exercise several times before stopping.

2. Body twist: begin by sitting on a stool, with your back straight, and a
broom or mop handle across your shoulders. While holding the handle on your
shoulders slowly twist your body from one side to the other. Repeat this exercise
at least 8 to 12 times.

3. Hamstring toner: for this exercise you need to have a 5 pound ankle
weight and a chair. Attach the weight to your ankle, lean on the back of the chair
and use it for support, and bend your knee to bring the weight up toward your
back. Repeat the process at least 8 to 12 times per workout.

4. The dumbbell row: here you will need two dumbbells (either one or two
pound weight is fine), and that is all. Take one dumbbell in each hand, with your
feet spread about shoulder width, then bend forward slightly at the waist and
rotate the dumbbells in small circles (first forward circles, and then backward circles). Also repeat this exercise at least 8 to 12 times.

As you can see these exercises can also be done by pregnant women as
well as by those who are planning to become pregnant. So don't ignore the exercise plan if you are already pregnant, and don't stop doing it once you have

become pregnant. Almost up to the time you deliver your baby you can continue to do exercises that will help your pregnancy to be successful. These can also be good exercises for those who have no interest in having a child, and anyone should be able to perform them just by following the instructions given here.

4 Secrets to a Healthy Pregnancy and Baby

Let us say you are in your first pregnancy, although it can also be your tenth, and you ask yourself if you are doing everything you can to have a healthy pregnancy and a healthy baby? If you have any doubts at all then you need to read our 4 secrets and see if you have covered all of the bases. Normally of course you can pick and choose your information as far as health goes, but when you are pregnant it is best to know that you have done everything you can to ensure that your pregnancy is successful and a happy experience.

Secret 1. The first secret is to make sure that your diet is all that it should be. If you are undernourished it is a good bet that your baby is going to be under-nourished too. Undernourished babies are light weight at birth, grow slowly, and are more prone to mental retardation and problems with metabolism. If you are overweight then you may be causing more problems for yourself than for your baby. Overweight mothers are more prone to having C-sections because their babies are too big, as well as a greater risk that they will develop diabetes, tox-emia, and phlebitis. The most important things you can do is to get a well balanced diet, take vitamin and minerals supplements, cut out all alcoholic beverages. This can cause birth defects.

Secret 2. Now that you are eating as you should you need to follow the next secret, which is exercising. Exercise is best begun well before you are pregnant, and if it isn't then keep it light and easy, such as walks. But if you have gotten an exercise program before you get pregnant you can and should keep it up. While exercise won't help your baby directly, it will make it much easier for you to endure the stresses of labor. In your exercising you do not want to get overheated, or chilled, you can reduce exercise time to 15 minutes at a time, that is convenient, and cut the intensity of the individual workouts so that there is less chance that you will hurt yourself or strain something. Also to avoid overheating you should give up both saunas and hot tubs until after delivery.

Secret 3. You now need to control the world that you walk in as well as other things that go into your body. Dangerous chemicals that you might wander into include weed killers, pesticides, household chemicals, and X-rays. If any of these are being used around the house or your work where you might get a heavy exposure you need to consider changing the way you are doing things. Remember the flap about video display terminals and how they cause birth defects, well that hasn't been proven, but the danger from X-rays have. So avoid the sides and back of computers and microwave ovens to cut your exposure to these sources. About things you put into your body, there are two, smoking and recreational drugs. While smoking is something you usually do yourself, and you can stop that, side-stream smoke has also been shown to be dangerous and you need to eliminate that as well. And while you are at it get rid of all recreational drugs, since you never know what they will do to your baby, and find out how many of your prescription drugs you can stop taking for the duration of the pregnancy as well.

Secret 4. These are the medical things you need to do before you get pregnant: get a check-up, get a pap smear, and find out just how healthy you are. If you are being treated for any chronic diseases such as high blood pressure or diabetes, both of these have to be under control before you become pregnant. In fact a doctor will want to watch you for any changes in a chronic problem all through your pregnancy much more intensively than they would for your normal treatment schedule. And something every potential mother should know is if she is immune to rubella, that is the old German measles. Surveys have found about 15% of women to lack this immunity, and the children of women who get rubella during their pregnancies are almost always born with birth defects. If you are not certain that you have been vaccinated for rubella you must get it done before you get pregnant. Doctors will not vaccinate you during pregnancy because of the danger that the vaccine will cause birth defects, and don't depend upon a childhood diagnosis of rubella by your family because they might be wrong.

Those are the 4 secrets to being and staying healthy during your pregnancy. Follow them and they will help to keep your baby as well as you healthy at this time. There may be many other things you can do at this time, but here is a good place to start.

A Simple Way of Preventing High Blood Pressure During Pregnancy

All pregnant women worry about high blood pressure during pregnancy, along with a lot of other things. Anything that you can do for yourself to make your pregnancy more worry free will help you to have a more pleasant and successful pregnancy, and a healthier baby. A wonderful discovery, reported by the American Medical Association, is that 65% of high blood pressure problems in pregnant women were solved by taking low doses of aspirin during pregnancy. Before taking any medication while pregnant it is always wise to check with your obstetrician, but a low dose should not cause danger to yourself or your baby. It is also interesting that aspirin also decreased the risk of Ceasarian section by 65%, so talk to your doctor today if you are pregnant, or are thinking of getting pregnant soon.

A Vitamin to Help Morning Sickness

Most pregnant women have morning sickness, and some have it so severely that they seem to be sick every morning for months. The University of Iowa has been studying a simple treatment for morning sickness which can decrease the nausea and vomiting, and in a safer manner than taking the prescription antivomiting drugs. This natural cure is vitamin B6, and it should be taken at 25 milligrams every 8 hours. At this level, and it was tested on women with severe symptoms of morning sickness, about half reported complete relief from symptoms of nausea and vomiting. While this may not be for you, if your symptoms are severe you have at least a 50% chance that it will help. However, as a warning, since vitamin B6 is only recommended at a daily allowance of 2.2 milligrams, you need to consult your obstetrician before taking a 25 milligram dose. Also, the women in the study only took it for 3 days, so taking it for a longer period also depends upon some assurance from your doctor that it will not be a problem, as well as judgment by you that it is doing some good in alleviating your morning sickness.

Avoid Lead Poisoning Your Baby by Avoiding this Natural Nutrient

This may come as a surprise to us when we think that it is always better to take natural forms of vitamins and nutrients, but some natural forms of nutrition are not as safe as man-made forms, because the natural forms can contain impurities that are dangerous.

If you are pregnant you have been advised by your doctor to take extra calcium supplements because of the growing baby. However, if you are getting your calcium from natural sources such as bone and oyster shell you may also be getting a dose of lead along with the calcium. In nature lead is incorporated into things like bone and shell along with the calcium, and anything that eats the bone and shell ends up with the lead in their bodies. If you are pregnant the lead will end up in your baby because that is where most of the calcium you are eating is going at that time. To avoid poisoning your baby with lead use synthetic sources of calcium like calcium carbonate. You can also increase the calcium level of many of the foods you eat by adding nonfat dry milk. This adds very few calories, but a good and safe dose of calcium.

Protect Against Birth Defects with a Nutrient

You can cut your risk of birth defects related to the spinal cord by taking folic acid supplements. This is what a study of 22,000 pregnancies by the AMA found. Folic acid is a nutrient found in foods as far as your normal needs go, but this study suggests that pregnancy puts a great stress upon our use of this particular nutrient.

The best natural sources of folic acid are fruits and vegetables. To protect your baby you only need .4 milligrams a day, but because it is not found in high concentrations in any food, you will have to have five servings daily of the fruits and vegetables. Beans are also a good source of folic acid, as well as supplying protein. For your general health even before you are pregnant, this is about the same amount of fruits and vegetables that everyone is recommended to eat, but for some reason many Americans seem to ignore. Be smarter than the majority and eat your fruits and vegetables.

PREMATURE EJACULATION

One Drug to a Better Sex Life

Premature ejaculation can ruin a love-making session by finishing off the man before he is ready. You may still have the desire, but be unable to do much about it for hours, or even longer. If it is a chronic problem, you may never feel quite satisfied when you do get the chance for sex. Of course there is also the fear of ridicule by your partner that premature ejaculation may bring on, and this could prevent you from even trying to have a sexual encounter.

Well there is good news, the common antidepressant drug Prozac is also effective against premature ejaculation. The Prozac stimulates your body to produce more serotonin, which in turn lowers your level of excitement, and allows you a longer time before ejaculation. Studies have confirmed that this treatment is effective in curing the problems of premature ejaculation.

Prozac must be obtained by subscription from a doctor, but since it is already licensed for depression, there is no reason it could not also be prescribed for premature ejaculation. While there are some bad side affects of Prozac therapy, this application usually takes only 6 months or less, after which the dosage is reduced or eliminated. Under this short course of treatment no side effects have been observed.

PRESCRIPTION DRUGS

10 Most Used and What to Watch Out For

Although doctors are usually very good at warning us about the risks of prescription drugs (because they fear malpractice suits), we should still take an effort to educate ourselves as to what is safe for us to take. Taking the wrong drug may not only not make us well, it may kill us. So as you look over this list of drugs, if you recognize any you are taking now, or that you will probably be prescribed for a medical condition, check very closely for the risks and side effects to make sure that you are not in one of the special categories who shouldn't take it at all. Even though there seems to be a best drug for every illness, there are also alternatives to every drug that anyone takes for anything. The possible complications from the drug should be no more serious than the disease or you are in more danger from the cure than you are from whatever the disease may do to you.

1. Alprazolam, which is also sold as Xanax, is prescribed for depression, and it acts as a central nervous system antianxiety medication. Risks: you should not take this drug if your are already taking any other antidepression drugs. Also not if you are nursing, and don't drink alcohol while taking it since alcohol is also a depressant. You should not take it for more than 3 months at a time, and don't stop taking it suddenly on your own since this can give you seizures. In regular use watch out operating a car or machinery because it can leave you drowsy and light headed.

2. Amoxicillin, which is also sold as Amoxil, Biomox, Polymox, and Wymox, is an antibiotic which is widely used for bacterial infections of all kinds. You may be given it for any thing from gonorrhea to a sinus infection, so expect to see it some day if you haven't already. Risks: avoid it if you are allergic to penicillin or have repeated attacks of illness in your intestinal tract. If you have a penicillin allergy you can go into anaphylactic shock, which can result in hospitalization or even kill you. Otherwise there is not much to worry about except that some people get skin rashes.

3. Cefacter, also sold as Ceclor, is a cephalosporin-type antibiotic which is used for bacterial infections of the lungs, middle ear, and urinary tract. Risks: do not take it if you are allergic to any cephalosporin antibiotics, repeated digestive system illnesses, or if you are pregnant or breast feeding. Danger signs include fevers, skin rashes, and digestive problems or pain which would indicate an allergy. Although some forms of cefacter can be used if you have a penicillin allergy, you have to be careful and work with your physician to find one that won't

cause an allergic reaction.

4. Conjugated estrogen, sold as Premarin, is the female hormone estrogen. It is used to relieve the symptoms of menopause, to prevent osteoporosis, and to treat prostate cancer. Risks: include any problem with blood clots including phlebitis, as well as pregnancy or breast feeding. If you are taking this drug you should also have progesterone or there is an increased risk of uterine cancer, especially after menopause. Watch for side effects of vaginal bleeding, tenderness of the breast, water retention, or intestinal upsets.

5. Digoxin, sold as Lanoxin and Lanoxicaps, is a heart stimulant which is used to treat heart failure or heartbeat problems such as atrial fibrillation. Risks: only the basics of pregnancy or breast feeding. The real danger in digoxin is of an overdose, and you may need your blood monitored to keep it within a safe range. Signs of overdose, or drug toxicity, are blurred vision, intestinal pain, headaches, general weakness, and even heart palpitations and arrhythmia. Since you would be taking it to control your heart rate, obviously you don't want to overstimulate your heart or you could bring on damage or a heart attack.

6. Enalapril meleate, also sold as Vasotec, is an antihypertensive drug used to treat hypertension and heart failure. Risks: avoid if pregnant or breast feeding, and watch out for fatigue, low blood pressure (hypotension), cough, and intestinal upsets. Stop taking it if you get swelling of the face, arms, legs, lips, tongue or throat. Do not take it at all if you have kidney disease or collagen disease. Watch your white cell blood count. This is obviously a very strong medicine that should only be taken under the supervision of a physician who knows what he is doing.

7. Levothyroxine sodium, sold as Synthroid, Levothroid or Levoxine, is a synthetic thyroid hormone used for hypothyroidism (an insufficiency of the thyroid gland). Risks: be very careful if you have heart disease or diabetes. Also be especially careful if you are on any anticoagulation medicine or are breast feeding. Signs of problems are a rapid heart rate, palpitations, or insomnia. Signs of danger that should be reported to your doctor include chest pain, palpitations, or an intolerance to heat (these are signs of thyroid problems). If it is used to lose weight it can cause heart failure and damage your thyroid.

8. Nifedipine, sold as Procardia and Adalat, is a calcium-channel blocker which is to treat angina and high blood pressure. Risks: avoid if pregnant or breast feeding. Signs to watch out for include heart palpitations, dizziness, nausea, and flushing. These could indicate low blood pressure. Low blood pressure can also result if you have been taking other blood pressure medication before you take the nifedipine.

9. Rantidine hydrochloride, sold as Zantac, is a stomach acid blocker which is used to treat ulcers in the duodenum and stomach. Risks: avoid if pregnant or breast feeding, and watch for headache, dizziness, diarrhea, constipation or drowsiness. You should not smoke while taking this drug since it reduces its effectiveness.

10. Terfenadine, sold as Seldane, is an antihistamine which is used to treat seasonal allergies. Risks: avoid if pregnant or breast feeding, or you are taking erythromycin or ketaconazole, or if you have liver disease. Watch for intestinal upsets, skin rashes, insomnia, dizziness, headaches, or feel nervous and anxious. These can be signs of an overdosage or problems with your liver. Overdosages can also lead to irregular heart rates and heart attacks. Also be cautious if you have asthma or any other disease of the lungs or air passages.

PROSTATE PROBLEMS

Diet Changes that can Help

Prostrate problems are one of the most common medical problem of older men. But there is no need to wait until they develop, or treat them as inevitable, when you can make some dietary changes that can help to eliminate the problems before they happen as well as help afterwards as well.

The prostrate function is irritated by meat, dairy foods, coffee, tea, chocolate, colas, and sugars. You need to cut down on all of these, and that means bakery good too, since they are loaded with sugar.

To help the prostrate you need to increase your intake of essential fatty acids (like you find in fish and seafood products), fiber, vitamin C, vitamin E (the antioxidants), and magnesium, selenium, and zinc. While you are at it you should also start eating more vegetables as well. This is a good and healthy combination that you need to follow anyway, especially if you are having prostrate problems.

What to do If It's Cancer

The fear of cancer is the only reason men will get a prostate examination if they don't already have pain or discomfort in that area. The problem with prostate cancer is that it doesn't usually develop symptoms until it has spread in the body. By the time you notice that there is blood in your urine, or that you have difficulty in urinating or have to urinate much more frequently, there is not a whole lot a doctor can do for the cancer.

Because it is such a silent killer doctors have developed a way of detecting it early called the prostate specific antigen test or PSA. With this test prostate cancer can be detected 30% earlier than before. This would seem to be a good thing since you are always told that early detection of cancer is more likely to lead to a cure. The only thing wrong is that most of the men who get prostate cancer don't die from it, so detecting it earlier doesn't necessarily cut the death rate.

If you are found to have prostate cancer you will probably be over 50 years old, and treatment will include surgery, radiation, and hormonal control through drugs or surgery. The treatment you get will all depend on what stage the cancer is in, and your general health. If your cancer is in an early stage, and just in the prostate, the gland itself will be removed surgically. You will probably not get radiation, and you have a 50-70% chance of returning to sexual potency. Survival is more than 90%.

In a second stage prostate cancer it has spread to the outer shell of the gland, and you may or may not get surgery depending on age. Radiation is the standard treatment, and there is a 500-60% chance of living 10 years. This is a much more serious condition if you are under 60, but if you are in your 70's or 80's it is probably not going to kill you.

A third, or late, stage case is one in which there has been a wide spread of the cancer. Treatment here will be castration to stop testosterone production and you will be given the female hormone estrogen for hormonal control. It is the male hormone that helps to spread the cancer so it has to be stopped by some means. There are also forms of estrogen that won't cause the cardiac problems or straight estrogen. These are called lupron block estrogen, and if you are facing this treatment check this out with you doctor.

Before you decide that your life is over if you are a man over 50, remember that most men who get prostate cancer don't die from it. Each year 132,000 men are diagnosed, and 32,000 die from it. This means that about 80% of the men with prostate cancer don't die from it. While treatment is the most important thing, the older you are before you are diagnosed is just as important in determining whether or not you can expect it to kill you. If you have no family history of prostate cancer you are less likely to get it yourself, and except for cases in the third stage, you have a good chance for a cure or long term survival with proper treatment.

PSORIASIS

A Natural Oil that Can End this Skin Problem, and Available in Health Food Stores

Recent studies have shown that the lack of omega-3 fatty acids in the diet, and the over-abundance of omega-6 fatty acids, may be responsible for skin problems such as psoriasis. Both type of fatty acids are available in plant foods, but the way our food is processed in the United States tends to remove the omega-3 fatty acids, giving us a deficiency, and increasing the amount of omega-6 fatty acids, giving us an over-abundance. This combination of imbalances affects the skin and can cause sores and diseases of the skin.

There is a simple remedy available which does not involve changing your entire diet, you can take flaxseed oil in health food stores. This is available as fortified flax, and is rich in omega-3 fatty acids. The flaxseed comes in a liquid form, and one or two tablespoons should be added to your diet each day. Do not change anything else in your diet, and it takes about three months before you will be able to be sure of your results.

Other good points about taking flaxseed is that it has been found to decrease tumors in rates, increase cancer fighting compounds in humans, reduce bad cholesterol and increase good (HDL) cholesterol in humans, reduce blood sugar, lower blood pressure, and help the immune system. These may not all be the result of omega-3 fatty acids, but flaxseed has many other nutrients in it as well.

In tests using rats, massive doses failed to find any bad effects of taking flaxseed, and no warnings are necessary. The recommended dose is one to two teaspoons a day, spooned over other foods. Flaxseed is also available as a cereal which can be mixed with juice or water, and all of these products are available without prescription at your health food store.

A Nutrient that Moisturizes Flaky, Cracked, Callused, and Itchy Skin "Magically"

This is a pretty big order for one nutrient, and there are several that are used for this collection of skin problems, but the one that stands out is vitamin A. In every nutrition book you pick up vitamin A is noted as a skin healing nutrient. Of course it doesn't hurt that it is also good for the eyes, works to control and prevent cancer, and if effective in controlling acne. In fact all of its effects have to do with keeping the surface of your body healthy.

It may also be that the reason we have so many of these problems in our country is because not enough people eat the foods which are high in vitamin A. It is also ironic that as we get older, and presumably our bodies need extra nutrition to fight off disease, we also tend to have poorer diets, which makes us more likely to get diseases and problems. Of course it is also possible that one causes the other. So if you want to stay healthy at all ages, eat a good balanced diet which is high in fruits and vegetables. But if you are suffering from skin problems anyway, then add vitamin A supplements to your diet until they clear up. Afterwards make certain that your diet is well balanced in natural foods, and you may not need the supplements again.

RECOVERY SECRET

Doctor's Proven Way to Imagine Yourself Healthy Again
It Works

Do you every wonder why some people die from diseases that others seem to get well from very easily? It's not all controlled by the quality of medical care they get, you know. A lot of it has to do with their self image as well.

No matter what your illness, if you can imagine yourself as healthy and active again, your chances of being that way grow immensely. A positive attitude about yourself translates into a healthier immune system, and a better recovery from practically any disease. Those who feel loved and supported, who feel that they are needed in the world, are much more likely to be in it a few years from now than those who think that they have nothing to live for.

The inability to imagine ourselves beyond our present troubles is pretty good evidence that you aren't helping yourself to recover. This imagining technique is also being used to treat cancer, and has always been used as a way of dealing with depression and stress. How could we get through the day if we couldn't imagine ourselves out doing something that we really want to do later on. The same thing goes for other illnesses as well. So give yourself over to imagining being well, and doing something you want no matter how fanciful, and your chances of being out there will be greatly improved.

RELAXATION

7 Relaxation Methods for a New life

Many times relaxation is not as easy as it sounds. Just look at those who are newly retired, it seems as if many of them don't have any idea about how to relax. And think of yourself on a busy weekend, when your time is limited you may not be able to relax and enjoy your time off. The truth of it is that relaxing must be learned many times, and a reminder of what you can do to relax can be a wonderful place to start when you feel the need to relax, but don't know quite what to do.

These 7 methods of relaxation are proven to work, and one or more of them will be perfect for you. For some you need someone else to help, but for most you can do them in your own home and in a limited time period. Give them a try and see what happens.

1. Massage is a fantastic way to relax, and although you can do some massages yourself, it is even nicer if someone else gives you the massage. A professional is the best for getting a perfect massage, but don't ignore an amateur if someone volunteers to give you a massage. For a nice back massage lay on your stomach in a comfortable position—let the masseuse work up and down your back kneading the muscles and stroking from the spine out toward the sides. Start with this, and then extend to a gentle massage to the back of the neck and the arms and legs.

2. Foot massage has been separated from a body massage because the benefits of type of massage can be almost as good, and you can do a very effective job of it yourself. According the Chinese medicine the soles of the feet are connected to all parts and all organs of the body. After you have had a good foot massage you will believe it. Because each area of the foot is so important to relaxation you will need to have every bump and crevice of your foot massaged to get full benefits. This should also include the toes and in between the toes. Because the feet do not tend to be the cleanest part of the body, it is good to start this massage by a warm washing or soaking, which will get you on your way to relaxation.

3. Progressive relaxation is a technique that you do for yourself, even though a tape or another person can help guide you. It is best to lie down for this, although sitting in a comfortable chair is acceptable. When lying or sitting comfortably, with nothing in your hands, begin by consciously relaxing the muscles in your hands and feet, work up the the legs and arms, the stomach and chest, and finally the shoulders, neck, and face. You must concentrate on what you are

doing for this to work, and you can repeat it for any areas of your body that still seem to be tense. Breathe slowly and focus your attention in the process as well.

4. Meditation is much the same technique, except it is mainly the mind that is relaxed, and the body will follow. You need to place yourself in a comfortable position, clear your mind of the days activities, and concentrate on a neutral picture, such as a candle flame or water in a brook. Do this with the television off, and in a quiet space of your home, although in the country away from the city will give you a new appreciation for nature and life.

5. Visualization is a way of relaxing that is very close to meditation. In visualization you begin by seating yourself comfortably, as you would in meditation, and then imagining a setting that you find enjoyable and relaxing. When you do this place yourself in the scene, and include the smells and feeling of the setting that you place yourself in. This method has recently been recommended for busy executives who have trouble getting away for vacations, but who are under high degrees of stress for long periods of time.

6. Controlled breathing is a relaxation technique which does not require you to think of anything in particular, but simply to concentrate on the control of your breathing. This is a part of many other relaxation methods, but can work quite well by itself. You need to focus your attention on your breathing pattern, and work to make it slow and deep, with long inhales and long exhales. After you inhale you should also retain the breath for five to ten seconds before you begin to exhale. This is also a good technique to use in a dentists chair, or for women having babies.

7. Biofeedback is a method which often uses a machine, at least when you are learning it. In biofeedback the objective is to put your brain into an alpha rhythm, which is a relaxed state, and when you have a machine attached there will usually be a light that lights up when you are in the alpha state. When you are experienced you can put yourself in this relaxed state without the aid of the light, at almost any time. If you don't have access to the professional equipment you can get some of the same effects by listening to instrumental music, or even by watching television if it is not a mentally demanding show. When you enter relaxation through biofeedback your entire body and mind relaxes without specifically working to relax them, the brain transfers its relaxed state to the rest of the body for you.

10 Second Secret for Tension Control

Do you need to relax before doing something important? Or is it just that you have had a long day and feel a little tense? In any case it is always good to tackle jobs in a relaxed manner, and this is just as true if all you are doing is trying to deal with your own family. The 10 second secret for relaxing is a breathing exercise, much like the yoga's do, only much simpler, and in a way that anyone can learn and use in a few minutes. At first just try this in private, but when you have gotten a bit used to it you can use it anywhere and at any time to help you relax.

First take a deep breath, then exhale slowly and let the muscles of your body relax at the same time. You can repeat the deep breaths and slow exhaling a few times if it is convenient, but if it isn't, then before you begin your activity take another deep breath and go back to work. You will find that your whole outlook has changed for the better. If you feel tension starting to build up again, just repeat the exercise each time and you will get through the day feeling better all the way.

SEXUAL DESIRE

2 Foods that Will Increase Your Sexual Desire,
or Your Partner's

Remember the old stories of the Romeos who would have a large meal of oysters before going out for a sexual adventure, or of how red meat would turn a man sexually aggressive, well they weren't all just stories. Both red meat and oysters are good sources of zinc, which is important in sex because it affects testosterone production. It is also helpful in controlling prostate problems in older men, and that would also help keep the sexual apparatus in good working order.

But these foods are also important for women too. Good zinc levels are necessary for a healthy pregnancy, and women also need a small amount of testosterone for healthy sexual desire. The relationship might not be as direct for men, but zinc is involved with both our desire and out ability to function happily as sexual animals.

So the next time you want a romantic dinner, with a good chance of love afterwards, a little red meat, or oysters on the half shell are good choices. If you aren't happy with either of these, look up some other foods with a good zinc level, and make up any meal you like.

8 Secrets For Better Sex After Age 40

While sex at any age can have its complications, after the age of 40 most of us have to do a little more planning to make it a completely rewarding experience. Good sex requires the attention of the mind and the ability of the body. As we grow older the mind wanders a bit more to the responsibilities we have in life, and the body takes longer to respond in sexual situations. Nevertheless, people can be sexually active, and find it entirely enjoyable throughout their lives. If you are older than your partner, then you can spend a great deal more time in foreplay as you get yourself ready for a satisfying climax. If you are younger than your partner, then use all of the powers of your youthful sexuality to bring them along and you will be completely satisfied sexually. In either case the 8 secrets discussed here might be of help in keeping sex alive and satisfying in your relationship.

1. One of the great enemies of our sexual equipment as we grow older are the free radicals. These free radicals tend to build up in our body over the years and produce many of those things we think of as the aging process. To counteract the free radicals, and rid our body of them, you can take anti-oxidant nutritional supplements. The most common vitamins which counteract free radicals are vitamin C and vitamin E. Others which need to be included are beta carotene, zinc, and selenium. They can also be gotten naturally from raw fruits and vegetables, and whole grain foods. Eating these raw is important because cooking destroys many of those things we want in the foods. As daily supplements you should take:

2-4 grams of vitamin C

400-600 units of vitamin E

200 mcg of Selenium

40-50 mg of Zinc

2. The big stimulus in sexual desire are the male and female sexual hormone levels. In men they peak at about age 17 and start to decline afterwards, and in women they peak in the mid 30s and decline till menopause. The falloff in sexual desire and performance is especially noticeable in men over the years. The sexual hormone is testosterone for both women and men, although this is not realized by most people. Women often get estrogen therapy which include a small amount of testosterone to help them with menopause and to control osteoporosis, so many women will not have a change in sexual desires and activities for many years after menopause. But most men do not receive testosterone therapy, and it is not used very often. The lack of this therapy usually speeds the drop in male sexual activity in later years. If you are interested in testosterone replacement therapy you will need to consult a physician, since there can be side effects, and it is only available by prescription.

3. To have a good sexual experience at any age the desires of your body have to get up to your brain. The substance which carries these desires is called dopamine. Dopamine is called a neurotransmitter because it transmits thoughts around the neurons of the brain. As we grow older, dopamine levels in the body decrease, and sexual desire along with it. Although the drop in dopamine level over time happens to everyone, it is possible to correct some of the loss by using certain foods and medicines that add outside dopamine. The most direct medical method of increasing dopamine levels is the drug L-dopa. L-dopa is available only by prescription, and is normally used for Parkinson's patients, so if you are interested in it as a sexual stimulant you are going to have to find as doctor who does that. L-dopa has not been widely used for this purpose, and it will take some effort to obtain it to improve your sex life.

4. If you cannot find a doctor that will prescribe L-dopa for sexual stimulation, or you would just rather not go to a doctor if you can help it, there are other sources. L-dopa is found in high concentrations in fava beans, which are cheaply available in the market, and are a good source of fiber too. One 16-ounce can of fava beans supplies a near clinical dose of L-dopa, and it you are reasonably active sexually anyway, a 1/4 can of fava beans a day is good insurance. Beans are recommended for the diet of vegetarians as well as a good source of protein to replace red meat in the diet, so using fava beans for L-dopa therapy will give you many benefits in addition to your main reason for taking it.

5. Another medical treatment of L-dopa decline is a drug called Eldepryl. Eldepryl is normally used for Parkinson's disease, and so is only available through a physician. Most physicians will not be familiar with this use, and you are going to have to search one out, but it might be worth it. Eldepryl does not add L-dopa to your body directly, what it does is help your brain to make all of the L-dopa your body needs. The beauty of Eldepryl is that the proper dosage can stimulate a man to a sexual activity level about the same as when he was 17 years old. This is amazing to most men who are older, and might just be worth the trouble of finding a way to get it. If you are considering Eldepryl as a sexual stimulant, you will not have to take the same amount as do Parkinson's patients. In Parkinson's they take 10 mg. per day, but for sexual activity it ranges from a low of 5 mg. every three days to 5 mg. each day. Because the doses are lower than in Parkinson's, the cost is a lot less too.

6. This next drug comes from Africa, and has been in use for hundreds of years as an aphrodisiac. It is called yohimbine, and works by promoting the stimulation of the nervous systems to cause more and stronger erections. Yohimbine doesn't seem to be quite as strong a stimulant as the other drugs in this list, but it still works for 50% to 75% of those taking it. Yohimbine has the advantage of being cheap, although it must be gotten by prescription, and simple to take. A 5 mg. tablet with each meal will keep you primed, and a one or two tablets just before sex will help in having an enjoyable time each time.

7. Now assuming that you have gotten everything working, but you are still interested in making it the best experience you can, you might consider have

a dose of vitamin B-3 (niacin), when you go through your own personal preparations. What niacin does is sensitize your sensitive area so that they respond strongly when being touched or stroked. Niacin has been called a sex pill, but it is really just a vitamin, so you can get it in supermarkets and health food stores. The main benefit of taking niacin for sex is that it seems to increase the pleasure of the orgasm. Of course niacin can be taken by both men and women.

8. If in spite of everything that is tried, there is a problem in keeping an erection, something a little different must be tried. An erection depends upon keeping the blood engorging the penis from leaking away before you have a chance to make love. When the muscles at the base of the penis become too weak to hold the blood where it belongs, it leaks away and the penis droops. This can make sex difficult and unpleasant instead of stimulating and fun. There are a couple of ways this can be handled; one is by putting what is called a constriction ring around the base of the penis after you have gotten an erection, to keep the blood from leaking back into the body. There is also a small vacuum device that men can use that engorges the penis at will, and can work pretty much any time. If you are looking for something with a little more dramatic effect, you might consider injections of the penis. What is injected is a smooth muscle relaxant, and it is put into the base of the penis. The problem is that you will have to do this to yourself just before you have sex. The reason for doing this, and not something else, is that those who have done it say they have had the best sex of their lives after getting pineal injections. While this might be a problem for most people, if you are looking for a great sexual experience it is certainly worth trying. If you want to try the injection method, you are going to have to go to a doctor to get prescriptions for the medicine and for the needles, as none of these will be available over-the-counter.

Male Sexual Performance Too Low
This May be Why

Think how sluggish you feel just after eating a heavy meal. There is now evidence that men's testosterone levels drop significantly for 1 to 4 hours after eating a meal high in fats. The study measured men from the ages of 23 to 35, which should certainly be peak years of sexual performance, and found that a meal in which over 1/2 of the calories were from fat lost 1/3 of their testosterone. So going out for a big steak dinner before a night of romance will probably prove very disappointing for men, and may lead some to wonder if their interest in women is real. Anytime you are considering a sexual encounter eat meals of less than 2% fat, and you should be at your best. Also, if you have been having some troubles lately in your sexual performance, try a couple of days of a vegetarian, or non-red meat, diet, and it is a good bet that you will be feeling a greater interest in sex, and that your partner will notice the difference as well.

SEXUALLY TRANSMITTED DISEASES

The Forgotten Disease that 30 Million Americans Have

It's true, 30 million Americans have this forgotten disease, and can give it to you, and nobody seems very concerned about it any more. The disease is herpes, not AIDS, after all, only 1 million Americans have HIV that gives AIDS. But herpes should not be forgotten even though it can't kill you. Before the AIDS epidemic people were afraid of herpes, and there was even research to see if herpes gave women cervical cancer, but that doesn't seem to have gone anywhere either.

You also should keep in mind that if you have cold sores, then you have oral herpes. Oral and genital herpes are called by different type names, but if you have one you can transmit it to the other. Someone with oral herpes can give someone else genital herpes through oral sex. The popularity of oral sex in America may be a clue as to where some of the 30 million cases of genital herpes came from. Of course you can also transmit genital herpes directly through vaginal sex.

Herpes, even if it does no permanent damage to you, is not something desirable to have. No one yet knows what the effects on men and women are of carrying around this lifelong infection. And no, there are no cures. Once you get it you keep it. You can take a drug called acyclovir which will speed healing, and maybe eliminate attacks, but that doesn't cure the disease. You will still carry the virus in your body.

The signs of herpes, if you get it, are a tingling around the genitals followed by a sensitivity and open sores. This is followed by a gradual healing process with closing of the sores, scabbing, and discarding of the scabs. The skin will appear normal at this point, and you probably can't give or get herpes if there are no signs. But herpes is a sly virus. In some people it produces no symptoms, and yet they can transmit it. It is those of you who are lucky enough to have no symptoms who are also cursed enough to be able to give it to someone else without either you or they knowing that you have done so. The recommendation, if you or your partner have herpes, is to always use condoms and vaginal gels. This is the best protection to use if you don't want to get, or give, someone else herpes.

If you still aren't sure that it is worth taking any notice of, there is also a legal aspect you should keep in mind. The courts are very much on the side of the infected partner when it comes to giving someone else a sexual disease. Just remember that if you haven't known someone for a long time, no matter how nice or desirable they are, if they want to have sex with you they will probably lie to get it. Of course there are lies and lies. If you have herpes, but it isn't active, you may tell your lover that you don't have it, and be telling at least half the truth. Of course they might be doing the same thing to you. You may be giving them herpes, and they may be giving you AIDS. To protect both of you, all new relationships should make free use of protection. The world will not give up sex, but it can take precautions.

SHINGLES

What You can do About Shingles
Can You Prevent It?

If you have ever had shingles you will never forget it. The sensitivity of the skin over your stomach, buttocks, legs, arms and face, followed by a rash and blisters is spectacular as well as painful. At its worst, and that can be for several weeks, you have been in agony, and had little to fall back on except to wait until it passed.

Well, there are a few things you might have done, and if haven't, then there are some steps you can take to relieve some of the symptoms. First, if your case is mild it will clear up in a few weeks anyway, so you will have to make a decision as to whether you want to take more direct action or not. For severe cases especially you should try pain relievers and cool compresses on the affected areas. Some physicians will also prescribe acyclovir, which is an antiviral medication. Even in severe cases the actual rashes and blisters will probably disappear quite rapidly, but the pains and aches can be one for several months. Because you don't want to get too dependent on any pain relievers you should keep to the lowest dose possible, and use more than one form so that you don't build up a tolerance and have to keep increasing your dose to get relief.

Prevention is another problem. Shingles is caused by the chicken pox virus (herpes zoster), but not when you have the disease. You probably had chicken pox as a child and pretty much forgot about it. Sometime later, usually in your 40's or much later, you developed shingles. Shingles at this later time of your life happens because your immune system isn't working too well at that time. This can be due to treatment for cancer, or AIDS, or any illness that makes you very sick. When your immune system isn't working as well as it should, the virus becomes active again and you get shingles.

The only way known to prevent shingles at this time is to keep yourself as healthy as possible. Eat right, exercise, and if you are sick, then be very careful about your diet. Not everyone who gets sick gets shingles, but even some young people who are unhealthy do get it. Taking care of yourself is the best prevention you have.

SINUS PROBLEMS

Runny Nose Bothering You
Drug Free Way to Control It

While there is nothing dangerous about a runny nose, it can be one of the most bothersome things about an allergy or cold. Cold medications are fairly good at controlling it, but there is always that dry tingle you have at the end of your nose, and the problem of keeping the dose just right to keep your nose in a fairly normal condition. Well there is something else you can do that doesn't involve drugs, and that is available in the market instead of the drugstore. Put 3 or 4 drops of Tabasco sauce in a glass of liquid, water is fine, and drink it. This should take care of the runny nose within 5 minutes, and can be repeated as often as needed.

Sinus Pain
Natural Relief Without Drugs

Chronic sinus pain is very difficult to deal with. We often take medicines which do little good, and it seems to go on and on. Now, however, there is a new way of dealing with this problem which doesn't depend upon drugs, and which can virtually guarantee success. The difference in this treatment and others people are familiar with is that the doctor is able to actually see what is causing the problem. He does this by putting a tiny fiber-optic camera up into the sinus and looking directly at the cause of the discomfort. Using this method doesn't require anesthesia, and that takes away one of the problems of minor surgery, and recovery when there is surgery is much faster, usually within a couple of days. Of course most sinus problems do not require surgery, but when there are polyps in the nose causing a blockage they must be taken out, and this is also done with a miniature forcep which doesn't damage other tissues.

Your Cold Might Really Be
A More Serious Sinus Inflammation

So your cold has given you a headache and runny nose, and you have so little energy you can't do anything. While this sounds almost like a common cold it is really the symptoms of sinusitis. To be reasonably sure though before you go to the doctor you should wait a week or two. Sinusitis is a chronic disease that can go on for months, while most colds should last only around a week. Also the headaches give away the cause. While you may have an occasional headache with a cold, sinus inflammations tend to make the headaches come back over and over. The most common time of day for these sinusitis headaches is in the morning, and this is unusual too since most stress headaches happen in the afternoon or evening.

But once you have accepted the fact that you have sinusitis, and not a cold, what can you do about it? Well, you can go the doctor, because he can not only diagnose the problem for you, he can also prescribe antibiotics that will help to cure it. Unfortunately if your sinusitis isn't cleared up with drugs the next step is an operation.

But let us say that you do not yet have a chronic case that needs these medical methods for a cure, what can you do to prevent the sinusitis in the first place? Although infections do play a part, much of the sinusitis is started by allergies. And the most common things people are allergic to that attack the sinuses are found in household dust. Dust contains microscopic mites, pollens, cast off cells, soil particles, metals, rubber, and anything and everything you can see around you. If you are allergic to anything, you will also be allergic to the dust in your house.

To get rid of the dust you need to vacuum and clean regularly, and for the most part use an air conditioner with a filter and keep your windows closed. For more local help in your home you can get a small device called a negative ion generator that takes all charged particles out of the air and leaves the immediate vicinity clean. If you have pets that go in and out of the house they need to be bathed regularly, and their sleeping areas kept clean.

SKIN PROBLEMS

Better Skin Care From Your Refrigerator

Some of the most popular stories of Cleopatra speak of her taking milk baths to keep her beauty. In the days of Cleopatra milk was a luxury which was both costly and rare, and it was an insult to her subjects that she should take baths in. But did it really do something for her beauty in the dry climate of Egypt?

As it turns out Cleopatra was practicing good nutritional skin care with her milk baths, and the reason it was good then has not changed in 4,000 years. Living where she did Cleopatra probably had a problem with dry skin, and today most of us have dry skin at one time and another. As it turns out milk contains proteins and fats that softens and moisturizes the skin while you bathe. Furthermore, a milk bath does not have to be a bath tub full of milk. Just add a cup of milk to your bath and it will do just as good a job as soaking in ten dollars worth of milk, and will add smoothness to the water as well. When you have finished bathing and before you are completely dry, apply some lotion to your body and it will keep that softness in your skin for several more hours. If you do this whenever you get dry skin you will be much more comfortable, and if you do it once a day or every other day, maybe you won't have a dry skin condition to begin with.

Dry Skin? A Nutrient that Almost "Magically" Moisturizes Dry Skin

Bothered by dry skin that you just can't seem to get rid of? If you think you have tried everything, and nothing is going to help, then you might just have a very pleasant surprise when you start using flaxseed oil. Flaxseed oil contains large amount of the nutrients called omega-3 fatty acids, which tend to be deficient in American diets. Omega-3 fatty acids are one of the essential nutrients in developing a healthy skin. Without a sufficient supply of this nutrient you are proven to develop dry and cracked skin, which may also be flaky, and which is worst when you come into harsh conditions such as winter dryness or summer heat. Since flaxseed oil is such a good source of this nutrient, and is so readily available, it is very highly recommended. Another excellent source is fish oils, and these can be taken as pills or in the form of fresh fish. These sources of omega-3 fatty acids are available in your health food store, without prescription, and doses should consist of one or two teaspoons, or capsules, daily.

Some Hints to Get Rid of Freckles

Freckles never seem fair. Light skinned people who would love a tan often end up with freckles, and other than a skin coloring application, cannot really get the sort of tan they might like. While there is no way you can get a good, natural, tan if you tend to freckle, there are some things you can do to at least cut down the problem of the freckles.

Freckles are caused by the same process that give you a tan. So to get rid of your freckles you need to keep your skin out of the sun, and the freckles will fade over time. The best ways to do this are to either keep your skin covered when you are in the sun, or to use a good sun screen (an SPF 15 or above), and that will usually solve the problem. If neither of these methods works to your satisfaction, you might have to go to a dermatologist for a dermabrasion.

The dermatologist might also do a chemical peel, or give you a prescription for a cream, but you should not use over-the-counter fading creams because these can have hydroquinone as a bleaching agent, and it has been found to cause cancer in lab animals.

Natural Wrinkle Removers and Why They Work

If you go to a dermatologist for treatment for wrinkles, there is a good chance you will end up with a skin removal process that will take off the wrinkled layers of skin and leave new, fresh skin underneath. This type of treatment often uses glycolic acid at 40% to 70% concentration, and is very effective if there is wrinkling or scaring which is not too deep.

This acid is one of the alpha hydroxy acids (or AHA's), and is found naturally occurring in foods and fruits. Natural sources of AHA's are sour milk (lactic acid), soured wine (tartaric acid), and glycolic acid (sugar cane). While they are being used by dermatologists and marketed expensively in cosmetics, they are also available in these natural substances.

To get the same benefits without the price, use the forms that have been in use for thousands of years. Allow some milk to sour and use it to bathe, or wash your hands and face in, as did Cleopatra two thousand years ago. The women of the French court of two hundred years ago washed their faces in old wine, and the Polynesian islanders continue to this day to rub their skin with sugar cane.

These natural sources are much weaker than the reformed types, and so there is no danger of overdosage. These acids also work better if used along with Retin-A, which is derived from vitamin A. Both of these wrinkle removers work best when used together, but their benefits take time to show up (up to a year), and last only as long as you continue to use them. So if you have used any of the natural, or pharmaceutical, sources of these acids and have achieved results, continue to use them if you want to stay wrinkle free.

There is also a good topical wrinkle remover that will help with the problem on a daily basis. Go to your health food store and get some almond oil. Gently massage this oil around the eyes and mouth twice a day and it will help to soften and smooth the small wrinkles in these areas. While this works much like any commercial cream, you don't have to worry about other things in the oil to which you may be allergic. You could also try opening a vitamin E oil capsule and massaging that into these areas, as another alternative.

SLEEPING PROBLEMS

2 Natural Secrets for Good, Restful Sleep Every Night

In order to fall asleep comfortably each night we have to relax both our mind and our body. If your mind is continually focusing on one problem or another when you go to bed you may lie there for hours tossing and turning before you are overwhelmed by sleepiness and fall asleep. Sometimes our mind refuses to relax at all during the night and we toss all night long, waking up so often that when we get up in the morning we feel that we haven't slept at all.

Being unable to relax our body is just as big a problem in falling asleep. If your body is tense from emotional strain, or sore from physical activity you may find it impossible to get comfortable during the night, and you can even wake up feeling just as stiff and sore as you went to bed.

To get a good and restful sleep you have to overcome these two problems. Relaxing your mind is best done by diverting your attention from your days activities and concerns—never take your work to bed with you. This can be done by reading something for pleasure, or by watching television, or even by putting on a clock radio for a half hour of soothing music when you go to bed and concentrating on the sound.

To relax your body you must use your body. A walk of 15 minutes before you go to bed will do it, but so will some simple stretching exercises, with 5 or 10 repetitions to be sure and warm up the muscles. The other secret you may want to use is to take a nice, warm shower for 10 or 15 minutes before you start the exercises, and that should take care of any problems in relaxing physically.

If you do the physical relaxation followed by the mental relaxation you should have no trouble getting the type of nights sleep you need, and being fully refreshed in the morning.

Use Daily Rituals to Overcome Sleeplessness

Often having trouble getting to sleep is just a problem of not knowing how to get ready to go to sleep. If you have no particular routine to go through before going to sleep your mind and your body may not be ready for sleep when you go to bed. And if things are too unsettled you may end up lying in bed for hours and getting up in the morning feeling exhausted.

To overcome at least the basic problem of teaching your body that it is time to rest from the day's activities you need to establish some daily rituals through the day, and particularly just before retiring. In many cases this will take care of the problem of sleepless nights and no medication, or further treatment, will be needed.

The most important rituals are those you do just before going to bed. You will have to decide exactly what you should do to put you body and mind in a relaxed and quiet frame of mind, but there are some suggestions that may be helpful. To prepare your house go through it in a regular way closing and locking doors and windows, and turning off lights. This will quiet and calm your sleeping area. Then clean your face, and brush your teeth to give you a clean feeling. A short warm shower can also help greatly to relax you. If you have trouble falling asleep after lying down then read a book or turn on the radio to a quiet, instrumental, music station. And don't get into any serious discussions with anyone when you are in the process of lying down to sleep.

Other important rituals during the day can also help with your goal of getting a good nights sleep at the end of the day. In the morning get up at about the same time each day, and don't let yourself lie around for hours in the morning even if you don't have to get up for a job. This will help to keep your body on an internal calendar of sleeping and waking. And if you feel tired enough to take a nap during the day, keep it short (no more than 30 minutes), and be active afterwards.

During the day you need to exercise both your body and your mind, neither should become bored and stiff from non-use. If you do not have a job that requires a lot of your mental effort, then find a project that does. This can be as a volunteer, or something done with friends. For physical activity, and this will also help to keep your emotions calm and your mind clear, you can do almost anything. Walking is fine, but so is bowling, or biking, or jogging, or whatever you enjoy that is physical. For best results, and you should do something almost every day, have several activities that keep your body moving and healthy.

Establish these rituals and you will not only sleep better, but you will feel better and be more productive during your waking hours as well. Good health requires a balance of both sleep and activity, and you can do all of these with a little planning. Remember that you are doing these things for your own health and well being, and you can be a lot more productive and kind to others if you are happy and healthy yourself.

What to do If Body Pain Prevents Sleep

Painful conditions from sore muscles to chronic illness can prevent you from getting a good nights sleep. In many cases regular sleep medications are not even of much use if you depend upon them for too long. In these cases you need to do some extra preparations before going to bed to ensure your rest. To put yourself into the proper mood for sleep you need to put your body into the same pattern it follows during a normal nights rest. When you sleep your body temperature first falls, and then begins to rise as you get to the time you wake up. You can imitate this pattern by warming your body up an hour or two before bedtime with a hot bath, and then relaxing for the rest of the time before going to bed. As your body temperature falls you will become sleepy and fall into a natural rest. The hot bath will also relieve you of minor body ache by relaxing your muscles and the surface of your body.

SMOKING

5 Alternative Ways to Cure the Addiction

If you don't believe that your smoking is an addiction just as strong as any narcotic, you have already failed to control it in your mind, and you will fail in your body as well. Nicotine is one of the strongest addictive activities that man has, and if you smoke you are addicted to nicotine. What makes it hard for you to give up nicotine is the same thing that makes it hard to give up any addiction, your body craves it almost any time you aren't using it, and you go into withdrawal after just a few hours of restraint. Your addiction to nicotine is both physical and mental because not only does your body crave it, but your mind knows you can relieve that craving by just a single cigarette. Of course nobody stops at just one of something they are addicted to, so if you have one to relieve the craving you usually have 10 or a 100 to satisfy yourself. The level of satisfying your addiction is much higher than the level at which you get the craving. If just satisfying the craving was all that was necessary then nobody would smoke more than a few cigarettes a day, and no one would be an alcoholic or fat either. Addictions take much more care than just relieving the worst craving to achieving real satisfaction. So with this in mind, and if you are looking for some alternative treatments to your smoking addiction that might suit you, here are 5 for you to consider.

1. Behavioral modification is an indirect method to stop smoking. The tobacco companies always try to put the best image they can to smoking, and we try too. A cigarette after sex, or with the morning coffee is too good of a scene if we want to stop this habit. Smoking is bad for you, and even if you do it in ways to make you enjoy it, it is still harming your body and your life—this is what you have to focus on if you want to quit. Start with the process of smoking itself, it makes the breath stink, dirties up your home and workplace, and leaves stains on your fingers and furniture that can never be removed so long as you smoke. Next look within you and you will see the disease and cancer that smoking causes many smokers (get a picture of lungs destroyed by smoking and keep where you keep your cigarettes. Finally force yourself to change your smoking habits. If you have always smoked in the most pleasant social situations, then start smoking in places that aren't pleasant, and the new smoking laws around the country should help some in this. Smoke in the alley and near the garbage—you will still get your fix of nicotine, but it won't be fun. Also change brands, and if you like the one you changed to, then change again. Get something that gives you the nicotine but doesn't give you the other positive feelings you are used to getting. If you keep this up long enough you will either give up the cure, or better yet give up the smoking.

2. If behavioral modification seems to put too much of the responsibility on you personally, try hypnosis to get some help. Hypnosis requires someone else to do, and sessions don't come cheap with up to $100 for a group treatment, and $500 for a private treatment. Hypnosis works with your subconscious, and during the session you are given instructions about how unpleasant it is to smoke or what you should do to avoid smoking. For many people this works just fine, but if it doesn't work for you, you may feel you have been cheated by paying all of that money and not getting anything for it. The truth is that hypnosis just doesn't work for everyone. Some people can't be hypnotized, and many just won't follow hypnotic suggestions no matter how much they say they want to when they are not hypnotized. If you know that you can be hypnotized successfully, then hypnosis may be your best choice. But if you have never be hypnotized, you are taking a chance. If you have never been hypnotized successfully, in spite of trying, then skip hypnosis and try something else.

3. Nicotine chewing gums are another alternative that might satisfy your needs. These gums are not meant to get you off of the addiction to nicotine, but only to break the habit of smoking to get the nicotine fix that your body craves. While nicotine itself might do damage to your body, at least you can avoid all of the other problems that go along with smoking. The things you will avoid in not smoking include the damage to your lungs, the heat to your lips and mouth that is associated with mouth cancers, all of the contaminants that are in tobacco (including formaldehyde and arsenic, the fouling of your breath and clothing, and the filth of wherever you live or go from the remains of smoked cigarettes. If you

use a pipe or cigars you have about the same effect on everyone and everything around you that cigarette smokers do, so don't use your method of smoking as a reason to continue a habit that will probably kill you.

4. Acupuncture is a new method of treating smoking, but an old method of doing medicine. In acupuncture your body is poked with needles in certain parts to achieve medical reactions, in this case to stop smoking. Because acupuncture has been in use for 3,000 years in China, the effects of an acupuncture treatment are pretty well known. To get an acupuncture treatment you need to go to a licensed acupuncturist. but the fee is only about $35, and that is a lot cheaper than most doctor visits. The results of a acupuncture treatment are usually good on the short term, you don't feel like smoking after you have had a treatment. The problem is that the effects may not last very long, and you will have to go back for at least several treatments before you will lose your craving for nicotine. If this is no problem for you than acupuncture may be the best choice for you. If you have a problem with needles, but are still interested in this non-drug method of treating addictions to smoking, there are variations that may work just as well, and without needles. A very popular method with acupuncturists is called acupressure therapy, and this uses just a message-like technique to get about the same effects as the needles. One other, and some American doctors even use it, is acupuncture with an electric current. In this method a low-voltage current is put to the acupuncture points, and the same affect is achieved. Try the one that you feel the most comfortable with, and you have a cure for your smoking without drugs or violent cravings.

5. The last of the five is an alternative to acupuncture, and it is called laser therapy. In laser therapy a laser beam is directed at specific acupuncture points on the ears and hands. When the laser hits chemicals called endorphins are released in the brain that stop the craving for nicotine. These are the same chemicals that are produced in acupuncture, but without the needles. The endorphins, which are also released during exercise such as jogging, give the same satisfaction as does nicotine, and relieve the need to smoke. Because this treatment does not require you to do any changing of your behavior, or to take any drugs, it may be a first choice as a stop smoking treatment plan. The drawbacks are that it can cost as much as $300 for a treatment, and because it is so new the results cannot be guaranteed. But sessions only last about 20 minutes, and if you can afford it, then why not use it.

5 Step Plan to Break the Tobacco Habit

Do you smoke? Do you really enjoy smoking? Then why do you want to quit? If you answered yes to the first two questions, then you must have a very good reason for wanting to quit. And if you answered no to the second one, then you already have your reason for wanting to quit. Now don't get this wrong, but quitting smoking is not going to be the most pleasant experience that you have ever had. Nicotine is one of the most addictive substances that man uses for pleasure, and far exceeds some of the narcotics that we spend our nation's wealth in locking up. But the effects of tobacco are so bad for the health of our citizens that it would be branded a dangerous narcotic if introduced into our country today. This is not to say that an occasional cigarette is going to kill you, but because of its addictive nature, a few cigarettes a year usually ends up with a few packs of cigarettes a day sooner or later. The outcome of that level of smoking, eventually, is cancer, heart disease, emphysema, bronchitis, high blood pressure, stroke, and on and on until we hit upon the one you are most prone to get. So follow these 5 steps and quit smoking.

Step 1. The first thing to do is to take whatever definition you have of smoking, and redefine it by what it does to you. Smoking is an expression of an addiction to tobacco and to nicotine. And once the addiction gets started, it also becomes a self-destructive compulsive behavior. And in terms of the legal actions you can do in your own name, it is the single most destructive thing you can do to your health, It increases the risk of every degenerative disease we suffer from, and will attack your lungs with cancer and emphysema all on its own. It does you no good, and now many people won't even have you in their homes if you smoke because they don't want to risk the effects of second-hand smoke for themselves or their families. Think of these things every time you think about smoking, and write them down on a card and look at it if that helps.

Step 2. We now have you thinking right, but you are still smoking. Perhaps you've cut down some, but what is the next step to actually get you to quit. Now we have to do a little analysis of the contexts in which you smoke, and plan some strategies to get around them. While you may eat a lot of vegetables here, just make up your mind that it is going to work. Now when do you smoke, and in what circumstances: after sex, chew some gum; in the morning with coffee, have some toast; at work under pressure, start doodling. These are only suggestions, but you should get the idea. And now that you have stopped, at least for the most part at the moment, use anything you can to take care of the craving. This includes nicotine gums, patches, or even acupuncture. Whatever you do, except smoking, is acceptable.

Step 3. You've quit, but what is going to make you stay quitted, you have to have a big incentive. For this step you need a friend and an enemy. The friend is going to help you, and so is the enemy. What you are going to do is make a bet with yourself that you will stop smoking for a specified length of time, not forever, but say 6 weeks. You are going to back up this bet with your money, enough to hurt, but not all out of range of your ability to pay (100$, or 500$, or some such similar sum is good). Should you lose your bet, and smoke again before the time limit is up, the money will be sent to one of your enemies. I do not mean personal enemies, but more philosophical enemies. If you are a right-to-life advocate, the money will be sent to the nearest abortion clinic. If you are a conservative Republican, it will be sent to the Democratic party, or the ACLU. But you get the idea. Because this is money changing hands you need to write this out in a contract and have it signed and witnessed. Then give your friend a check and the contract and instruct them to send it out as specified should you fail to carry out your end of the contract, and refrain from smoking for the specified period.

Step 4. Now that you have made this commitment and have stopped smoking for a while, you are in a period of great temptation. In fact you may be tempted to the point that nothing is so desirable to you as having a smoke, but you hate the idea of sending the money to your enemy. Now comes a new point of decision, and it is just as important as the others above. If you stick to the period of time you have set, and not smoke, you have won and there is no further problem on that point. Or should you go ahead and smoke and pay the money. You get your satisfaction from smoking, but you pay the price. This is an honorable, though not a desirable, outcome, and you would have failed to quit smoking. Or should you smoke, but deny it to your friend, and refuse to send the money to your enemy. This is not only failure to stop smoking, it is also a blot on your character as well. If you choose either of the first two alternatives you still have a chance to quit smoking, but if you choose the third then you have shown yourself that you have too little will power to quit on your own, and you had better take the money and sign up with a clinic to stop smoking. But before you make this fateful decision, no matter what it is, give it at least 24 hours at the time of your greatest temptation.

Step 5. To get to this step you will have to have been successful in not smoking for your contract period. Now you may have lost the craving to smoke, and essentially be a non-smoker. If so then your fight is over, and you can go about the business of ignoring tobacco for the rest of your life. But if you have gotten this far and you still have a craving to smoke, it is not necessary that you immediately set up a new contract. You have demonstrated to yourself that you can stop smoking, so that part is proven. What you have to do now is to re-examine yourself to see if you still have the commitment to stop smoking. For this I would take a month, and if you smoke occasionally in this period you know that you can still stop. If, at the end of this time, you still wish to stop then go back to step 1 and go through the entire process again. If you can do this until the craving has stopped you will have beaten smoking, and helped yourself to a longer and more healthy life. You will also have been a non-smoker for most of the time involved in going through these steps. But if you decide to go back to your old habit, then at least you will always know that you have the will power to stop, and that you can do so when you do make up your mind to stop.

A Painless 7 Day Plan to Stop Smoking

Even though most of the people who smoke want to quit at some time or other, they don't, at least not for very long. Smoking is one of the most addictive habits we get into. It can, and often does, start out as just an experiment with cigarettes. But within a few weeks we are dependent, and might even hate ourselves for it. When you ask yourself why you keep smoking, most of the time you say because quitting is too hard. Of course it is on many plans, but not on the one we have here. If you just follow this simple 7 day plan, you can be smoke free in 1 week. It can save your life, your health, and your self esteem. But before you start find someone who will support you in stopping to smoke, and who you can call and talk to when you need to. The plan works by having you say a pledge each day. The pledge is the words quoted for the day, plus all of the other quotes from previous days. This will remind you of what you are trying to do, and reinforce your resolve to carry it out.

Day 1: "I don't have to quit forever, but I am quitting for today." Quitting is something you have to take care of every day, and if you smoke one day and not the next you are still a smoker. Win this battle today and for today. If you fail tomorrow, then start over again the next day with this day 1 quote.

Day 2: "All that I have to quit for is today, but the todays will add up to many." Not smoking for one day makes you a non-smoker for that day, and you are successful. Focus your attention on the good you are doing for yourself by not smoking today, and do that as often as you need to.

Day 3: "I am a non-smoker." Admire yourself as a non-smoker. Remember all of the reasons that you want to be a non-smoker, and of the dirty and smelly mess that smoking leaves you in. There is nothing good in smoking, but there are many goods in not smoking. By not smoking you will be one of the clean ones. You will be admired by your friends and family, and accepted by all other non-smokers. Even smokers will admire you for having the will to stop, especially since many of them wish to stop but don't feel that they have the strength to do so.

Day 4: "I am changing myself for the better and taking control of my life. Smoking doesn't control me, and I like it that way." This is a positive declaration that you have taken control of your life. Since you no longer choose to smoke, smoking does not influence how you conduct your life. This is a positive life statement, and shows that you are in complete control of how you live.

Day 5: "I will avoid those situations where I have smoked in the past to the best of my ability." This may require stopping some rather innocent activities that you enjoy, like have a cup of coffee in the morning, for at least several months. Some things you may have to quit entirely if the temptation is too great. Such things as having a drink in a bar may seem to demand also smoking, and only stopping the action of entering a bar may work. In some cases, such as at work where you have to be every day, you might have to declare your particular workspace smoke-free to keep co-workers from coming around you with cigarettes. This is a necessary action so that you will break all habits that were part of your smoking pattern.

Day 6: "If I feel like smoking I will direct my attention to something else, and ignore that feeling." When you smoke your body becomes so dependent upon nicotine that you will feel the urge to within just a few minutes after you have finished a cigarette. This is what turns occasional smokers into chain smokers and 5-pack a day smokers. If you are quitting you can't be an occasional smoker too. When you do get the urge to smoke, direct your attention to something else, and if that doesn't work all of the time then call your support person. This is where you might really need the outside support. Make an agreement with yourself that you will talk to your support person whenever you get the urge to smoke. By handling these urges one at a time, and learning that they will pass away, you will be able to see that they can't control you, and that they will get weaker over time.

Day 7: "Being a nonsmoker is now part of my life, and shows that I am responsible for my life and my health. I have changed who I am by changing what I do." You have now been a nonsmoker for 7 days, and you have passed through the hardest part of stopping smoking. Smoking is just like any other habit, when you stop doing it you start to build new actions what become your new habits. It is these new habits, as a nonsmoker, that now make up your life pattern. While many nonsmokers begin to count the days since they stopped smoking, this is not necessary. If you are a nonsmoker each day, then it is that day that is most important, not the past and not the future. As long as you do not smoke today, you are a nonsmoker.

SNORING

10 Cures to Snoring So You Won't Go Crazy

Snoring, when its loud enough to wake others in your family, can make them do irrational things. Spouses get divorces over snoring, and snorers can become the butt of jokes that are more cruel than kind. Snorers themselves are innocent because they don't snore on purpose, and usually aren't even aware they have been snoring. But no matter what is said about snoring, nor how long its gone on, it is always caused by something that can be cured. Some cures are simple and painless and others require surgery. If you are in need of a cure for someone in your family who snores, then you will have to decide just how far you, and they, are willing to go to stop the snoring. If it drives you crazy you are going to be a lot more interested in doing everything possible then if it is just something that happens on a rare occasion. Read over the 12 cures and try those that seem to fit the best, but don't do anything too violent to the snorer, because they probably want to stop just as much as you want them to stop.

---

1. Short term infections and problems that you take cold medicines for antihistamines especially, or tranquilizers, or sleep aids can cause snoring. If the snorer has been taking any of these then consider stopping, but if they are really needed look for alternatives, or talk to your doctor. The reason cold medicines are taken is often colds or the flu, and without some sort of medical relief during the night, the sick person may not be able to sleep either. Snoring then makes the innocent companion of the sick person go through a sleepless night, and that is not fair either.

2. Because snoring caused by sickness, such as colds and flu, is usually a result of the nose and throat being clogged up, simply elevating the snorer's head with an extra pillow might stop the snoring. This will open the breathing passages more, and might solve the problem. Using extra pillows to help breathing has been used for hundreds of years as a home cure to night time breathing problems, and it still works just as well.

3. Another way to cure the snoring of the sick snorer is to use a decongestant containing ephedrine. This is also an old remedy, and it will not only clear the throat but will also help the muscle tone in the throat so that no snoring takes place. There are several brands with ephedrine, and even herbal teas, so just check the over-the-counter brands and health food store and you should have a good selection. One problem with decongestants is that they cause insomnia in some people. If you try a decongestant to stop snoring and get insomnia instead, then try a different brand, or one of the other methods of handling snoring.

4. A lot of snoring is also a result of the changing seasons. If you have allergies at certain times of the year, it is a good bet that those are also the times of the year when your snoring is worst. To cure this kind of seasonal snoring you need to get rid of the things you are allergic to. If it is seasonal pollens and weeds, then putting an air cleaner or air conditioner into the room you sleep in may be all that is needed. If your snoring is tied to an allergy to a shedding pet that spends time in your bedroom, the pet should be removed, at least at that time of year. And if the thing causing your snoring allergy is in your bedding, pillows, or carpets, all of these need to be cleaned or removed to get relief. If you just aren't sure, then start with the bedding and pets and continue until you have taken care of everything. This is something you can do entirely in your home, and which doesn't require any doctor's opinion or involvement.

5. Besides the infections and allergies already talked about, anything that causes irritation or swelling of the throat can be a cause of snoring. Sometimes the cause is something we are just born with, but which can be controlled with various medical treatments, or a doctor's care. But in most cases snoring is caused by something that is temporary, and which will pass away all by itself if just left alone. If you are pretty sure that the cause of the condition is one of these temporary problems, and you can't think of any easy way to treat it, the best way might be just to remove the snorer from other people who are trying to sleep. While this might be a problem for some people, the solution is quick and effective. In fact it is 100% effective, and doesn't even require much of a sacrifice by any-

one if the time required is short enough, and doesn't need to be done very often.

6. For the chronic snorer, becoming more athletic might help out. This is something of an indirect method of controlling snoring, but being more athletic will probably cut down on weight and help to improve muscle tone. While this does not guarantee that snoring will stop, both being overweight and having poor muscle tone are common in chronic snorers. If you have not been very active for a long time, but would like to try this method then it is best to see a physician before starting. Exercise programs, especially at their start, put a lot of strain on the body. If you have a heart condition which you do not know about, starting to exercise without watching your blood pressure could result in a stroke or heart attack. Don't be discouraged though, if this is something that you want to do. Doctors often prescribe exercise as a treatment for heart and blood pressure problems. You just need to take the right precautions.

7. The next thing to watch is your eating habits. Having a large meal just before bedtime is going to cause you to have a poor nights sleep, and can cause snoring. If you have a schedule that prevents you from having your dinner until late in your day, the best way to go might be to have larger meals early in the day and just a light snack at night. Many hard working people around the world use this kind of an eating pattern, and find that the larger meals early in the day gives them energy for their days activities. Then at the end of the day, when they are tired, they eat just enough for comfort, and always have a nice and quiet night.

8. Many times snoring is done in just one position. That is why having a snorer turn over often stops the snoring. But it can also be a little more complicated than just turning over. People sleep in a certain way because they have gotten used to it. If they snore in that position they don't know it, so they just continue, and the snoring gets worse. If you are a snorer and haven't tried changing the position that you go to sleep in, even slightly, then do it tonight. Roll to your side, or your other side. Or even get a special anti-snoring pillow (if you look around they can be found in some department stores).

9. Back to the physical problems, the uvula is a flap of skin just in back of the palate in the throat, and the soft palate is the top part of the mouth where it is soft. If the uvula is too long, or the soft palate projects a bit into the air passage it can cause chronic snoring. And if this is the cause then nothing in position, or medicine, or exercise is going to do much good. The only way to really cure snoring that is caused by a tissue problem like this is surgery. What the surgeon will do is go in through the mouth and just cut off the extra tissue. The cure is nearly 100% effective as long as the problem was correctly defined. Because this involves surgery, and the dangers of even simple surgery, you should make sure that this is the problem and that surgery is what you want to do to correct it. The actual danger should not be any greater than what you would have for having your tonsils out, and you never see anyone dying or seriously disabled from a tonsil operation.

10. If nothing else works, including surgery, then the only solution left might be for the snorers sleeping companions to wear ear plugs at night. This

might seem to be putting all of the problem of correcting snoring on the victim, who can't sleep because of the snorer's snoring, but if people want to sleep in the same room it may be the only remedy left. If just using separate sleeping areas is acceptable to those involved, then that will certainly work as well or better than ear plugs.

Snoring is not an incurable disease, and it is not something snorers do to bother every one around them. If someone snores and knows it bothers some-one else, it is a good bet that they would like to stop, but just don't know how. Unless someone is told that they snore, there is no way to be sure that you snore. If you are try to stop someone else from snoring, be kind, and they will do what-ever you want. If you are trying to stop snoring yourself, then take all suggestions from those tired loved ones and see if you can come up with a good solution to your snoring that will work for everyone.

Some Simple Cures to do at Home

Most snoring does not require either surgery or medication to cure, but simply a change in your sleeping habits. For one thing most of the time you snore if you are sleeping lying on your back. This is corrected by sleeping on your side or your stomach. If you can't change your sleeping position without some kind of help, then sew tennis balls to the back of your PJ's, and you will find that you have to get off of your back to get any sleep at all.

If rolling onto your side doesn't cure the snoring then it might be caused by something other than your sleeping position. Snoring is also caused by drink-ing alcohol, and increases with weight gain. If you drink in the evening and snore, then cut out the alcohol. If you are overweight, you may need a longer range solu-tion, but at first just try changing your sleeping position because it may help a lot anyway.

SORE THROAT

On What to do, and Why You Shouldn't Let it Bother You

While you can get a sore throat almost anytime, it is the ones you get with the flu, and that hang around long after everything else has cleared up, that really bother you. But you will be happy to know that doctor's don't recommend any particularly difficult treatment for sore throats. All that they will tell you to do is take linctus. Now while that seems easy enough, you might be asking just what is linctus. All that linctus is is cough drops. While you shouldn't take them for more than 3 days at a time, that is what you should do first.

If you have gotten to the end of your 3 days and the sore throat is still there, you might want your doctor to take a look at it. If he doesn't find anything, you can go back to your own natural remedies.

The only reason you take cough drops is to keep your throat moist. Cough drops also have a mild anti-pain medication (such as licorice), and a mild anti-bacterial substance to discourage infection. But all that they do 99% of the time is keep your throat from drying out. So naturally the alternative to cough drops is just cool water. Get yourself a glass, or a sipper bottle, and anytime that your throat bothers you take a little sip. This works just as well as the cough drops, and there is no time limit. If you get tired of the water you can make some lemon, or licorice tea. Add a little honey to coat the throat and sip that instead. So long as you don't have any diseases of the throat, these home remedies will work just as well as anything your doctor will give you to clear up your sore throat.

STOMACH PROBLEMS

9 Causes and Cures of Stomach Pain

Stomach pain is so common that just about everyone suffers from it on occasion, and as many as 1 in 5 Americans have it as a chronic problem. While the occasional attack can be bothersome, chronic sufferers may have weekly or daily attacks of bloating, diarrhea, and constipation. They just never seem to have a comfortable stomach, and nothing they do helps very much. If you have this problem don't decide that you have to live on stomach medicine, or that you just have to live with the pain and discomfort, until you consider the suggestions here. If one or more of them apply directly to you, you may be able to cure or control the problem in the future. Even if none are directly part of your life, you might be able to get an idea of how to go about solving or controlling your own problem. Here are the 9 most common causes and effective cures for stomach pain.

1. The most common reason for stomach pain and gas is eating foods that trigger poor digestion. Sometimes you will be bothered by beans (the classic cause of gas), or onions, or vegetables in general. In any case, whatever the reason for your stomach discomfort you will need to find out exactly what it is and try to avoid it. If you have a diet which varies a great deal from day to day, finding one food that triggers stomach problems might be a rather large problem in itself. To help look over the list below and see if any of these are part of your basic diet. If they are, then watch when and how much you eat of each one and you may discover the cause of your own stomach pain.

The most common food triggers of stomach pain are:

dairy products

wheat

corn

citrus fruits

food additives (such as monosodium glutamate (MSG))

If the problem is dairy products it could be an inability to digest milk sugar, which is called lactose deficiency. Lactose deficiency can be cured by switching to a non-dairy milk, giving up some milk products such as cheese, or taking lactose enzyme tablets on a daily basis. Using non-dairy milk is a common method of dealing with this problem when it occurs in babies.

2. Besides choosing the wrong foods to eat, many of us also eat too fast and too much when we sit down to a meal. If you are eating too fast then you are probably not chewing your food thoroughly enough before swallowing. This is a problem with many foods, such as vegetables, that benefit from being thoroughly chewed before entering the stomach. Look at yourself when you are out eating with others. If you are the first one through, or part of that group, much of the time, then all that you have todo is slow down, take smaller bites, and take a few moments to chew each one. However, if you have decided that your chewing is just fine, but you get up from every meal feeling overfull, then your problem may be overeating. Think of holiday meals, and if you feel the same way after every meal, then you need to cut down on your portions if you want to help your digestion. If you overeat at your evening meal then you are probably not getting a good night's sleep either, and that should be another clue that overeating could be your problem.

3. Now that you have decided that the foods you eat are not a problem, nor how much you eat at a meal, the next question that comes up is do you eat the right things. For your digestive system to work well it needs fiber to work on, and if fiber is low in your diet then your digestive system will work more slowly. The longer it takes for food to pass through your body the more likely it is that you will have chronic stomach problems. The best, and almost the only, sources of

fiber for your diet are vegetables and fruits. While they have to be fresh for some vitamins, they work just the same fresh or cooked as far as fiber goes. Fiber can come from onions, beans, corn, peaches, apples, bananas, or any other fruit or vegetable. There is a difference in the fiber content between different ones, but remember that meat, refined flower, and sugar have almost no fiber. Every meal that you have, day or night, should include fruit or vegetables, and most should have both.

4. Drinking late in the day, and this means water, juice, or milk, as much as alcohol, can cause pain in the stomach. When your stomach gets overly full an hour or two before going to bed, you can be pretty certain that you will feel about the same when you go to bed. In fact it is a good idea to have your evening meal at least 5 or 6 hours before bedtime. Many people have their largest meals at breakfast, and have very small meals at the end of the day. This sounds like a very good idea for everyone, but especially if you are having any problem with your digestive system. Food normally takes from 8 to 12 hours to pass through your body, so that drinking, or eating, a lot an hour or two before bedtime will probably give you pain. If you do feel the need to have more than a light meal in the evening, then snack—and use vegetables and snacks for the snacks as much as possible.

5. If you are one of those people who likes to keep everything on schedule, including your bowel movements, you may be contributing to your own digestive difficulties. In general the rate at which food moves through our bodies is not something we can willfully control. Whether it takes 8 hours or 24 hours for a meal to pass through our bodies is more a peculiarity of how our bodies function, and of what we eat, than of what we would like it to do. We also are fooled in this by the many schedules that we are forced to follow in our daily lives. If you have a lunch break from 12:00 to 12:30, then that is the time to use the restroom, and not before or after. We even expect children in elementary school to follow this same rigid plan. The problem with this cultural attachment to schedules is that our bodies do not always want to follow them. When our digestive system is ready to expel waste, it does not care if it is 9 O'Clock in the morning, or 1:30 in the afternoon. We have let our culture and ourselves tell us when we need to use the restroom, and not our bodies. If you don't want the bathroom to contribute to your digestive problems then use the restroom when you need to, and stay away from schedules as much as possible. The motto to follow is "Never Hold It In," and if you can follow that you will eliminate a lot of real and potential digestive problems.

6. Worrying about every little thing is a major cause of stomach problems. Stressful situations can come up for anyone, but if you seem to be stressed-out every day, then you might have an answer to repeated attacks of stomach pain. There are a couple of reasons that stress will do this to you. The first is that when you have stress your body gets you ready to fight, and to do this it stops the stomach from having its normal digestive actions. The other reason is that stress makes us contract the muscles in our digestive tract and restricts what is able to pass through. Our bodies put getting rid of stress over having a normal digestion

since the cause of stress (and worry) might be something that can kill us. If you can't get rid of the root causes of your anxiety, worry, and stress, then at least get rid of them around the time you have your meals. Some deep breathing exercises before mealtime and a 30 minute walk afterwards will give your digestive system a good chance to work. If the cause is a problem of time, where you are always late for something, then change your schedule around enough to have some time to eat and relax each day. Chronic stomach pain under stress is more likely to lead to an ulcer than to a promotion in your job.

7. A more local problem, but one that can sneak up on you and cause bloating is the use of candy and gum. The candy and gum do not cause stomach problems directly, but the air you swallow while eating or chewing them can. Air, or gas, in the stomach is the main cause of bloating in the stomach. If this has been a habit of yours, then cut down on your use, or cut it out altogether. Regular use of carbonated beverages does the same thing. Go to teas, or herbal teas as an alternative, or fresh fruit juices,

8. Other activities which are usually harmless can also irritate your stomach, and alcohol, caffeine, and nicotine are the main culprits. Alcohol, particularly on an empty stomach, can irritate the stomach violently and produce painful abdominal cramping. If you have this problem then only use alcohol with meals, or change the form of your drinks by going from regular wines to light wines or beers. Caffeine is not such a direct problem since coffee is often taken with meals, or with milk, but when nicotine is used at the same time it can cause painful colon cramps. The solution is to not use these at the same time, and not to drink coffee on an empty stomach either. If coffee in the morning helps you with a bowel movement, it might be the liquid rather than the caffeine that is giving you the benefit. Using herbal teas could give you the same effect but cut out the caffeine.

9. Strange to say, but some of the products you are using to help keep yourself regular may be contributing to your problems. If you are using laxatives and enemas on a regular basis, say once a week or more, then it is very probable that they are irritating your system. You can become so dependent upon them with overuse that nothing seems to work until you use them. You can wean yourself off by a better use of natural sources of roughage. Increase your use of vegetables and fruits. Add bran to your diet. Rhubarb and squash are very good high roughage foods. By including these foods in every meal you should have no need of extra medical items to stimulate your digestive system. This brings us back to the most common cause of digestive pain and problems in our country, many of us just eat too much white flour products, sugars, and fats to have a good digestion.

If in spite of all of these suggestions your stomach problems persist, and have for more than a few weeks, then you need to see a doctor because there might be something more serious going on. Colitis and ulcers cannot be self-treated any more than a lot of other things. Although the odds are that your problem is not one of these, any condition that persists more than a few days needs medical diagnosis to either treat you for the problem, or to clear up the risk that what you have is more serious. You need peace of mind as well as painless digestion to be healthy.

STRESS

3 Exercises to Relieve Your Stress

Instead of reaching for medication the next time you have strained nerves, take a few minutes out for some simple exercises which can leave you relaxed and comfortable, and free of concern from drug side-effects. These exercises are part of a beginners program for yoga, and have been in use for many years. The purpose of each one is to attain a state of complete relaxation, so you will have no aerobic effects such as deep breathing or perspiration, except as instructed.

1. Seated breathing technique: for this you begin by sitting on a chair with your hips touching the back of the chair, and your feet flat on the floor. Now relax your knees, raise your arms over your head, and take a deep breath through your nose. Lean forward and slowly exhale, and as you are breathing out push your chest forward toward your knees. When all of the air is out of your lungs your body should be lying on your knees, with your arms extended below. Hold this position for 5 to 10 seconds, and then breath in slowly, extending your arms above your head, and calmly sit upright again. After 5 to 10 seconds fully upright, begin the process again, and repeat it two more times.

2. Seated spinal twist: again sit fully back against the chair, and with your knees drawn up, feet flat on the floor, so that your knees form a 90% angle. Now place your right hand on your left knee and turn your upper body to the left, breathing in before you begin and slowly breathing out as you turn your body. After holding this twisted position for 2 to 3 seconds return to the forward position, breathing slowly in and out all of the time. Then repeat this exercise to the other side, doing the complete exercise 3 times to each side.

3. Arm rolls: these can be done seated or standing. First raise your arms directly out to the sides of your body. Rotate your hand so that your palms are facing away from your body, and slowly rotate your arms forward a few revolutions, and then backward. After 3 or 4 repetitions shake your shoulders out, and make smaller and faster circles with your hands. Do 5 repetitions and you will find your neck and back muscles well relaxed. Also keep a nice, even, deep breathing rate throughout the exercise.

13 Natural Stress Reducing Secrets

1. **Anger**—find a healthy way to express your anger. Don't let it build inside of you until you blow up. Its that explosive release of anger that is dangerous to your health, and can cause you to do things you don't want to do. Try going for a walk, or going bowling, when you become angry. Doing something physical often helps to calm us down.

2. **Stress**—this is often brought on by particular events or situations, such as a run-in with a particular person. Identify these situations and try to avoid them in the future.

3. **Overwhelmed**—at times we all get to the point where we just cannot handle everything that we have to do, and we have too many responsibilities and demands upon our energy and time. This is when we must find someone to talk to; a counselor, friend, or family member is ideal, but if there is no one to confide in, then write them down. That often works just as well. The key to surviving these times is to have a group of people who support us without question, and who will listen to our problems.

4. **Goals**—to avoid stress we need to set attainable goals for ourselves. If the goals are too far below our ability, we are bored with them, and uninterested in what we are doing. If the goals are too far beyond our immediate abilities, then we can never see the progress we are making, and become frustrated and stressed out. Most goals should be something we can do in a day or two, with only a few going past a year.

5. **Task**s—it is by performing the tasks that we attain our goals. If all of the tasks are stressful, we will suffer stress. To avoid stress from our tasks alternate stressful jobs with interesting and relaxing jobs. Also budget some time to relax and reflect in the days work routine, and at home plan some time for yourself when no one will bother you. By setting our tasks creatively we can seemingly move through impossibly stressful situations with hardly a problem to ourselves.

6. **Doing Nothing**—getting away from it all is one of the best ways of relieving stress. It can be done on a vacation, or just by taking a long lunch break occasionally. An even shorter version can be fashioned by taking a few minutes to read each day, or meditate, when no one can bother you and you can forget all of your other duties and responsibilities.

7. **Sleep**—not getting enough sleep is one of the main reasons people become irritable and feel unable to handle their daily stress. If you are tired all of the time from a lack of sleep, you tend to forget things, and you are often unable to take care of the boring tasks that are often required during a normal day. If you seem to feel sleepy and tired during the day try to get an extra 30 minutes or hour

of sleep during the night, and then see how you feel.

8. **Recreation**—it is said that recreation is actually re-creation. We re-create ourselves when we take time out to have fun. It can be at a hobby or a sport, but it should involve actually doing something, or making something. While reading or watching television can be a grand recreation, our activities should also include going out into the air and walking, hiking, or working in the garden. For an added bonus it is also good to do a new recreation every once in a while; it could be once a year or once a month, whenever we feel the need for something new in our lives.

9. **Meditate**—this is a good stress reliever for many people in the world, Although it takes some practice to learn to meditate, it is often the only stress reliever that is needed, and it can be used by anyone, no matter the age, physical condition, or place where they live. The idea is to go into a quiet place, close out outside stimulation by closing the eyes, and concentrate on a neutral object or word for a few minutes. It often helps to repeat a word over and over at this time. A few minutes of meditation each day can often be as beneficial in relieving stress as several hours of other activities which can only be carried out once or twice a week.

10. **Muscle Relaxation**—this is the direct approach to relieving stress, and is based on the idea that whatever the source of our stress it results in our bodies becoming tense and tight. Muscle relaxation is best carried out lying down, but can be effective while sitting if that is all we can do. What we are going to do is relax the muscle from the head down to the feet; first relax the muscles of the face, then the neck, torso, arms and fingers, legs, ankles, and feet. This takes a little practice, but it can leave you feeling refreshed in just a few minutes. Don't try this when driving because you may also fall asleep before you finish.

11. **Deep Breathing**—remember the old saying that when you are mad count to ten. This is based on the same general idea; when you are under stress, if you can take a minute or two out and simply breath deeply, your whole body will be oxygenated, and you will feel better. This activity doesn't require any real practice, and can always help a bit. It works especially well if the source of your stress is something that has happened but has stopped, like someone nearly hitting you with their car or saying something upsetting to you personally. When we come under stress our breathing gets shallower and shallower until eventually we are nearly panting. If you get into a stressful situation, or find yourself breathing rapidly for no particular reason, then consciously take deep and regular breaths, with slow exhalations.

12. **Social Support**—we need to have close relationships to live happily as humans. A social support network of friends and relatives gives us people we can relate to, complain to, and share our problems and theirs, as needed. Having the right kind of people close to you is the best insurance you can have that someone will be there to help lighten your load of personal stress, no matter how bad it is. Social isolation is a major factor in heart disease, and serious illness in many areas. If you don't have any friends or family near where you live,

then go join a club, or volunteer at a hospital or school, and those who appreciate your efforts will give you the social contacts you need to handle your own stressful situations.

13. **Alcohol and Drugs**—these are to be avoided as ways of dealing with stress. Alcohol is a depressant, and can simply make you feel worse than you already do about your problems and responsibilities. Even caffeine will speed up your heart rate, and may add to your stress. Work on the twelve ideas above, and you can relieve your stress naturally without relying on drugs or doctors, but only on yourself and who and what you are.

STROKES

The Antioxidant Vitamin
that Can Help You Prevent a Stroke

It has been found that one of the ways of protecting against stroke is by taking antioxidants. One of the best, and safest antioxidants, is vitamin E, which has been found to be a stroke preventive. While vitamin E is one of the very best of the antioxidants, others that might be taken include vitamin A, vitamin C, beta-carotene, and selenium. If you decide to take one of the other sources you be be careful with vitamin A, since high doses of this vitamin can be toxic. Vitamin E is a good, safe, and available source of antioxidants which can be taken over an extended time without side-effects.

The Vitamin Supplement that Cuts the Risk of
Dying from a Stroke

In a study at the Free University in Belgium it was found that stroke victims who had a high level of vitamin A in their bodies had a much lower risk of death than those with a low level. The difference was that only 1/7 of the high vitamin A group died compared to the low vitamin A group. Not only was the risk of death much lower for this group, but the risk of having a stroke, or heart attack, was also much lower. Vitamin A protects your body against having strokes, and against dying from them.

While it is not known exactly why this works, it has been found that a

5,000 IU dose daily was effective. If you are taking your vitamin A as a supplement you should not go over the 5,000 IU level. High doses of vitamin A can
make you sick, and are unnecessary anyway as a protectant from stroke.

If you want to use natural sources of vitamin A instead of supplements
you should eat foods with a high vitamin A content as part of your daily diet.
Vitamin A foods include carrots, leafy green vegetables, and fruits like apricots
and peaches. These should be part of your daily diet anyway for many other reasons, but now you know that they can also help to protect you against one of the
major killers in American society.

SUMMER HEALTH

10 Summer Health Hazards to Watch Out For

Summer is a time of fun and relaxation, and no one likes to think of it as
a time when we have to watch out for our health. In spite of this outlook there are
ten problem areas that we need to be especially careful of each summer, and this
is a handy guide to finding and avoiding them, and what to do if you run into one
or more.

1. Sunburn: after a winter mostly indoors you can get a severe sunburn
in just a few hours of putting your skin in the direct sun. Besides the usual problems of pain, blisters, and peeling, sunburns are dangerous because getting a
severe case boosts your chance of skin cancer, and even getting a good tan can
have the same effect. To avoid a burn, cover up, put on sunblock, and if you want
to be out in the direct sun during the day, restrict your exposure to the morning
before 10 A.M., or the afternoon after 3 P.M. If you do get burned treat it with cold
compresses and aloe vera, and take some aspirin or ibuprofen.

2. Yard work accidents: after a winter mostly indoors it is surprising how
often you can get injured just mowing your lawn (60,000 accidents in one year),
or trimming trees. Since you can't avoid this type of work without hiring someone
else to do it, take your time when you do the job. If you are mowing the lawn clear
away rocks and sticks from the area before you start so they won't be thrown up
into your face. If you are trimming a tree get a good ladder and wear some protection over your eyes. Also keep your pets and small children out of the way
when you are doing any of these jobs.

3. Playground injuries: this very common source of accidents for children
had 250,000 injuries in one year. Kids fall off of swings, loose and corroded equipment breaks or has sharp edges or protruding metal, falls off of climbing equipment

ke monkey bars can break arms or cause head injuries, and other junk around a play area can lead to easily preventable injuries that shouldn't happen with a little bit of care. Before letting your children use any play equipment take a look at the area around it to see if it is clean; also look at the equipment itself to see if it is in good shape; and finally don't let your child play on something that is beyond his physical ability.

4, Insect stings and bites: stings from bees, wasps, mosquitoes, and bites from spiders and ants can come at the times we least expect them, and happen to anyone. Most of these scare us more than they hurt us, but remember that many of these stinging and biting insects also carry diseases and poison. A few simple precautions can protect us from most of these attacks. Watch out around old wood piles where spiders hide, and be careful early in the evening when most mosquitoes come out to feed. Also don't wear bright clothing when bees are around because bees are attracted to bright things. Finally, if you have a problem with any of these biting insects that you can't prevent by being careful then put on an insect repellent. Most of these work very well when you keep a good dose on all exposed skin.

5. Animal bites: summer always seems to bring a lot of stray dogs out into the streets, and dogs you don't know are always liable to bite if you get too close. Cats also go out to hunt mates or just to protect their territory on the long warm summer nights, and it is good never to try to grab a cat that is in the process of having a fight with another cat, even if it is your cat. For either of these problems a handy garden hose can take care of the problem without putting you into any danger, and your cat or dog will forgive you afterwards anyway.

6. Head injuries: the big danger most kids and adults have with head injuries are in falling off of bikes or motorcycles, but these can be almost completely protected against by using a good helmet when you are doing either of these activities. The other big risk, and where you don't usually see helmets, is in skateboard riders. For some reason people do not use helmets when skateboarding unless they are some sort of professional. The idea is to look professional while you are still an amateur and wear a helmet whenever you skateboard. Head injuries are too serious to mess around with.

7. Swimming accidents: the biggest danger in swimming is drowning, and drowning is the 3rd leading cause of accidental death in the United States, with 4,500 victims in one year. To protect yourself while swimming don't swim alone, don't jump into water when you don't know what's underneath the surface, and don't swim so far out in any area to where you will become exhausted and can't get back. It is also a bad idea to swim in areas with riptides, people are drowned every year in their friendly neighborhood rivers after rain storms when the rivers aren't friendly any more.

8. Heat exhaustion and heat stroke: working in the sun on a hot day can make anyone feel a little light headed, but most people don't realize that they could be minutes away from heat exhaustion or heat stroke. On days like that you can lose water from your body much faster than you think, and as you lose water

your body temperature can go up. If it goes up a few degrees you will suffer heat exhaustion, and if you lose too much water you will have heat stroke. To avoid these problems don't work in the middle of the day on very hot days, drink lots of water at these times, and if you feel at all strange on this kind of a day then sit down in the shade even if you can't get water. For anyone with heat exhaustion you must cool the body down, and jumping into a shower and then letting the water evaporate off of the body helps a lot in this. For heat stroke, get the person to the hospital because this can lead to death, and the danger is too great to take care of yourself.

9. Lightning: while not everyone is exposed to lightning each year, there is a lot of danger in those summer thunderstorms. Lightning kills about 100 people every year, and has killed people in groups as well as alone, so being in a group is no protection. The danger of lightning is that it can strike you anytime there is a thunderstorm in the area, so any time you are around one of these storms take some precautions. Don't play golf, walk across or stand under a tree in an open field, or go swimming at a time like that. The best protection is to be in a building or a car, and at least stay out of the open if you are out hiking or biking when a thunderstorm develops.

10. Tick bites: these are a special kind of insect bites, and can be much more dangerous. Ticks are not usually found around houses, but any time you are out in the woods or fields there is the chance of running across ticks. Ticks move about on birds and the coats of animals, and ticks can carry serious viral diseases like Rocky Mountain spotted fever. Protect yourself from ticks with repellent, and long sleeved clothing. If you do get a tick apply some alcohol to him, or a little heat to his rear end to get him to back out. If you try to remove him and the head breaks off, then try to work it out carefully as you can. If a tick bite gets red and swollen see a doctor.

Have a careful and fun summer, but watch out for these ten hazards to good health.

SURGERY

How to Tell If You Need Surgery Or Not:
20% of All Surgery is Unneeded

Yes, it's true, 20% of all surgery is unneeded, but for some surgeries even more than 20% can be avoided if precautions are taken before agreeing to surgery. If your doctor recommends surgery for you, you need to be able to ask some questions which will help you make up your own mind whether or not you really want to have the surgery, and this even includes surgeries for life threatening illnesses.

In order to find out if you really need the surgery your doctor is telling you to have, begin by asking for all of the information he can tell you about it—most doctors will be glad to do this because it is how they usually go about convincing patients to have the surgeries they are recommending. Make sure to also ask about complications, and the statistics on complications and errors. Even if your doctor doesn't know this information himself he will probably give you some information to read.

Next get a second opinion from a specialist in a closely related field. A lot of conditions for which you might have a surgical procedure are often treated with medicines, so an internist would be a good choice. You might also go to a special center where the problem you are having is studied, and new advances are made. There are centers like this in many parts of the country, and they treat cancer, heart conditions, the brain, skin diseases, and many others. But be sure to find out if there is something you can do other than surgery that has just as good an outcome since once something is cut out or fused together its going to be with you like that for the rest of your life.

The surgeries to watch out for most closely, those which have the highest rates of unnecessary surgeries, are hysterectomies (20% unnecessary), tonsillectomies (27% unnecessary), and coronary bypass and Ceasarian sections, which are also high but are still under study. Any surgery should be considered to be serious no matter how safe you are told it is, and you should always think it through before agreeing to have it.

Is Your Surgeon Experienced Enough
to Operate on You?

This is rather a silly question isn't it, if your surgeon weren't qualified to operate on you, then what is he doing offering to take out your gallbladder to solve your problem? The truth is that your surgeon is simply exercising the right of his medical degree. A medical degree gives a doctor the right to diagnose you, prescribe drugs, and if he decides to do so, to operate on you for anything that he thinks is wrong.

Of course he can't operate on you just to make money, or to get practice so that he can operate on other people better latter on, but it does happen. America does not require that a doctor be qualified as a surgeon before he operates on your body. And even if he is qualified by the surgical boards, he will have a lot more experience after he has done 100 operations of a particular type then when he has only done 5 or 10. It takes time to learn surgery, and you don't want to be anyone's learning tool. You want the best possible surgeon for any procedure that you have to go through, and the best way to ensure that is to get someone who has been around for a while. Preferable 5 or 10 years, or more.

And how do you do that? This takes some action by you. You should write to the medical board of your state and see if any, and how many, malpractice suits are filed against this doctor. Also how long they have been practicing. Certainly 1 or 2 a year should not concern you if the doctor is an active surgeon. But if he has 100 lawsuits a year for the last 2 or 3 years, then you had better think hard about him cutting up your body to fix anything.

But aside from the numbers of malpractice claims filed against a doctor, the most important reason for choosing him should be the number of years he has practiced, and the number of operations of the type you are going to have done. If he is in his first year, your chances of a bad outcome may be 10 or 20 times greater than if he has been doing this for 5 or 10 years, and done at least 100 of them.

THYROID PROBLEMS

Alleviate Thyroid Problems and Disease
Without Harmful Drugs

Because thyroid problems can come in three forms, you need to be aware of three natural approaches to dealing with them if you want to avoid, or minimize, your use of drugs. The thyroid can either be defective as a result of not having the nutrients it needs, or it can underproduce or overproduce its hormone, thyroid stimulating hormone (TSH). In any of these cases you will be sick.

To ensure that the thyroid gets the nutrition it needs, you have to have enough iodine in your diet for its needs. If you look into any old medical books you will see people with goiters, these swellings on the neck are the result in inadequate iodine in the diet. For this reason iodine is now added to most of the salt that we buy, although you can get it in foods without the salt as well. The main iodine supplying foods are seafood, vegetables, meats, eggs, dairy products, breads and cereals, and fruits. As you can see, any diet which includes a variety of foods will have no problem supplying you with all of the iodine that your thyroid needs to run properly.

But suppose your thyroid gland is overproducing hormones. This results in Graves' disease, like President Bush and his wife have, as well as other illnesses. The extra hormone accelerates the metabolism of the body and can also lead to a breakdown of the body's cells as well as contribute to osteoporosis. Medication for hyperthyroidism will consist of antithyroid drugs, although until the thyroid returns to normal function you are going to have to increase your nutritional intake to prevent your body from destroying itself through its accelerated metabolism. Your diet may go to 4000 or 5000 calories, and your protein to 125 grams a day. Calcium should be increased to 3 grams, and vitamin C, vitamin D, vitamin A, and vitamin B complex all needs to be increased. Drinking large amounts of milk will supply many of these nutritional needs.

If your problem is hypothyroidism you have a problem which is even more difficult to solve. Your thyroid is just not putting out enough hormone to take care of your body's needs. In this case you will be given a medication consisting of desiccated thyroid to replace the function of your own thyroid, and you must watch your diet closely. Because you will be decreasing your total intake of foods, you have to be especially careful to have a balanced diet. It is very easy in this situation to end up malnutritioned, and thereby weaken your body even more so far as susceptibility to other diseases is concerned.

What are They and What

Some of the Best Treatments Are

It is entirely possible for you to have a thyroid problem and not know it. In many cases thyroid is long mistaken for the effects of aging, psychological depression, skin disease, cardiac irregularities, or Alzheimer's related memory loss. This is a real tragedy because thyroid problems are nearly always treatable, and treating these other symptoms without treating the thyroid problem may actually cause you more danger and more disease rather than less.

To try to find out if you have a thyroid problem you need to know the most common forms, as well as some of the other symptoms you might have if it isn't well defined. The most common forms are goiter, Grave's disease, and Hashimoto's disease. Goiter is rather easy to diagnose since it always shows up as an enlargement of the skin on the neck. A goiter is treated with surgery, but it should always be treated because sometimes it is a sign of cancer.

Grave's disease is the thyroid problem that George Bush and his wife had. The most easily seen symptoms are irritation and bulging of the eyes. It might also show up with heart rate variations, impotence, menstrual problems, and weight loss. If you have this disease you may also feel warm and sweaty in cool weather. For this disease you may have to take a pill to block the action of the thyroid, or have your thyroid removed and take thyroxin afterwards to replace what the thyroid was secreting that your body needs.

Hashimoto's disease is caused by too little secretions by the thyroid, and shows up as a slow pulse, constipation, constant cold feeling in the body, weight gain, hair loss, and depression. The memory may also be affected, and decision making become difficult. Treatment is to take pills of thyroxin, and the blood should be checked every couple of years for the level of thyroid secretions.

This covers the basic ways you may see a thyroid problem in your body, but just as a last note, iodine in the diet does not either cure or prevent problems with the thyroid. Iodine was originally put into salt to prevent goiter in people with very poor diets. If you have a normal diet, which doesn't consist of only one or two types of food, then you are getting all of your nutritional iodine in your normal diet anyway, and extra additions are not going to do you any good.

TOOTHACHES

Herb that Relieves Toothache Pain

There are many chemicals sold which are meant to relieve toothache pain, but there is also an herb that will do the job just as well, and is no more difficult to use than any of the others. It is oil of clove, and you can get it in health food stores or markets. The application is simple, just apply a dab to the tooth that is hurting and you will ease the pain. Then keep up the applications as needed until you can get to your dentist.

How a Slice of Cheddar Cheese After Meals Can Prevent Plaque, Tooth Decay, and Gum Disease

Diseases of the teeth and gums start with the foods we eat, and while everyone is advised to brush after every meal to prevent these diseases, you can also eat a slice of Cheddar cheese at the end of your meals and get the same results. The Cheddar cheese works by changing the amount of acid in your mouth, and leaving you with a more normal level than you would otherwise have. If you combine your cheese with a piece of fruit, like an apple, then the fruit will take some of the food particles off of your teeth, and help in the prevention process.

How to Whiten Your Teeth Without a Dentist

Teeth can be badly stained from smoking, or drinking coffee or tea. The acids in coffee and tea have even been used to tan animal skins, and they color your teeth in the same way. Stains can be caused by chemicals soaking into the enamel of your teeth, or by coating the outside of the teeth with the chemicals in things that you eat or drink. In either case your teeth will take constant care to keep them white, as well as special treatments for certain types of stains. Because you have to know something about your teeth to remove stains, you have probably gone to a dentist to remove stains. This often isn't necessary, if you follow the suggestions given here.

Plaque is the most common problem we have with our teeth, and the first ones anyone notices as discoloring your teeth. A layer of plaque, which comes

---

from the food you eat, can build up in a day or two and will stay there until you remove it. Plaque is usually whitish or yellowish, and not only discolors the teeth but makes the breath smell bad too. The heaviest areas of plaque build-up will be near the gums, but it can also cover the whole surface of the teeth. The easiest way to remove plaque is with a good toothbrush, and flossing. A good toothbrush is of soft or medium stiffness, and not one of the stiffest ones you can find. Flossing is necessary because you can't get plaque out from between the teeth or around the gums with just a toothbrush. While you should brush 2 or 3 times a day, flossing once a day, or every other day, is sufficient depending on your diet.

Now that we have gotten your teeth clean and plaque free, what should we do about the stains? There are several different ways of removing stains, and we will look at the ones you can do yourself first. If they don't work you can always go to the dentist for the others.

The first method of removing light stains is with a whitening toothpaste. These are sold along with the regular toothpastes, and will remove stains that are not too noticeable anyway. Their big advantage is that they can help to keep your teeth white if they are not now stained, and their use can be part of your normal toothbrushing pattern. The downside of these toothpastes is that they can also make your teeth sensitive to heat, cold, and sweets. Because they are giving your teeth a chemical bath every day, over time they may result in irritating the nerves around the teeth, and make you think you have abscesses or cavities. Try them, but if you have a problem like this, then give them up.

The next method you can do yourself is bleaching. As the name indicates, bleaching means that you use bleach to whiten your teeth. There are 2 household products you can use for bleaching, and they work just as well as what a dentist would use to whiten teeth. The products are household bleach, and hydrogen peroxide. To use them safely all that you will need is some Q-tips, or something similar, and the chemicals themselves. Put a little of the bleach or peroxide into a bowl, touch the Q-tip to the liquid, and then put it onto the stained spot on your tooth. The Q-tip should not be do damp that it drips, but needs to be quite dry. Do this on every stained area that you can see on your teeth and you will whiten them up. If you are careful, there will be no problems with getting the chemicals into your mouth. For areas that you can't reach, you will still have to have a dentist do the job, but this should handle almost everything. Bleaching is probably the most effective way of treating discolorations of the teeth, and one of the simplest that you can do yourself most of the time.

For problems that are more severe, you will need a dentist. If your stains are in teeth that are also cracked, or chipped, you may need bonding or capping to cure the problem. Of course you are also curing the problems of the cracking or chipping along with the stains, and those are much more serious. In bonding the tooth surface is cleaned an a layer of new enamel-like material is put over the tooth. In about an hour the procedure is finished and you have a new tooth surface. In capping the tooth is ground down to a base and a new, artificial, tooth is glued onto the natural root. If you have either of these procedures done, and they

won't be done just to remove stains, you will still have to carry out the same procedures to keep them clean and unstained. So keep brushing and flossing, and
use home bleaching whenever you need to. In a normal cleaning your dentist will
not only remove any plaque or tartar you have missed, but you will also get a polishing. Toothbrushing also gives you a polish, but not at the same level that you
get with a cleaning by your dentist.

What A Gum Surgeon May Never Tell You

Gum surgeons, like any surgeons, don't like to talk about cures for their
specialty area that doesn't involve surgery. And because there are non-surgical
ways to treat some of the problems they operate on, few of them will be willing to
discuss them with you.

One of the non-surgical ways for treating gum disease uses what is called
a phase-contrast microscope. With this microscope it is possible to distinguish
between types of bacteria on the teeth, and then design a non-surgical treatment
which will get rid of the bad ones before they cause a permanent loss of teeth.
You are unlikely to have this idea even discussed by a gum surgeon since a paper
by the American Academy of Periodontology attacked the microscope in 1991 as
being unable to distinguish bacterial types, and therefore of no use in treating
gum disease.

Natural Ways to Save Your Teeth Without Surgery

If you have just read the words above, about the microscope, you will
know how wonderful an opportunity this is for anyone who suffers from gum disease. The reason it is wonderful is that it was found that gum disease is caused
by particular bacteria, and not just by what you eat or whether or not you brush
after every meal.

The discoverer was a dentist named Paul H. Keyes, who decided that
bacteria was the problem and found the phase-contrast microscope both in the
late seventies. With this new tool he devised a way to save teeth without surgery,
and that is what we want to look at.

This is a procedure you are going to have to get from a dentist who knows
it. If you go to ask, it is called the Keyes Treatment, after the man who discovered it. To begin the Keyes Treatment the dentist will take a scraping from the
part of your mouth that is giving you trouble. It will be put under a phase-contrast
microscope so that the disease causing bacteria can be seen. Then you will be

treated until you get rid of the bacteria, and you are cured.

The actual treatment to your teeth begin with the standard tartar and plague removal by scraping and polishing. Then the cleaned areas are flushed with a strong medication to kill the disease causing organisms. This will cut out most, but not all gum surgery, so if your disease has gone too far don't be surprised if treating the bacteria doesn't cure everything. It is also common for this type of treatment to take several visits over 6 months to keep the bacteria under control.

Besides the treatments at the dentist's office, you will also have some responsibilities at home. You will need to floss regularly as well as brush your teeth with a combination of baking soda and hydrogen peroxide. This is a bacteria killing combination which is available in your supermarket. If this seems like a lot of trouble just remember that 95% of those who follow this plan can avoid gum surgery, and if you have ever had your gums scraped by a surgeon almost any trouble is worth it to avoid that kind of treatment.

TOXINS

5 Natural Ways to Purify Your Body, and Get Rid of Toxins that Cause so Many Diseases and Illnesses

Toxins are everywhere around us, in the foods we eat and the air we breathe, and on the grass our children play on and that we lay on. Toxins are so common everywhere that we live that we can't escape them, so we must have some ways to rid our bodies of those that we come in contact with. To get to that place of purity and good health there are 5 natural ways you can go about it, and if you do you can be at least reasonably sure that you will have avoided the worst affects of the toxins around us.

1. The first way to purify your body is to cut down on the amount of toxins that are entering it. This may be a bit hard seeing that they are all around us to begin with, but doing a few simple things around where we live can help. For heavy metal toxins like lead, don't live in a home with lead soldered water pipes or lead paint on the walls—if you have these things already you may have to move or have them redone in non-lead forms. Also don't live near any factory area that handles lead, like a battery factory. With this start you should also avoid living in a farming area where toxins are sprayed on crops every year, or even a

orest area where there is an active weed control program going on using weed killers. This should give you a basic idea of what to do to avoid toxins in the first place: find out what the sources are and avoid them or get rid of them.

2. Other than avoiding toxins completely, you can also counteract their effects by blocking them once they have gotten to your body. For any toxic substance to hurt you it has to get to the place in your body that it attacks. Your skin protects you against most of these toxins, and just keeping your skin clean and not having open cuts will help a great deal. But if toxins, such as heavy metals like lead or mercury, get into your body they will go to the bones and into the brain and attack you that way. However, the way that they attack you is by replacing trace elements that your body really needs. If you take high levels of these trace elements you can largely protect yourself against attacks by the heavy metals. The trace elements you want to take supplements of are zinc, copper, iron, manganese, and chromium. These are all used in your enzyme system and keep the chemical reactions in your body working properly.

3. The third level of protection is the taking of antioxidant supplements. The antioxidants will work to neutralize the free radicals that do the damage. Our bodies do not produce these vitamins, so the only way you can get what you need is through the food you eat or through supplements. The main antioxidants are vitamin E, vitamin C, and the B-complex vitamins. Since vitamin C and the B-complex vitamins are the most important antioxidants against toxins they will make up the last two subjects for discussion.

4. Vitamin C is recommended for many things, and it is not surprising that it is also recommended as an antioxidant to fight toxins as well. Vitamin C seems to reduce that amount of lead which we absorb as it goes through our digestive system. To get this effect you will need 2,000 milligrams of vitamin C daily. Along with the vitamin C you should also take zinc, which is one of the trace elements your body needs. The supplements level for zinc is 60 milligrams daily. These effects of vitamin C and zinc were proved in a study in New Jersey where 39 workers at a battery plant were watched for 6 months. Of 22 of the workers who completed the study, all had much lower levels of lead in their bodies than those who did not take the supplements.

5. The other supplement of major importance is the B-vitamins. It has been found that treatment with vitamin B1 (thiamine) can reverse the effects of lead poisoning. In an experiment a veterinarian from the University of Tennessee gave doses of B-1 to a deer suffering from lead poisoning, and the deer made a complete recovery. Thiamine apparently protects the body against lead deposition in the kidney, liver, and brain. Studies in India have also found the other B-vitamins to protect against heavy metal poisoning and toxicity. You don't have to worry about overdosing on the B-vitamins since extra amounts are excreted by the body . If you want to protect yourself from the toxins around you, take supplements of the trace elements, and of the antioxidant vitamins.

Harmful Toxins from Your Dishwasher?

How to Eliminate Them

Toxins in your dishwasher, that can get into your food and drinking water are more likely to come from the detergent you use than from the leftover food on the plate. Of course the detergents have to be strong or they wouldn't be able to cut through food that has been left on dishes for days, and they are also needed to kill food bacteria. But to make sure that you don't end up with some of these detergent toxins in your diet you need to occasionally check the quality of the dishes coming out. For instance, if you take a drink of water from a just washed glass and it tastes a little soapy, then your dishwasher didn't do a good job of rinsing the dishes. And the same goes for the dishes you eat off of as well.

But what can you do? If you have an old dishwasher the best thing you can do is to replace it. After about 10 years the belts, pumps, and motors of a dishwasher will wear out and repair costs will be higher than total replacement. Also the new dishwashers are more efficient than the older ones, and can be trusted more to leave your dishes without a residue of soap and chemicals. Other actions you can take include shopping for a dishwasher detergent which has a better rinsing agent, so that it gets rid of its own contaminants, or even going to hand washing if that can be managed.

In any case it is possible to get rid of these contaminating toxins if you take some time to think about it, and shop for better products.

ULCERS

Does Aspirin Cause Ulcers?
Sometimes

Studies have shown that a heavy use of aspirin can cause ulcers. This is especially bad for you if you are taking aspirin to cut your risk of heart attack but maybe there is something you can do about it. If you take some precautions to protect your stomachache when you take the aspirin you may not have any problems, even if you already have a problem with your stomach.

The reason your stomach might have problems with aspirin is because it can be irritating to the stomach, because it decreases blood clotting, and because it suppresses some of the things the stomach secretes. If you have an ulcer the secretions can be irritating, but if you do not have an ulcer they are more likely protective, and help you to digest anything that you eat.

Because aspirin changes your stomach chemistry it can also cause you to have problems with your stomach. The best way to protect yourself from any ill effects of aspirin is to not take the aspirin, but if you are worried about heart attacks you might be giving up more than you want to. The risk from dying from a heart attack is more of a problem than the risk of getting an ulcer (at least to most people).

If you are someone who feels the danger of a heart attack is worth the risk of an ulcer, then there are still a few things you can do to protect yourself as you take your daily aspirin. The first thing is to keep your aspirin dose as low as possible (the lower the dose of aspirin the less your risk of getting any problems from it). To do this go with minimum daily doses of aspirin, after all, no one has said that high doses are necessary to prevent heart attacks.

The next thing you can do is to never take aspirin on an empty stomach. When an aspirin tablet enters your stomach and begins to dissolve it creates an area of very high aspirin concentration. In this little area, around the dissolving aspirin, you can start an ulcer or give your blood a big dose of aspirin and affect its clotting action in some other part of the body. If you take it with milk, or just after a meal, then you know it will reach a high concentration in any part of your stomach and will probably not cause you any problems.

Finally you can just make it a point to use buffered aspirin whenever you take it. Buffered aspirin costs very little more than plain aspirin, and it will help to protect your stomach when you do not have the opportunity to eat before taking your dose of aspirin. Aspirin is a funny medicine, since you can take it for any aches and pains as well as colds, and there is no telling just when you may decide that you need to take one. If you are sure to take buffered aspirin as a rule, then you will always have the minimum protection possible from any side effects.

There is a warning that should be given here though. If you already have ulcers, or a blood clotting problem, never take aspirin because it will make those problems worse. Do not take aspirin just before you go to your doctor for a look at your fever and body ache, since aspirin will decrease both of these. And never take high dosages of aspirin on a long term basis (more than a couple of weeks) under any circumstances. High doses of aspirin over a long period of time can cause ulcers, as well as other problems, and it doesn't matter what precautions you take, or what good effects you may be getting over a short term.

Heal Chronic Ulcers With this Combination Treatment

Chronic ulcers are often caused by infections, and although you can relieve them with over-the-counter stomach medications, you can't cure them that way. Also taking drugs to reduce stomach acid, which is a common treatment, will not work either. The best way to heal these ulcers is through a combination treatment that used stomach soothing medicines, stomach acid decreasing drugs, and antibiotics. Even if you don't actually have ulcers, but suffer from chronic gastritis you may have the same cause, and need the same treatment.

This treatment was reported in the Annals of internal Medicine in 1991, and a 98% cure rate was reached. The treatment took 16 weeks, and consisted of Rantidine to decrease stomach acid, over-the-counter bismuth preparations to soothe the stomach, and two antibiotics to kill the infection. This treatment isn't for everyone who has an ulcer, but only for those who have an infection along with their ulcers. It may even be that the infection comes along after the ulcer has formed, and keeps it from healing up with the regular Rantidine treatment. If you have a chronic ulcer, or chronic gastritis condition question your doctor about using a combination treatment as a cure.

How Licorice Tablets Can Help You Get Rid of an Ulcer

Ulcers can be one of the most painful, treatable, illnesses we can develop. Early symptoms are easily mistaken for simple upset stomach, and by the time we go to the doctor the medications we are given have to be so strong that they can cause side effects. I think that it is much better to use a natural substance that can be purchased anywhere, and that has no side effects.

Of course I am talking about licorice. Licorice has been used in China to treat stomach problems for thousands of years, and is sold in health food stores in United States in several forms.

Recently licorice has been studied as a treatment for ulcers, and it has been found to be better than Tegument. It also has no side effects, like Tegument and Zantac, and is certainly less expensive than either one. Licorice works mainly by helping the stomach lining to heal, and by keeping it healthy afterwards.

For licorice to work most effectively it needs to be taken as a chewable tablet, and one of the best is known as DGL, for deglycyrrhizinated licorice. For most people it is best to use this form because the ingredient taken out sometimes raises blood pressure, and does not affect the treatment for ulcers. This DGL form of licorice is called Rhizinate by the manufacturer, and your health food store can order it from Phyto-Pharmica if they don't already have it on the shelves.

UNDERWEIGHT

No Sympathy and Little Help
Here's Some

Underweight people get no respect or sympathy for their problem, even though they are just as much at risk for health problems as are overweight people. In the United States we have half a population that is overweight, but only a few percent who aren't actually in poverty who are underweight. So what can you do about it?

The first thing to consider is that if you are underweight you are probably deficient in essential fatty acids, and both vitamins and minerals. Furthermore if you have a simple illness, like the flu, you can come out a few days later looking like a skeleton. But unless you have some problem in getting enough calories in your diet you must have some underlying medical problem for being underweight.

Those that you should be checked for include thyroid malfunction. Either an overactive or underactive thyroid can leave you underweight, but this can usually be treated easily once diagnosed. If your thyroid is in good shape then have your digestive system checked out. Intestinal parasites in many countries cause malnutrition, and you have to have medication to get rid of them. One of the most common in this country is Giardia lamblia, which you can get from untreated water anywhere, and can give you flu-like symptoms along with weight loss.

If you check out medically then look to your own diet. If you have a generally poor appetite it may be because you are missing some trace elements in your diet. Taking 30-50 mg of zinc picolinate daily can restore a sense of taste and wake up your appetite. Once you have gotten your sense of taste, and your appetite back, set a diet for yourself which is 500 calories above your daily needs. This will add one pound to you each week, and for most people will cure an underweight problem in 3 to 6 months.

Above all don't give up since being underweight by more than 10% of your ideal weight is a dangerous physical problem that needs to be corrected.

URINATION PAIN

A Test You Can Use in Your Home to Prevent Infection

Painful urination is usually caused by infections, many of which are from yeast. Yeast infections are a more common cause of women, but many men may have them as well without being aware. By the time you know you have urination pain your yeast infection is beyond the point where you can really treat it at home, and then you must see your doctor for relief. There is hope, however, if you are willing to give yourself a monthly screening test. This test will allow you to catch yeast infections at an early stage when you can treat many of them yourself. Of course if you have a positive test, and the infection in beyond the preliminary stage it must be treated by the doctor.

The test is called the Biotel home screening test, and all you do to take it is collect some urine in a cup and immerse a Biotel dipstick. The color of the stick indicates whether or not you have a yeast infection. If you want to be reasonably certain of catching any of these infections at an early stage you should perform this test every month. The test is also quite reasonably priced, and should cost under $15 for a kit.

Secrets to Prevention for Women

A cause of urination pain unique to women is the disease called cystitis, a urinary tract infection, which 1 out of 5 women will have, and many of them repeatedly. In fact 4 out of every 100 women will have 3 or more cystitis infections in a year, and the infection comes from your own body. The bacteria causing cystitis is called E. coli, and originates in your digestive system. Actually it comes from the anal area and gets to the bladder by going through the vagina. As you can see, it is quite easy to contaminate yourself, depending on your own habits and digestive health.

But before we tell you how to avoid cystitis, let's first make sure that is what you have. The symptoms include painful urination, an inability to empty the bladder completely (it makes you get up in the middle of the night), and sometimes blood and the urine, and strong smelling urine. Now these symptoms are not unique to cystitis, but are shared with vaginitis (which is a non-bacterial inflammation of the urethra), but which often accompanies the venereal disease of gonorrhea and chlamydia. To get a full diagnosis, and as well as clear up the cystitis and venereal diseases, you are going to have to see a doctor. If you have cystitis you will be given antibiotics, and of course penicillin or a penicillin-type drug if you have a venereal disease (but this is not about how to avoid this type of dis ease, and we will stick to cystitis from now on). Most of the time the cystitis will be cleared up within 48 hours. If you don't get it treated, the cystitis can spread eventually to the kidneys where it can be fatal, so get treatment if you have the infection.

But how to prevent it in the first place? Well, there are several steps you are going to have to take to cut down the chances of getting cystitis. The first of these is urinating after having sex. There are several theories of where the bacteria come from in sexually active women, but it is known that the more frequently you have intercourse the more likely you are to get cystitis. Also that urinating afterwards results in a lower risk of getting the cystitis.

If you use a diaphragm and have cystitis attacks, it is possible that there is something wrong in the way you use the diaphragm that is causing the cystitis. Try another method of birth control in these cases. Of course it might not be the diaphragm that is the cause of the problem, it could be the spermicide. Spermicides are thought to kill off protective bacteria in the vagina and allow the E. coli to increase so as to cause an infection. While it is not known which of these two are really the culprit, it is best to consider them both guilty and switch to other brands and other methods as a means of preventing cystitis attacks.

There is one further preventive, which may be the best of all, but you will need to work with a doctor to use it. This is an antibiotic therapy that gives you regular doses of antibiotics to kill off any infection at such an early stage that you never get cystitis. This is a somewhat less common way of dealing with this disease since taking any antibiotic daily increases the chances that you will eventually get a resistant strain that can't be easily cured, and besides, there are several variations you should consider that will avoid this problem. The first is to take a dose of antibiotic from 3 to 7 nights a week before going to bed. The antibiotic will get into your bladder and kill any bacteria that have gotten in there before it can do any harm. For the sexually active, a dose of antibiotic right before or after sex will do the same thing.

If your attacks of cystitis tend to be very intermittent, and you aren't pregnant, diabetic, or elderly, you can also take a single large dose whenever you do feel symptoms coming on. The effect of this treatment is just the same as when you are treated by a doctor for cystitis, so you should expect symptoms to continue for up to 2 days afterward. If this is the treatment you are using, then you are deciding that you have cystitis, but because of the possibility of the venereal diseases, you need to go to the doctor for a follow-up visit every time you do this. If you don't have faith in the large singe dose method, then dose yourself for 3 days when you have symptoms. At least you will be getting medication as long as you have symptoms, so it may make you feel better whether or not it does any real good medically.

For very persistent cystitis you can dose yourself for 7 to 10 days, or more, and this is a very effective method. However, it can also lead to yeast infections and allergic reactions. Any time you extend the dosage period you also increase the chances that you are going to have side effects from the treatment.

But, all in all, one of these therapies should be ideal for you, and any of them should work for most people. Don't let your cystitis go untreated or you risk serious disease rather than just pain and discomfort.

Your Pain May be the Price
You are Paying to Treat Your Cold

Painful urination can occur when the prostate enlarges, or when the penis is irritated from any urinary infection. What is not well known is that you can cause the symptoms of a urinary infection by taking cold medications. Cold medicines all have decongestants to stop your runny nose from bothering you. They do this by cutting down the flow of blood in the nose, which is fine. What they also do is cause the blood vessels in other parts of the body to also cut down their blood flow. When the blood flow to the bladder is decreased, it's not able to completely empty out and you find yourself straining. Unfortunately this narrowing of blood vessels also takes place in the prostate, and as you try to urinate you develop a bout of painful urination. These things can happen every time you take cold remedies, and if you do have occasional painful urination there are some things you can try when you have a cold.

First, of course, you could just live with the runny nose, although you may not want to do that. If you really feel that you need to take a cold medicine than at least cut down the dose you take as much as possible, and remember that you are probably only going to need it for a few days. Try taking a 1/2 dose to see if it works in controlling the runny nose, and whether you have any urination problems. If the nose is controlled and there is no pain, than stick with this level of medicine. If there is pain then cut down some more, and if there is no pain and no relief then increase your dose. At some point you will probably find a dose level where your runny nose is controlled and there is no problem with urination.

If any dose of cold medicine results in painful urination then you are going to have to live with one or the other, a runny nose or painful urination. Of course you could also try to find a cold medicine that doesn't have antihistamines, and that may do the job. The problem with painful urination is limited to the antihistamine type of cold medicines, so you could still take aspirin or motrin to relieve bodyache.

VACCINATION

Shot and Test Reference Guide

A List of Vaccines and Screening Tests
You Should Get, At What Ages, and How Often

1. Flu—if over 65, have impaired immunity, or chronic heart or lung problems, an annual flu shot is needed. If you are allergic to eggs you should never get a flu shot. Flu vaccine is grown in eggs, and a flu shot will be just the same as eating an egg, only worse because it will go directly into your blood stream. If you have been exposed to the flu, but don't yet have symptoms, look into getting a shot of amantadine from your doctor, it can lesson the symptoms, and might prevent it completely. Remember that you can get the flu every year, so you must get a shot every year if you want to avoid the disease.

2. Pneumonia—if over 65 you should be vaccinated for pneumonia; also if you have chronic heart or lung problems you should be vaccinated at an earlier age. Only one shot is needed, so you don't have to worry about pneumonia again after you have had your shot.

3. Tetanus/diptheria—most people receive shots for these when they are children. A booster every ten years will keep your immunity at a high level, and keep your defenses secure.

4. Checkups—a regular checkup will help to find diseases at an early stage, when it can be cured, and ensure good health. The checkup should include a complete blood count, weight, blood pressure, and cholesterol measurements. The best schedule for the checkups is:

20-29	every five years
30-39	every three years
40-49	every two years
50+	every year

5. Women—age 20 to 39 should have a Pap smear and breast exam at each checkup, and should do a breast self-exam each month. Women die from cervical cancer and breast cancer because they are found too late, not because they kill everyone who gets them.

6. Women—age 40 and above need an annual mammogram rather than a simple breast exam. The risk of getting breast cancer increases after the age of 40.

7. Men—age 20 to 39 should have a testicular exam with each checkup, and should perform a testicular self-exam each month. As in women, men die from cancer of prostate because it is not caught at an early stage, not because it kills everyone who get it.

8. Men—age 40 and above should also have a rectal exam with each checkup to look for rectal cancer. Risk increases after the age of 40 for men.

9. Men and Women—age 40 to 49 should have an eye exam and glaucoma test every two or three years, and after age 50 they should be done every one or two years. These are important because the eyes can indicate other serious diseases in the body, and glaucoma is the main cause of blindness in the American population.

10. Men and Women—age 50 and above should have a sigmoidoscopy every ten years to check for colon cancer and other serious diseases of the digestive system.

11. Oral Health—at all ages everyone should see their dentists every 6 months for a checkup and cleaning. The loss of teeth, and diseases of the teeth and mouth, can often lead to serious illness involving the whole body.

12. Skin—everyone should do a monthly self-skin exam to look for changes in moles and lumps which might indicate cancer. This is especially true as you become older. Be especially concerned for moles that are irregular in shape, have variations of color in them, are larger than a pencil erasure, or are growing in size.

VAGINAL INFECTIONS

Ever Had a Yeast Infection?
Here are a few Diet Hints

Yeast infections are usually caused by an organism called candidiasis. For women who have them frequently they can be a very painful and persistent problem that seems to always need care. Luckily, however, yeast infections, and candidiasis in particular, do respond to particular diets, and you can help control how often you get them by changing your diet, but what diet do you need?

The first step to take on this anti-yeast infection diet is cut down on refined carbohydrates (sugars), alcohol, milk, fruit, fruit juice, yeast (why give it to yourself on purpose), coffee and tea. This will get rid of the main list of foods that are likely to promote yeast infections, and is a good start.

Now the next step is to add some foods that promote your immune system and prevent yeast infections. Begin with garlic, vitamin B, raw green leafy vegetables, stick to vegetable oils, and use natural and unpasturized yogurt. There you have it, a list of foods that will help you in one way or another to control and cut down on your yeast infections.

WEIGHT LOSS

7 Questions and Answers to Help Lose Weight
While You Eat Fast Foods

A big problem for anyone in American culture who needs to lose weight is just which fast foods are best, or can I eat any of them. As it turns out some fast foods are perfectly good diet foods, while others that seem like they would be good diet foods actually have some of the highest calorie counts in the restaurants. Since you will probably be dragged to a fast food restaurant in the near future, what can you choose that will satisfy you, and yet have the least calories. To be in charge of your own diet, you must also answer this question on your own. But you can always have some help. As an aid to choosing fast foods, there are 7 questions and answers which will help you think on your feet, and avoid having a diet buster when you only meant to have a snack.

Question 1: First let's take care of your protein, so you tell me which of the following three items has the highest protein value (and no peaking at the answer below): a wing from Church's Fried Chicken, an Arby's beef N' cheddar sandwich, or two slices of Domino's veggie pizza?

Answer 1: Since protein is usually thought to mean meat, you probably chose one of the meat dishes, but you would be wrong. The veggie pizza has 31 grams of protein, the sandwich has 25 grams, and the chicken wing has 22 grams. What you need to keep in mind when choosing protein foods is that cheese has a lot of protein, and even vegetables supply some of our protein. But grains, from which the pizza crust was made also have protein. The pizza wins because the chicken wing is smaller than two slices of pizza, and the Arby's sandwich simply has less meat than the pizza has cheese. If you are trying to eat light, then cheese is a better choice for protein than are many of the meat dishes that tempt you, but which come along with a lot of extra calories too.

Question 2: *Since we have taken care of protein, it is now time to consider iron, a necessary nutrient for healthy blood. Which of the following fast foods gives you the most iron: a honey dipped yeast ring doughnut from Dunkin Donuts, hash browns from Jack-in-the-Box, or a 6-inch-club sandwich from Subway?*

Answer 2: In what might be a big surprise, the doughnut has the highest amount of iron (remember it was a yeast and honey doughnut), with 4% of your daily requirement. The next best choice was the hashbrowns with 2%, and the worst was the sandwich with 0%. Now although you are getting a little iron in these foods, even the best is not a good choice as a source for iron—have you ever tried eating 25 doughnuts in one day. Doing so to get iron would also put a pound a day of weight on you. Nevertheless, this does show that a sandwich is not necessarily a better source of a nutrient than is a donut, which is good to keep in mind when you are looking at food values.

Question 3: *For this question want to know which of these fast foods has the least amount of (remember that fat can have most of the calories in many foods). So which of these is lowest in fat? Is it seafood gumbo from Long John Silver, chili from Wendy's, or a hard shell chicken taco from Taco Bell?*

Answer 3: The lowest in fat is the chili at 29% calories from fat, the second is the chicken taco at 47%, and the highest is the seafood gumbo at 60%. In choosing between these three you have to keep in mind what goes into each one. Chili is thickened mainly with tomato sauce, which is low in calories. The chicken taco has meat, which is going to have some fat, and is cooked in oil, which will add more calories. The gumbo, which is the villain here, is made up of several high fat fish, and may have fat added to the sauce to make it thicker. For any kind of a low fat diet, go with the choice that has ingredients with the least fat, tomato sauce, if you are unsure of which is lowest in fat.

Question 4; *Let's say you are looking at a limited menu of items, all of which have a lot of fat, and you want to choose the one with the highest amount of fat so you can rule it out. Here are your choices of which is highest in fat, is it the chef salad from Burger King, the junior roast beef sandwich from Arby's, or a Personal Pan pizza from Pizza Hut?*

Answer 4: While lettuce doesn't have many calories, salad dressing does, and the chef's salad is highest in calories at 46%, the roast beef sandwich s next at 44%, and the pizza is lowest at 39%. Now 39% calories does not make omething a diet food, and the servings would have to be of equal size to compare, but it is as easy to eat an 8 or 12 once salad as the same weight in pizza. f you like salads heaped on a plate with plenty of salad dressing, then you might eally be better off with a couple of slices of pizza. Since the roast beef sandwich omes in the middle, it is kind of a tossup over the other two. Roast beef sandwiches come with high calorie dressings, and Arby's invites you to add extra (oil ased) horseradish dressing, or barbecue sauce, so the total calories from fat in he roast beef might even be higher for many people.

Question 5: *Now getting away from fat, let's just look at calories, since hat is what many of us are really concerned with anyway. Which of these has the owest number of calories (we are going to order just one), is it a banana nut muffin from Dunkin Donuts, a croissant from Burger King, or a fat-free apple bran muffin from McDonald's (it sounds like the best choice, doesn't it?).*

Answer 5: If you made the best sounding choice, the fat-free muffin, you jet 310 calories, while the other two are tied at 180 calories each (about 1/2 the at-free muffin). To see how this can be true you need to look at the ingredients f the baked goods and the size of the serving. All are made from basically the ame ingredients, so you may just be getting more in one serving than in another. In general apples and bananas have about the same calories, so the differ- ance does not lie in those ingredients. Just remember that if you get a more sat- sfying serving of any food you are probably also eating more calories to get that atisfaction. The only way to guard against this is to eat foods you know have few alories like raw fruits or vegetables.

Question 6: *Looking at the other side of the question, which of the fol- owing choices has the most calories. Is it a Whopper with cheese from Burger King, a scoop of jamoca almond fudge ice cream from Baskin-Robbins, or a homestyle shrimp dinner from Long John Silver's?*

Answer 6: Not too surprisingly, the shrimp dinner has the most calories vith 740 calories, and the Whopper is not far behind with 706 calories. The least alories are in the ice cream, which is only 270 calories. This is, of course, a question of serving sizes. A scoop of ice cream, no matter how large, does not nave the overall size of a dinner (even a small one), and a Whopper is pretty arge. Even 740 calories for a dinner is not a very large number, although nearly hat many for a sandwich seems like a lot. A meal in a fast food restaurant based on the large hamburger, fries, and ice-cream, can easily go over 1,000 calories, and that may be too many for you if you have three of these kind of meals a day.

If you have one meal a day, it is probably not even large enough, and the same goes for the shrimp dinner. The ice cream should be just a treat, or a dessert, and the calories are not out of line with many dessert items you are going to run into.

Question 7: *For the last question we will get away from calories and fa a bit, and look into a needed nutrient. Which of the following choices has the mos vitamin C. Is it a King garden salad from Burger King, a baked potato with sou cream and chives from Wendy's, or a, apple shortcake parfait from Kentucky Fried Chicken?*

Answer 7: The best choice, for vitamin C, is the parfait with 83% of the recommended daily requirement, the second is the potato with 75%, and the last is the salad with 58%. Now 58% is not too bad, and even 83% is not a lot if you are interested in a high vitamin C level, but it is still good to know. This question is really thrown in as a little reminder that just because one food is based on ice-cream, and another on vegetables, it does not mean that one is necessarily better than another. If you want a really high vitamin C food you would go with something with citrus in it. And if you are eating foods to get a minimum requirement then two serving of any of these foods would do just fine. Take supplements i you want high vitamin C, and don't worry about it if you want minimum recommended amounts, and you eat a variety of foods.

10 Ways to Lose 10 Pounds

If you thought that there was only one or two ways to lose weight suc cessfully, you are pleasantly mistaken. Here we have 10 ways that can work fo you, if you want them to. The secret behind losing weight on a diet is that you rec ognize every time that you go off the diet, and give yourself time to correct what ever overeating you have done. Other then that you naturally have to stay on the diet all of the time. If you go off of it for any uncounted length of time, and ther go back on you will be surprised how much weight you have gained, and how long it will take you to lose it on any diet. Of course all that we offer here is a chance to lose 10 pounds, which is fine if that is all you have to lose. But if you have more than 10 pounds to lose, then just use these ideas as starters, and go onto a long term plan afterwards. This will make you feel good about what you are trying to do, and get you committed to working over a long time to get to your goal. Also remember that if you can't lose the first 10 pounds, then you certainly aren't going to lose anything more than 10 pounds either. Without further comment, here are 10 ways to lose 10 pounds.

1. Exercise can help you to lose 10 pounds even if you don't do anything else. With the right amount of exercise you can eat the same diet you have

always eaten, and lose 1/2 pound a week. At that rate it will take 4 1/2 months to lose the 10 pounds. Of course you will need enough exercise to do this, and that means 5 days a week. Walking 45 minutes at a time will do it. The nice thing about exercise is that after you have done it for a few weeks you will feel like doing more than the minimum amount each time, then the rate that you lose weight will increase, and you will lose the 10 pounds in less than 4 1/2 months. A couple of other hints to help it work: if time is a problem then park a 15 minute walk away from work and get your 30 minutes in that way; and if your appetite starts to increase as you begin to exercise start snacking on fruit and no fat crackers so that you will stay away from high fat donuts and things.

2. For both weight loss exercising and diet reform try a combination program where you do a 45 minute walk, at least 3 miles, but cut back on your calories at the same time. Most people who are exercisers will add some dieting to lose pounds rapidly, and you can do it too if your exercise is walking. By taking off just 150 calories a day, along with walking, and you will lose 10 pounds in 3 months. If you cut 500 calories a day and walk you will do it in 7 weeks. While it sounds fast and easy, it's still work and you have to dedicate yourself to it for the time required. This is a good combination plan though since you are learning better eating habits while exercising, and improving your cardiovascular health at the same time. Your chances of keeping the weight off are very high if you keep up some of this program after you have lost the 10 pounds, and always keep it in your back pocket if you start to gain or need to lose some more weight.

3. If you are in a little better shape you can use aerobic exercises to get rid of the 10 pounds a little faster, and have your body stronger and in better shape afterwards as well. The big four low impact aerobics are jogging, dancing, swimming, and biking. Stay away from the high impact aerobics since the risk of injury is much greater, and don't put yourself in pain every time you exercise or you will get discouraged and quit. The way to do each of the four to lose your 10 pounds are: jog for 45 minutes, 5 times a week, and cover 5 miles and you will lose 10 pounds in 3 months; dance energetically for 1 hour, 6 times a week, and lose 10 pounds in 4 months; swim for a total of 4 hours a week and you lose 10 pounds in 4 months; or bike for 4 hours a week and lose 10 pounds in 5 months. As you can see, although some of these are faster than others, they all work just fine, and all give you the extra benefits of lower blood pressure and cholesterol.

4. Now that you have gotten your exercise program decided on, or maybe decided not to exercise, it is time to consider dieting. The easiest diet is just to cut down how much you eat at each meal, but to continue eating what you always have. If you cut your portions by 25% you will lose 10 pounds in 10 weeks. If cutting all of your portions is something you can't do regularly, then at least pick out the highest calorie food you eat most often and cut that down by 25%. This modified reduction diet will allow you to lose 10 pounds in 7 1/2 months, and it won't seem quite so strict and make it easier to stick to. Also follow the general rule that all diet doctors are giving, don't skip meals, it just leads to more extreme hunger and binging. If you fall off of the diet sometimes you will still reach your goal, only later, just so long as you are on it most of the time.

5. Now a diet that is a little more extreme, and one that you can't keep up over your whole life, is to replace 1 or 2 meals a day with a liquid supplement. These have been around for a long time, and you can get powders to mix your own, or premixed forms, in the supermarket. On the good side they are easy to use and effective. On the bad side even though you lose weight with them, you tend to gain it back very rapidly. To lose your 10 pounds with a liquid diet, and keep it off, you have to look at your regular diet and plan how to correct it before you have finished taking off the 10 pounds. Of course you still want to lose the 10 pounds, and all that you have to do is replace 1 meal a day with a liquid supplement and it will take 8 months, or 2 meals a day and it will take 5 weeks. If you want to replace 2 meals a day do it under a doctor's care to avoid nutrition problems. And just in any diet plan, don't skip meals since you just get more hungary and will have a greater chance of binging and losing all the benefits you gained in the diet.

6. Fat has 2+ times the calories per pound that protein or carbohydrate do. This means 3600 calories per pound for fat, and 1600 calories for carbohydrates and proteins. So how do you use this to lose weight? Since most American diets have way too much fat, if you cut your daily fat intake to 20 to 40 grams you can lose 10 pounds in 2 months. This isn't bad so far, but here is what you are going to have to replace in your diet, or cut out: regular ice cream, mayonnaise, hamburgers, processed meats, red meat, and pork. Don't let the low fat claims of some meats lure you into large meals of them. You only need one 3 or 4 once portion of meat a day to get all of the protein you need, and you need a lot of other foods in your diet to stay healthy. A final hint is that you need to buy a diet food guide that gives the grams of fat in different foods in order to keep your fat intake down as low as it should be.

7. We have looked at some specific diets that will take off the 10 pounds, but if you want a more general approach, then go out and shave calories off of your diet any way that you want, or even in many different ways. This is the old calories counting method, but it still works. To begin start reading the calorie per serving numbers on supermarket foods, that will give you most of the information you need. Then go to lower calorie forms of the foods you are eating. Taking 500 calories a day from your diet will take 10 pounds off of you in 2 1/2 months, and if you cut 800 calories you do it in 6 weeks. However, don't bring your diet down below 1200 calories a day, and don't fast without medical supervision. Too limited a diet for too long affects the function of the heart, and if you have a heart condition it could be life threatening. While you are counting your calories remember to eat as wide a variety of foods as possible to keep your nutrition in good balance.

8. Weight training has become more and more popular around our country, with many more women now involved, but can it help anyone lose weight? At first glance there does not seem to be any reason that it should. Unless you work very hard at weight training you barely break a sweat. But that would be a wrong conclusion. Take a look in a gym, or at a neighbor lifting weights in his garage, and you will see a people breathing hard and sweating plenty. Anyone on a seri-

ous program of weight lifting gets plenty of aerobic exercise. Weight lifting has the added advantage of adding muscle to your body as well. So if you want to do weight lifting to lose weight do it. Lifting for 45 minutes a day, 3 times a week will take 10 pounds off in 10 months.

9. Now that you know you can lose weight by lifting weights, you may still complain that 10 months is too long a time to take to lose 10 pounds. There is a simple solution that will cut your loss time by 2/3 and still let you lift weights, that is cut fat. You already know that cutting down on fat in the diet will also let you lose weight, but combining the two gives you the benefits of both. If you cut 20 grams of fat from your diet every day, and lift weights for only 20 minutes at a time, 3 days a week, you lose the 10 pounds in only 3 1/2 months. This is especially good plan to follow if you are not an experienced weight lifter, and it loses the weight faster too. Along the way you will build muscle mass, and learn better eating habits which will make it possible for you to keep the weight off more easily afterwards as well.

10. What is the perfect plan to follow to lose those 10 pounds and keep them off? That depends on you. While you can follow any of these plans to lose the weight, the only way you will keep it off is to change the habits that put it on you in the first place. If you binge on holidays, then step up your exercise and cut some of your portions at that time and you will gain less, or not at all. If you love chocolate and can't give it up, then cut your portions and exercise away the difference to maintain the weight loss. But to get into the habit of controlling your diet and exercising, which you will need in the future, also use it to lose the first 10 pounds. If you cut 100 calories by cutting out 2 cookies a day from your diet, walk 2 miles in 30 minutes 3 times a week, and lift weights for 40 minutes 2 times a week you will lose the 10 pounds in 5 months and learn some things about yourself that will help you keep it off.

Also do not worry excessively about how fast you are losing weight. There is no problem with losing as little as 1 pound a month on one of these programs. You probably gained the weight initially even more slowly although it might have come on in units of a pound or two at a time. To be permanent, weight loss has to be gradual just as weight gain is for almost every one. All of these plans will work if you stick to them, and they will all help even if you have problems sticking to them.

11 Foods that Lowers Cholesterol While You Lose Weight

The main culprit in being overweight is too much fat in the diet, at least for most people. But because fat makes many foods taste good to us, it is a real hardship to cut it down to just a few grams a day. On the other side, the saturated fats that come in most meats and baked goods also raise cholesterol in our bodies, and can lead to strokes and heart attacks. So we have two good reasons to cut down on all fats in our diets, and to cut out saturated fats entirely if we can.

There is an approach to doing this that does not require us to quit eating everything we have grown to love over our lifetimes. In recent years supermarkets have started carrying lines of food that are nearly fat free, but which taste very much like the regular high fat kinds we are used to. With the 9 food hints here you can keep a normal diet, but lose weight and cholesterol at the same time.

1. Cream cheese can be found in the market which carries a big "low fat" label, but which tastes just the same as the regular high fat form. Because several producers are offering this new form of cream cheese it is not necessary to recommend any particular one, and most taste about the same anyway. A cream cheese which lists 4% of calories from fat will save you 70 calories per once of serving, or 560 calories for an 8 once package. Saturated fat of this form is less than 1/2 gram per serving. Besides saving both calories and saturated fat, these low-fat cream cheeses are also available in flavors so that you can use them to replace flavored hard cheeses for snacking and party foods.

2. Cheese, which you may eat to get calcium, gets most of its calories from fat. Because cheese gets so much of its taste from its high fat content, you will have to taste test the low fat varieties to find ones that you like, but it will be worth it. A single ounce of regular Cheddar has a total of 6 grams of fat, which includes 4 grams of saturated fat. If you like cheese, you won't be able to lose weight unless you can control the fat you get from it unless you give it up entirely. Find non-fat varieties of the hard cheeses and you can save 70 calories per ounce, the same savings as in the low-fat cream cheeses. Independent taste tests have found a great variation in the acceptability of different kinds of cheeses, so don't get discouraged if you don't like one type because the next one might taste just as good to you as what you are used to. Also remember that many cheeses are high in sodium, so if you have any kind of a blood pressure problem you have to watch that closely as well.

3. Crackers, which go good with hard cheese or cream cheese, can also be a problem for fat and weight loss. The unsalted saltines are probably the winner as far as being fat free and low calorie, but if you also like the flavored crackers and wheat crackers you have a bit of a problem. These wheat crackers carry about 10 calories each, and 10 of them give you 2 grams of fat, 1 gram of which is saturated. Snacking wheat crackers for an evening can easily give you 200 or 300 calories and 6 or 8 grams of fat. Finding fat-free crackers is little harder than some other foods, and might require a trip to a health food store. But, Health Valley does have a line of fat-free, and herb flavored, crackers. Because they do not have fat, these crackers seem a bit dryer than the regular form, but if you use them with the low fat cheeses or other non-fat dip they are just fine.

4. Granola bars, as a popular snack food and sold in health food stores, as also a high calorie and high-fat food that needs to be avoided in its regular form. A regular granola bar has 8 1/2 grams of fat, and 1 gram of saturated fat. Health Valley has a non-fat form that cuts all of this fat out of the bar, and saves

ou 80 calories as well. You will need to check your supermarket closely, and very possibly go to a health food store to find these, but they are worth it if you like a candy bar sometimes. Granola bars are good sources of fiber, so they have their good points over the sugar type candy bars you find for sale everywhere.

5. Muffins have grown largely as substitutes for donuts over recent years, and are generally believed to be healthier for you than other morning roles. You can also find muffins for sale in all supermarkets and bakeries, but you must choose carefully if you want a fat-free muffin. While muffins are usually made with butter and oil, and have 11 grams of fat and 2 1/2 grams of saturated fat, there are several sources of fat-free muffins to choose from. MacDonald's has a fat-free apple-bran muffin that is very good, and Health Valley has several varieties of fat-free muffins on the market. Because of the variety of ingredients in muffins, even fat-free ones are not completely fat free, but have a little more than half of the fat of the regular muffins. Because of the fat and calories in even the fat-free types, it is not recommended that you make muffins a part of your daily diet, but having one of the fat-free ones a couple of times a week will do you no more harm than having a regular muffin once a week. The best advice is to use the fat-free varieties, and do not increase the number of muffins you eat each week, and you can cut some calories and cholesterol from your diet this way.

6. Mayonnaise, made from oil and egg, is almost all fat in its regular form. And regular mayonnaise has 11 grams of fat per tablespoon, along with 1 1/2 grams of saturated fat. Choose a fat-free form and save all of that fat, and the taste is the same as regular mayonnaise when it is blended into other foods like potato salad or tuna. Some food seem to require mayonnaise to be good, and you can both save the fat and have the mayonnaise at the same time with a little care.

7. Eggs are half fat and half protein. The white part of the egg is the protein, and the yellow part is the fat, 1 1/2 grams of saturated fat per egg and 75 calories. If you turn to egg substitutes you can save all of the fat and many of the calories and still have your morning eggs. The egg substitutes can also be used for cooking, and doing so lowers the calories in everything you bake.

8. Sour cream is similar to eggs and mayonnaise in having a lot of fat (3 grams per tablespoon), but even more saturated fat with 2 grams per tablespoon. Using the fat-free sour cream saves the fat and cuts the calories by 20 per tablespoon. These are all available in the market, and you should try a few to see which has the best flavor. Cost is about the same as regular sour cream, and they can be used for dips in the same way.

9. Frozen desserts, the favorite midnight snack of so many people, have ruined many diets and added many pounds to those who eat them. The typical high quality vanilla ice cream has 12 grams of fat and 7 1/2 grams of saturated fat in a half cup serving. That is only one scoop of ice cream, and if you like larger servings you can just multiply the problems. Going to a nonfat frozen dairy dessert will take some effort, but finding some flavors you can live with can save you all of the fat, and 75 calories per half cup along with it. These nonfat frozen

desserts are at the supermarkets in the same bins with the ice cream, and cost about the same.

10. Pudding, another of the alternative dessert choices, and popular in buffets, will give you 6 grams of fat per serving along with 3 1/2 grams of saturated fat. Fat-free puddings, and they now come in all flavors, will save you the fat and 70 to 90 calories per serving. Making your own fat-free puddings is easy too. Just buy instant pudding mixes and use non-fat or low-fat milk to make them, and you can get the same thing whenever you wish.

11. Cookies can be fattening. Home cookie recipes call for up to 1/2 pound of butter, and commercial varieties have just as much fat. While you don't realize it as you are eating 5 to 10 cookie serving to satisfy your late afternoon or evening hunger, you are getting 2 grams of fat in each cookie, and 1 gram of saturated fat. You are also getting about 50 to 70 calories per cookie, most of it from fat. While you may not be able to make good fat-free cookies at home, they are available in the market if you look. Health Valley markets some varieties, and others can be found. You might also consider trying fruit bars instead of cookies. Since these have a fruit base they are lower in fat.

This concludes the listing of fat-free foods, but it should give you an idea of some of the alternatives to the regular foods you have grown up with, and that now add weight to your body. If you don't eat any of these foods but still have a weight problem, then look at what you do eat and look for fat-free alternatives to each problem food. Start with the food that gives you the most calories and find a substitute. Do this for each of the problem foods and you will cut cholesterol and lose weight. Add some modest, daily, exercise and you will see results in a month, and great results over a year.

A Miracle Pill for Weight Loss
Is It Safe?

A miracle pill is being tested by the National Institutes of Health, which can cut 30% of the calories out of your diet, without you changing what you eat. It works by stopping some of the fat in your normal diet from being absorbed into the bloodstream. This can cut hundreds of Calories from your diet every day, and help you to lose weight slowly and naturally. The name of the pill is Orlistat, and it has already passed one test with humans, without side effects. An added advantage is that it also stops cholesterol from being absorbed, and can help to lower blood cholesterol levels. Ask your doctor the next next time you visit him, and keep your eye out for more bulletins on this new miracle pill.

10 Secrets for Getting and Staying Thin

If you have weight that goes up and down all of the time then you know what it is like to live on a yo-yo. One of the most frustrating things about losing weight is that it isn't permanent, and you can always backslide. It is obvious that you are going to need some guides if you are going to lose, and keep off, extra weight. You can't just lose weight, and then go back to your old way of eating and expect the weight to stay off. Follow this guide and you can both lose weight, and keep it off.

1. Take charge of your life. If you have a weight problem it is because you put too much food into your body. No one else can force you to eat too much of the wrong things, and only you can lose the weight you want. To help you realize the control you have over your self, just remember that every bite of every thing you put into your mouth is a decision you have made your self. When you take charge of your life you can begin to reject those things that are bad for you, and eat those which are good for you. While this may take some planning, you can do it because you have control of your own life, and your own diet.

2. Plan your future before you begin. For one thing don't consider this just a plan to lose some weight, but a plan to reform your life. The main parts of your life that you are going to have to reform are your diet and your exercise program, if you have one. Exercise is just as important as diet in losing weight because it uses up a lot of calories, and can help your body to look good as you lose weight. You may have to cut some things out of your diet that you like very much, but try to find substitutes that you can live with. Also give your self plenty of variety. The more varied your diet and exercise plan the easier you will find it over time. If you haven't exercised for a long time then start slowly, with walks, and build up to whatever you are comfortable with that has an interest to you. Remember, if you want to keep extra weight off than you must eat, and exercise in ways that will not put weight on.

3. Give yourself a trade-off, occasionally. You are going to do this whether or not you plan for it because of holidays and special dinners, but if you plan for it, then it won't hurt you. If you are going to a large dinner, and you know you will eat more, then cut down for a day or two before. What you need to remember is that every time you get one of these treats you must pay for it. The pay is in the form of extra exercise and cutting down on part of your weight loss diet. If you don't you will start to gain, and be back into that yo yo again. Finally, never skip meals, because a few skipped meals is the most common excuse used for binges than can't be easily made up.

4. Take your time. It took you a long time to get overweight, and it will take you a long time to get down to what you want. A weight loss of 1 or 2 pounds a week is just fine, but even 1 or 2 pounds a month will work wonders over a period of a couple of years. If you find your self losing more than two pounds a week, then cut back on your dieting because you are on something you can't maintain

for very long. It doesn't really matter how fast you lose weight, only that you are losing weight and not gaining or staying the same. With any diet where you have cut out the most fattening foods, and where you exercise at least 3 times a week, you will lose weight. If it takes longer than you had first thought it would, just remember that your friends will have all that much longer to remark on how slim you look each time they see you. The end result will be the same.

5. Treat yourself, but keep it under control. We all have our favorite foods, even those with the best bodies. If there are things you don't want to live without, then plan to give it to yourself as a controlled treat every once in a while. You may not be able to have it whenever you want, as you did before, but you will also not be doing without it forever. If your favorite food is something you only ate when you were depressed, then you were punishing your self with it. Make it a reward for a good week. Have a moderate amount of whatever it is, but give it to yourself on a regular basis. You will be surprised how you can go from week to week knowing that you have not given up every food you love forever.

6. Make your meals special. When you just go and grab yourself a bite to eat, you will only appreciate being full, but not the process of eating. If you make your meals special with a little preparation, you will enjoy them more. Use good dishes and glassware, and make a complete meal. The effort at planning and eating in a nice setting will make you take more care in choosing your foods, as well as in the dinning experience.

7. Don't make your meals come cheap. Get the best foods you can afford, so you are treating your self at every meal, and you won't be tempted to go out for something afterwards to make up for the poor meal you have just had. Even if you can't afford everything of the best quality, at least try to have something each day that is special, and something that you weren't able to have before your diet. Since you are cutting down on what you eat you should actually have a little more money available each day to make the meals worthwhile.

8. Don't binge away from home. When you go out of the door, you shouldn't leave your diet at home. For many people a business meal is a time to splurge a bit in the diet just to show you are as good as your companion, and even more so if they are buying. Instead find things on the menu that fit your diet and stick to those. Save the treat you want to have for a single item, or dessert, but not for the whole meal.

9. Don't depend on "diet foods" to lose weight. Many of these dishes are made up by diet organizations, and are their main source of profit. Besides they often don't taste very good, and they are not something you will want to live on indefinitely. Look at the packaging and see how many calories they have. With a little planning you can do at least as well in calories, and better in taste, by buying the basic foods and preparing it on your own.

10. Exercise. While you can lose weight without exercise, we all need to be active to be healthy. Exercise burns calories, tones the muscles, and can be fun if you choose to do something active that you like. If you don't know what to do then just take a half hour walk three or four days a week. Walking is recom-

nended for everyone, but if you want something more strenuous then bike, or swim, jog, hike, or play baseball. Getting out at least every other day will take off a pound a week all by itself, and with dieting too, you can even reach that 2 pounds a week that you may want. To exercise regularly plan ahead. Pick days and times of day, and vary what you do every day so you don't become bored. You may even find that the enjoyment you are getting from exercising is more important than the weight loss after a few months. You need to exercise through life to live longer and be healthier.

Lose Up To 14 Pounds in 7 Days
A Natural, Delicious, and Filling Eating Plan You'll Love

The number of pounds you can lose on this diet in the first 7 days depends on just how much overweight you are. You can't lose 14 pounds of fat in 7 days unless your body uses 7,000 more calories a day than you eat, and most of us have a daily diet that is less than 3,500 calories. So a reasonable fat loss, at the maximum, is no more than 1 pound a day, and that only for a few days at a time. Of course if you fast under a doctor's care, and you are very much over-weight, you might lose a pound or more a day for several months. But most of us are not that much overweight (usually no more 20 to 50 pounds), and we would rather do our own weight plan than put ourselves under a doctor's care for it. After all, if you are going to have to diet half of every year, or more, you don't want to be going to the doctor twice a month for a weigh-in.

So you see, this diet can't exactly promise that you will lose 14 pounds in 7 days, but some people have. If you are already on a diet and very active, this diet will not be as much of a change in your normal diet as it would be if you did not diet, and have a lot to lose. But if you fall into that group of those who have many pounds to lose, and you follow the diet plan for each day of the week, you too can lose 14 pounds in 7 days.

For each of these meals you can have tea or coffee, but no milk or sugar. You also need 8 glasses of liquid through the day, and water is better than either coffee or tea. Also no alcoholic beverages at this time, and go easy on the salt. All servings are single unless more than one is given. You may however use cin-namon or other spices, excluding salt, as you wish to add taste to the various fruits and dishes you are having this week. All cooking of meats, and so on, are to be done without butter or oils.

Sunday: Breakfast—1 piece dry toast, 1 scrambled egg, 1 glass juice. Lunch—1 small sandwich (200 calories), glass tomato juice, piece of fruit. Dinner—4 ounces chicken or fish, 1 serving vegetable, 1 glass juice.

Monday: Breakfast—1/2 roll, 1/2 cup cottage cheese, 1 cup unsweetened cereal with skim milk, 1 glass juice. Lunch—4 once serving of fish or chicken, 1/2 cup of yogurt, 1 baked potato. Dinner—4 ounces veal, fish, or chicken, 1 cup peas and onions, 1 cup fruit compote.

Tuesday: Breakfast—1 glass juice, 2 slices toast with butter, 1 dry cooked egg (boiled or poached). Lunch—1 cup vegetable and egg dish, 1 cup raw vegetables with yogurt sauce, 1 glass skim milk. Dinner—1 serving meat loaf, 1 medium baked potato with butter, 1 cup vegetables, 1/2 cup yogurt.

Wednesday: Breakfast—1 glass juice, 1 cup unsweetened cold cereal with skim milk, 1 cup cottage cheese with fruit. Lunch—chicken salad or tuna sandwich, 1 glass skim milk, 1 piece fruit. Dinner—4 once serving red meat, 1 cup cooked rice, 1 cup raw fruit or cooked vegetables.

Thursday: Breakfast—1 grapefruit, 1 dry egg, 1/2 cup yogurt. Lunch—1 sandwich, 1 cup raw vegetables, 1 glass skim milk, 1 small slice carrot cake. Dinner—4 once serving unbreaded fish, 1 cup potatoes, 1 cup cooked vegetables.

Friday: Breakfast—2 eggs, 1 piece fresh fruit, 1 slice plain bread, 1/2 cup cottage cheese. Lunch—1 cup pasta with herb seasoning and butter, 1 cup salad with dressing. Dinner—1 cup casserole, 1 cup cooked broccoli, 1 cup cooked rice, 1 piece fruit.

Saturday: Breakfast—1 glass juice, 1 egg, 1 ounce cheese on 1 piece of toast. Lunch—1 cup ceasar salad with yogurt dressing, 1 cup cottage cheese, 1 small piece of cake. Dinner—1 cup soup, 4 ounces of fish, 1 cup cooked vegetables, 1 cup cooked rice.

Some of the items in this diet are not strictly defined, but for a reason. Cooked vegetables are listed, but not usually cooked broccoli, and that is because if you are allergic to, or hate, the food listed you won't want to follow the diet. Also, the calories in most vegetables are pretty close, and so long as you get a variety you will have good nutrition. Also the diet works best if you also exercise at least 30 minutes every day. If you are not already an exerciser, then take the time and take a 30 minute walk each day, or two 15 minute walks, and it doesn't matter how far or how fast you go in that time.

An Amazing Herbal Tonic Tea to Lose Weight and More

Herbal teas can be very good for us. It seems like Chinese medicine uses these teas to cure about everything, and now there is one that can help with weight loss. The name of this wonderful herb is yerbamate, and when it is combined with honey leaf here is what it can do for your weight. When used by a variety of people in Hollywood on a weight control program, with no other changes in diet or activity, this group lost one pound each week.

The reason for this amazing result is that this tea has some very good qualities. It is a mild diuretic, mild stimulant, dries the mouth somewhat, and maintains the blood sugar level which helps to control appetite.

The other effects which make this such a desirable herbal tea are that its help with blood sugar can also help diabetics cut down on insulin needs, and its stimulant effects are an aid in stopping smoking. It should not be hard for you to find this tea in a health food store, or you can get it in bulk form to get its best effects. Definitely try it if you have any of these problems.

Chocolate or Carob Candy Which is Best?

While you are eating a piece of chocolate you may be thinking that you should be eating carob instead because it is healthier. In some ways carob is healthier than chocolate, but not as far as gaining or losing weight goes. Both chocolate and carob candy have about 135 calories per ounce, with up to 40% coming from fat. Also because carob fat may be in the form of coconut or palm oils it is high in cholesterol while the natural fats in chocolate candy may have no cholesterol. The fat is included in candy to make the candy melt when you eat it. If you have ever taken a spoonful of straight powdered cocoa in your mouth you know how dry it can be. That is the same reason that sugar and salt are added to candy too—they make your mouth water and make the flavor more like what you expect from candy.

Mineral Weight Loss Miracle Pill What is It?

Everyone who has ever wanted to lose weight has been hoping for a pill that would do the job for them. Well there is one, and its been here all the time. This pill works by keeping your insulin levels constant so that you don't get so hungry in the first place, and by raising your metabolism so that you burn fat faster. While scientists do not know exactly why it has those effects, they have concluded that you can lose up to 2 pounds a month without cutting calories or exercising, but just by taking a pill or eating certain foods.

Now, not to tease you any longer, the mineral that does this is chromium picolinate, which is actually one mineral and an acid that helps it work. But that doesn't matter since you need them together anyway. Chromium is one of those dietary minerals that you don't hear about very much because you need it in such small quantities. In spite of that most Americans do not get enough in their diets, and certain foods need to be included purposely, or you should take a supplement.

The recommended daily allowance for chromium is 50 to 200 micrograms, and no food has it in a high enough concentration that you can get to the weight loss level with just a couple of servings a day. While you probably got to around the 50 mcg minimum every day, you need to get up to 200 mcg for it to help you lose weight.

The best foods for chromium are whole grains, certain fruits, vegetables, meats and shellfish. As to what you actually get though, it is only 52 mcg in an ear of corn, 36 mcg in an apple, 34 mcg in a glass of beer, and 33 mcg in one cup of mushrooms. For most people these are not something that they eat every day, and then not in enough servings anyway to get much more than the minimum requirement. And that leaves supplements. If you do use supplements, use the chromium picolinate, since the picolinic acid is necessary for proper use of the chromium. As far as how strong a supplement, if you never seem to eat these foods, use enough to get 200 mcg a day of chromium. For most people, probably a 100 to 150 mcg chromium supplement is sufficient. Don't go overboard on this though, so don't take 1000 mcg thinking it will make you lose 5 pounds a week. You took time gaining the weight, and you should take some time to lose it. Also, 2 pounds a month takes off 24 pounds a year, and I bet that you didn't gain it that fast to begin with anyway.

Snacking Diet Lets You Lose 5 Pounds a Week

While you must cut calories to lose weight, you can cut and burn calories while still snacking on some of those things you love and lose weight. This will take some planning, but if you can get rid of 500 calories a day from your normal diet you can splurge on a dessert or special food 1 day a week. For snacks you will need to stick to low-cal foods like vegetables or fruit, but these will help to keep you from getting too hungry at meal times. The only reason anyone gains weight is that they take in more calories than their body burns. So if you are gaining weight cut what you eat and increase your physical activity. A 30 minute walk every day will burn 175 calories daily, and help you to lose weight evenly.

If you are overweight but not gaining, then at least you are not overeating for your weight. If you are careful not to increase your diet, then simply exercising will cause you to lose weight since you will be burning more calories. If you also cut down on the high calorie foods in your diet you will lose weight even faster.

Foods to cut down on are whole milk, pastries, red meats, alcoholic beverages, candy, ice cream, fried foods, and fast food meals. These are the foods most Americans gain weight on, but any others in your diet that are high calories should also be included. For the foods you are cutting back on, substitute fresh vegetables and fruits, broiled or baked chicken, fish or turkey, low fat or non-fat milk, low fat yogurt, and sugar substitutes. If you look around your market you should be able to find a low fat substitute for everything you are cutting back on. Also eat in moderation, don't try to get the same calories in the low calorie foods you were getting before, that just defeats the whole idea of the diet. Finally, if you have more than 5 or 10 pounds to lose check with your doctor first. Make sure that you don't have a blood pressure or diabetes problem before going on a diet that could be bad for you.

WOUNDS

Cure a Simple Cut on the Fingers With a Band-Aid

Is curing a cut on a finger as easy as just putting a band-aid on it? It sure is, and that isn't all, a band-aid, without any other medication can protect blisters, and rough and cracked skin that medications don't help. You do need to keep the area clean, so wash and dry it once a day. But even the nastiest little cut on the hands will heal more rapidly and painlessly if you cover it.

This band-aid cure works by trapping your own perspiration around the wound and preventing the skin from drying and cracking. It works the same way for blisters, and even where you have had a hole torn out of your finger or hand, if it isn't too deep. These painful little cuts and cracks will stop hurting in about a day, and you will be able to feel it healing by the itchiness it develops. If you leave the band-aid on for 5 days and then uncover it, the rest of the healing will take place in just a few more days, and be practically painless.

Wound Healing Secrets
How to Recover Faster from Accidents, Cuts, Scrapes, Bruises, and Even Surgery

Anytime we get the surface of our skin damaged we always have a risk of infection until it heals, and even in healing there is pain the problem of keeping the hurt area clean and protected. We also know that some people seem to heal much faster than others, but very few people know why. Now we have learned some of the secrets that control the healing of all kinds of wounds, including surgery, and what we can do to help our cuts and scrapes heal faster than ever before.

First I will tell you of some of the things you can do yourself, and these work especially well anytime we are not seeing a doctor for these problems. To heal rapidly the body needs enough of certain vitamins and minerals to build new tissue, and the closer we are to the optimal amount, the faster we will heal. The basic nutrients we need are zinc, vitamin C, vitamin B6, vitamin B12, vitamin E, and vitamin A. Others are very helpful too, but in smaller amounts and we can get those as a multivitamin.

While many of us are familiar with the vitamins some people might be surprised at zinc in the list. But zinc acts with many of the body's enzymes to speed healing, and should not be neglected.

As a caution though, for anyone with kidney problems, or who is in the hospital for surgery, be careful with vitamin C, because the kidneys have to work hard to excrete it from our bodies. If you are in a hospital it is best to talk over using vitamin C before taking supplements.

Now another secret which is a surprise. Insulin, such as diabetics use for their blood sugar, can be used to help us heal. Insulin in an anabolic, or tissue building substance, like the athletes use, and can be used to build damaged tissue. For healing purposes we don't use diabetic insulin though, but a long-acting form called protamin zinc insulin. You will need a doctor for a prescription, but if you can find one this insulin is known to shorten healing time dramatically.

X-RAY DEFENSE

Supplement Which Neutralizes Free Radicals

The problem with X-rays, and there are many good reasons to have them, but they also create free radicals in our bodies. Free radicals have been implicated in everything from being the cause of cancer to being responsible for aging. In any case it seems like it would be a good idea to avoid or neutralize free radicals in our bodies as much as possible. Then we wouldn't have to worry very much about what they did because we wouldn't have any.

Avoiding free radicals is mainly a job of avoiding X-rays, and only having them when we are convinced that there is a real need. It has now been found out that if you are a woman in your forties you should avoid mammograms, an X-ray technique, because at that age they cause more cancers then they find, and so will raise your chance of getting cancer—and this may be because of the free radicals they create along with the mammogram.

To neutralize free radicals, and we all have to assume that we have some, we need to take antioxidants. Antioxidants are things like vitamin E, and it would be good to take a regular dose of this exactly for the control of the free radicals in your body.

NOTES

_____

_____

_____

_____

_____

_____

OTHER HEALTH AND MONEY BOOKS

The following books are offered to our preferred customers at a special price.

BOOK   PRICE

1. Health Secrets	$26.95	*POSTPAID*
2. Proven Health Tips Encyclopedia	$14.97	*POSTPAID*
3. Foods That Heal	$14.95	*POSTPAID*
4. Healing & Prevention Secrets	$19.95	*POSTPAID*
5. Most Valuable Book Ever Published	$12.95	*POSTPAID*
6. Powerful Secrets	$12.95	*POSTPAID*

Please send this entire page or write down the names of the books and mail it along with your payment.

NAME OF BOOK_____PRICE_____
NAME OF BOOK_____PRICE_____
NAME OF BOOK_____PRICE_____
NAME OF BOOK_____PRICE_____

TOTAL ENCLOSED$_____

SHIP TO:
Name_____
Address_____
City_____ST_____Zip_____

MAIL TO: AMERICAN PUBLISHING CORPORATION
BOOK DISTRIBUTION CENTER
POST OFFICE BOX 15196
MONTCLAIR, CA 91763-5196